THE "GO ASK ALICE" BOOK OF ANSWERS

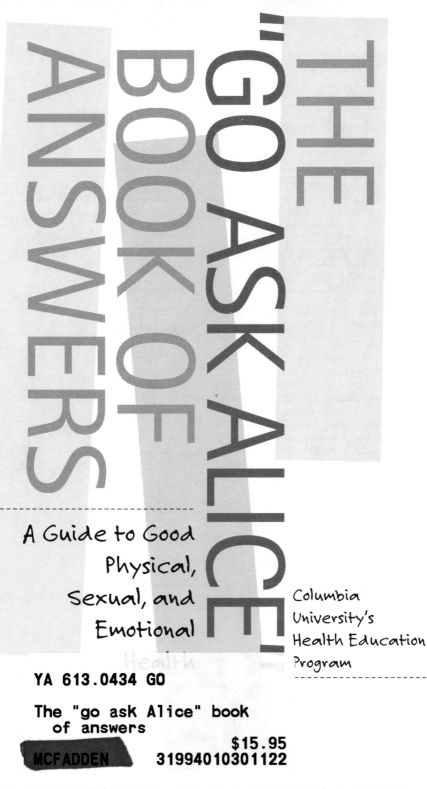

THE "GO ASK ALICE" BOOK OF ANSWERS

A Guide to Good
Physical,
Sexual, and
Emotional
Health

Columbia
University's
Health Education
Program

AN OWL BOOK | HENRY HOLT AND COMPANY | NEW YORK

The information in this book should not be considered specific medical advice. Please consult a health care provider for any serious and/or chronic health conditions. The authors and publisher disclaim any liability arising out of anyone's misuse of, or undue reliance on, any information provided in this book.

Henry Holt and Company, Inc.
Publishers since 1866
115 West 18th Street
New York, New York 10011

Henry Holt® is a registered
trademark of Henry Holt and Company, Inc.

Published in Canada by Fitzhenry & Whiteside Ltd.,
195 Allstate Parkway, Markham, Ontario L3R 4T8.
The lists of bulleted suggestions on pp. 247–48 are adapted from
The College Woman's Handbook. Copyright © 1995 by
Rachel Dobkin and Shana Sippy. Used by permission of
Workman Publishing Co., Inc., New York. All Rights Reserved.

Library of Congress Cataloging-in-Publication Data
The "go ask Alice" book of answers : a guide to good
physical, sexual, and emotional health / Columbia University's
Health Education Program.
—1st Holt ed.
p.   cm.
Includes bibliographical references (p.   ) and index.
ISBN 0-8050-5570-3 (PB : acid-free paper)
1. College students—Health and hygiene.   2. College
students—Mental health.   3. College students—
Sexual behavior.   I. Columbia University.
Health Education Program.
RA777.3.G6   1998
613'.0434—dc21   98-3318

Henry Holt books are available for special promotions and
premiums. For details contact: Director, Special Markets.

First Edition 1998

Designed by Debbie Glasserman

Printed in the United States of America
All first editions are printed on acid-free paper. ∞

10   9   8   7   6   5   4

To our wide world of inspiring and courageous readers and writers who share the healthy desire to learn about themselves, and without whom Alice wouldn't live here anymore.

The "Go Ask Alice" Book of Answers

Masturbation

Orgasms

SEXUAL HEALTH   85

(Questions about reproduction, contraception, and sexually
    transmitted diseases)

Reproduction

Contraception

Sexually Transmitted Diseases (STDs)

Men's Sexual Health

Acknowledgments

There's not enough memory anywhere to store the energy, dedication, support, and skill that lets Alice run. Nor is there adequate server space to express our appreciation to the people and organizations that make up the *Go Ask Alice!* team. From writing and editing to information sharing and uploading, and everything in between, thank you one and all (and anyone we've missed) for putting the *"Go"* into *Go Ask Alice!* and her off-line debut.

At the helm on Alice's voyage from cyberspace to the pages of this book were Jordan Friedman, MPH, Director of Health Education; Judith E. Steinhart, MA, Senior Health Educator; Janet Kim, MS, MPH, Health Educator; and Billie J. Lindsey, EdD, former Director of Health Education. Fortunately for Alice, this top-notch crew brought along their exceptional knowledge and experience, not to mention their outstanding creativity, composition skills, and production savvy.

The following "friends of Alice" were on board, too. Their many professions and passions, combined with their belief that *learning* leads to good health, were instrumental to this book's arrival: Beryl Abrams, Esq.; Jose Aguiar; Patricia Anders, NP; Sandy Angulo; Tim Baer; Daniel Bao; Lauren Becker; Jane Bedell, MD; Ben Beecher; Justin Braun; Amy Burke; Mark Burstein, MBA; Vito Cammarota; Anne Canty; Richard G. Carlson, MD; Allan Cassorla, PhD; Melissa Chappell Burns; Andrea Chernus, MS, RD; Eric D. Collins, MD; Kevin Doñe; Rachel Efron, PhD; Richard J. Eichler, PhD; Will Engelbrecht; Dick Glendon, MD; Jim Gossett, MS, ATC; Giselle N. Harrington, M.Ed; Miriam Hernandez; Stacey Hill; Jan Holland; Elizabeth Honigsberg; Jeff Hsu; Neille Ilel; Mihee Kim; Pamela Donofrio Koch, MS, RD; Alan Kouzmanoff, MD; Joan Lantz, RN; Lawrence Lerman, MD; Deborah Levine, MA; William Lloyd, MD; Franklin C. Lowe, MD, MPH; Brigetta Magar; Rachel Mazor; William McKoy; David Millman; Mary E. O'Brien, MD; Tchaiko Omawale; Taylor

Ortiz; Matt Pietras; Ruth Polanco; Amy Root; Suzette Sanchez, DO; Kathleen Sanders, NP, MSN; Istar Schwager, PhD; Michael Schwartz, MD; Harrison Schweiloch; Carin Seadler, BSN; Brenda Slade, Women's Health NP; William G. Sommer, MD; Andrea Spungen, MA; Tom Thai; Steve van Leeuwen; Michelle Vivas, MS, RD; Jared Wakeman; Jennifer Weiss, MA; and Jean Witter.

A special double-click of gratitude to the Trustees of Columbia University, our Student Services division, the Columbia University Health Service, the Academic Computing and Information Service, the Office of the General Counsel, and the Office of Public Affairs for providing the institutional, financial, technical, and moral support so that Alice *can* live here.

And because books are still an essential source of knowledge, we value our publisher Henry Holt and Company, Inc., for giving Alice to millions not yet on the Net, plus those who still prefer to reach for answers on their bookshelves and night tables. In particular, our immense appreciation and admiration goes out to Ray Roberts, David Sobel, and Amy Rosenthal for opening your doors to Alice and for taking such good care of her while she was down at your house.

Introduction

Dear *Go Ask Alice* Readers and Writers,

Teens and twentysomethings have *lots* of questions about their rapidly developing bodies and minds. Just as the perplexed Alice-followers in Jefferson Airplane's 1960s anthem "White Rabbit" grow and shrink in a mesmerizing world of altered consciousness, thousands of you have coped with hormonally charged sexual desire, evolving self-esteem, opportunities to experiment with drugs, and pressure to become more responsible for educating, housing, nourishing, and supporting yourselves. Peers may have replaced your parents, or one of their old self-help books on the shelf in the den, as sources of information, sometimes offering conflicting opinions and incorrect "facts." Maybe you've never had the facts and support you've needed. Whatever the scenario, the questions remain.

So, in 1993, Columbia University's dynamic Health Education Program combined this need for accurate, straightforward, and open-minded health information with the far-reaching, interactive, and anonymous Internet frontier. The match produced *Go Ask Alice!*, and, since then, the Net and the quest for better health have never been the same.

In the beginning, *Go Ask Alice!* was available only to Columbia students. With its growing success, Alice moved to the World Wide Web to provide greater access beyond Columbia's campus. Since then, Alice has received a phenomenal global response, including a comment from a Saudi Arabian reader who wanted to express gratitude for the Alice site, explaining that it is impossible—and, in some cases, illegal—to obtain certain types of health information through conventional Saudi resources, such as the library. During orientation, a new Columbia student eagerly expressed how he and his friends had been logging on for years from the Philippines, using Alice as their main source of information on sexual health. Across the United States, students read Alice in their school newspapers, and she's even been downloaded by teachers as a textbook supplement.

Alice receives hundreds of questions each week, with hundreds of thousands of readers logging on each month who discover that no matter how much they may differ from each other physically, emotionally, culturally, and in other ways, human beings have the same basic plumbing and wiring, and many of the same feelings and needs.

Alice continually works on improving the site so that it's easy to use and access. The service also has a huge, growing on-line archive of Q & A's from which readers can search for answers to questions they share with past readers. If they find that no one has asked their questions already, they can e-mail them along to Alice. You'll find that while Alice provides carefully researched responses, she encourages readers to get help from their local health care providers. Alice isn't a substitute for a doctor's visit. The Web allows more people than ever before to learn about their health, but it is *not* a virtual doctor's office or health service. **If you're having any serious or urgent symptoms, see a doctor, nurse, counselor, or some other live person.** Don't wait for on-line advice. One of Alice's most important prescriptions is to talk openly with your health care providers, and to use them to learn more about your health.

Nonetheless, the freedom to come to Alice anonymously (all readers' e-mail addresses are scrambled) enhances the site's appeal. Health questions are often so personal that we're afraid or reluctant to ask a health care provider what we really want to know—we're also reluctant to reveal an incident, or an ignorance, we'd rather not admit.

Besides anonymity, Alice also offers credibility: Alice users can be confident they've logged on to a team of professional health educators and health care providers from Columbia University's Health Service staff who review questions, research answers, and post information in a voice that millions have come to know, trust, and value as the one and only *Go Ask Alice*. From her own unique perspective, Alice provides much-sought-after information and facts. She encourages readers to use their own good judgment, confident that her help will enable them to make the best decisions possible for themselves.

This book comprises actual questions e-mailed to Alice from her readers. There were tens of thousands of questions to choose from—from hangovers to hand jobs—and Alice selected a mix of commonly asked queries, hoping you'll find not only answers, but also encouragement— to have a frank talk with your partner, become more aware of your body, and ask for help when you need it. And the asking and answering shouldn't stop here. Many of the responses include a symbol (icon) **RES** that will refer you to an extensive collection of hundreds of on- and off-line resources at the conclusion of the book. Additionally, at the end of each chapter you'll find a sample list of related questions available in the archives of the *Go Ask Alice!* Web site that offers you the chance to get even more information—because when it comes to health and health information, bigger is definitely better.

So, go read . . . and *Go Ask Alice!*

Alice

THE "GO ASK ALICE" BOOK OF ANSWERS

The rules of the dating game sound simple. Whether you're looking for a "hook-up" or a lifelong marriage, pleasurable encounters require both partners to identify what they want, let the other person know, and agree—or negotiate. For those boarding the Love Boat for the first time, the risk seems huge: yes, you may get tossed around on some waves of humiliation along the way, but the queasiness does subside with practice, and with the satisfaction you'll gain just from having survived.

What are the payoffs of intimacy? We can feel safe, understood, special, sexy, desirable, and physically ecstatic. We can also experience the pleasure of someone else feeling this way with us.

So, identifying what you want shouldn't be so tough, right? You want all the benefits of intimacy. But Alice has observed that the question many people ask—"what exactly are you looking for?"—can be a little trickier than it seems. What if you're attracted to someone, and you're not sure if the feeling is mutual? How do you toe the fine line between keeping your distance (and maybe missing out on the love of your life) and being pegged a stalker? Or, what if the object of your affection says, "Yes, I'm hot for you, too—let's get naked," and then you realize you aren't so attracted anymore? Maybe you love your partner, but don't feel sexual chemistry with her/him. Maybe the sex is great, and the love is great, and you still fantasize about being with other people (perhaps, even with people outside your usual sexual orientation).

Not all of the relationship mysteries are so hard to solve. One Alice reader wants to know how to cope with morning breath. Someone else needs to know how to approach his very first goodnight kiss (Where do the noses go? How do you know if your date wants to be kissed?). You'll also see the varied possibilities: long-distance relationships, deliberations about virginity, dilemmas faced by interfaith couples, and crushes on best friends. Alice will also talk about how to handle rumblings with roommates and other friends and acquaintances.

Another serious issue is nonconsensual relationships and abuse. Where most relationships build on trust, some men *and women* become dangerously harmful to their partners. Whether there is physical battery or emotional degradation, it's often hard to admit that a relationship is abusive, and it can be scary trying to get an abusive person out of your life. It can also be confusing to watch a friend or relative be abused—when the safest escape route is not clearly marked. Alice's information and resources can help a person change the dynamics in a relationship and the direction of her/his life.

By simply hearing others describe this wide range of personal experiences, Alice is confident you'll feel less alone if you run into a relationship snag. Also take advantage of the many other resources mentioned in this chapter. Answers are out there, if you are.

Relationship Stuff

Asking to Kiss Goodnight

Dear Alice,

I've always been a guy who has a lot of fun on dates, but performs absolutely awful when it comes to the kiss goodnight (or the first kiss with a girl). I just feel it is awkward and was wondering how a woman likes a guy to go about it. Whether boldly or just asking for a kiss?

Dear Reader,

Alice conducted a small, informal survey of friends to find out how they like the first kiss to happen. As expected, the responses varied.

Most of the women said they preferred to be asked first. Of course, there is an exception to every rule. If the moment feels right and you're pretty sure you know she wants you to kiss her, then go for it! However, you'll really need to hone your body language reading skills to know when the moment is right. If you're not sure a kiss is wanted, you're better off asking. Most women perceive this as a sign of respect and of your "gentlemanliness."

Sincerity is your best bet when it comes to the kiss question (it may also earn you brownie points with your date). Tell your date how you feel. "I had a great time tonight . . . I hope we can see each other again, I really like you . . . Would you mind if I kissed you?" Pause so that your date can respond to what you say. Hopefully, she'll say things like, "I had a great time, too." But if she is not very responsive, if she looks away, or if she just mutters something unintelligible, do not proceed with the kiss question!

It's possible she'll deny your request for a kiss. There's no harm in asking, right? But, if you try to kiss an unwilling kisser, the scene could be embarrassing. You could also harm your chances of a second date by kissing before it's time. Speaking of which, now that you've opened the communication/question lines, you can ask her if she'd like to go out again. If she says no, then you save yourself a phone call or two (or more). If she says yes, then you'll know that the next time may be the right time for kissing.

Not every date has to end with a kiss. Sometimes, it's better to go on a few dates and work up to the kiss—waiting until both you and she feel comfortable enough. And when you do finally kiss, relax and have fun! Kissing is not a chore—it's something that both of you can enjoy.

Alice

How to Kiss

Dear Alice,
Thank you for the useful information about a kiss to say goodnight. Could you please also provide some information about what I need to be careful of while I'm kissing her? (I guess that it's not just pushing my mouth to hers?!) Please help.

INEXPERIENCED TWENTY-THREE-YEAR-OLD GUY

Dear Inexperienced Twenty-Three-Year-Old Guy,
Learning to kiss is a bit like learning how to ride a bike. You are scared to try, but it looks like so much fun on TV! Eventually, the fear subsides and you give it a try. What a thrill that first ride is, and then . . . down you go! That's okay, you had fun, so you know you'll try again. Kissing isn't too much different. The best thing is, just like riding a bicycle, once you learn, you'll never forget. Also remember each kiss will be different, depending on who you are kissing and how you feel about the person.

But you wanted Alice to give you some kissing consideration: You are absolutely right, you don't want to "just push" your mouth to hers. It's probably easiest to begin with a peck on the cheek. Just pucker up, tilt your head a little to the side, gently plant your lips on the person's cheek, and follow through with the puckering motion. This might give you the confidence to try kissing on the lips. It's the same basic movement of your lips, only now the other person's lips are involved in the action, too, which may make it a little easier. A few things to bear in mind when going for the big kiss: do not open your mouth until your lips have reached the kissee's lips, avoid bumping teeth, and make sure there's no food in your mouth (as if . . . !).

Then there's the "French kiss," which involves your and the other person's tongue. Approach your French kiss gently, with no quick and sudden movements of your tongue. Avoid what some call "the frog" (sticking your tongue all the way out inside the kissee's mouth). Your tongue will most likely be met by the other person's, and both of you can go from there, figuring out what is pleasurable.

If you want to practice before trying a kiss on a person, try it out on your arm or your hand (by making a pair of lips with your thumb and index finger) to see how it feels, or practice with a pillow. Pay close attention to the face-sucking scenes in movies or TV shows (any soap opera will suffice).

You'll never know what it's like until you try it. When the opportunity presents itself, pucker up and go for it! You may be surprised at how easy and fun kissing can be.

Alice

Kissing with "Morning Breath"

Dear Alice,
I long to be able to spend the night in the arms of my boyfriend, but I'm too embarrassed to do so because I've noticed how unpleasant my breath smells in the morning. I've read your previous advice on this subject, but both my dental and general health are excellent (I've had recent checkups), and I clean my teeth and drink water before bed. How can I ever wake him with a kiss? I can't spend my life destined to leap out of bed before he wakes to clean my teeth! Please help me—I'm desperate for advice.

LONGING TO WAKE TO A KISS

Dear Longing to Wake to a Kiss,
Alice has a couple of additional breath and spirit-refreshing ideas that you did not mention. If you're not doing so already, brush your teeth and floss before you go to bed. This can prevent food particles from stewing for eight hours and adding to normal A.M. smells. Similarly, how about stowing some toothpaste, mints, or a piece of gum at your bedside? Then, when you wake up, you can pop one in and lay one on without ever leaving the mattress. You could also keep your mouth closed if a peck on the cheek or mouth is the extent of your wake-up call. Sacrificing the rewards from nights in your boyfriend's arms because of natural oral odor seems like a very high price to pay. "Morning breath" is about as common as bed-head, so a little mouth-to-mouth talk with your partner about your concerns probably won't come as a distasteful surprise to him, and just might help to clear your mind, too. Who knows, your beau's morning breath might make yours smell like a basket of potpourri—ooooooh, how pretty.

Alice

"Reading" My Date

Dear Alice,
I really liked my first blind date and thought we had much in common (even backgammon). He, however, was hard to read. Parting, he said,

"Really enjoyed meeting you, hope we talk again soon." But his body language and lack of follow-up hollered, "Don't bother me again, you fool."

WHICH TO BELIEVE: WORDS OR DEEDS?

Dear Which to Believe: Words or Deeds?,
Listen to your intuition. Actions usually speak louder than words.

Alice

Friends to Partners Possible?

Dear Alice,
I am a college student who has a big crush on a friend of mine. While we are pretty close, I am not interested in ruining a good relationship if he isn't interested. The thing is that I have begun recently picturing myself married to this guy in thirty years and seeing him across the breakfast table talking about our kids. I've never felt this way about a guy before. It has usually been more superficial. I keep meaning to tell him but I get really shy because of my fear of destroying our friendship. I think about him often. What should I do?

SINCERELY, LOOKING FOR A LITTLE ADVICE FROM A THIRD PARTY

Dear Looking for a Little Advice from a Third Party,
First of all, slow down. Thirty years is a long time from now—especially if you don't know if the feelings are mutual. Considering that you're good friends, how about talking with him about how you feel? Let him know that maintaining the friendship is your top priority, but that you're feeling attracted and interested in something more. Check it out with him—maybe he's feeling the same thing, or maybe he's not. But, if you emphasize the friendship, at least you have something to fall back on, if the interest is not mutual. And, Alice wouldn't bring up the breakfast table thing with him during that first discussion; it has major potential to scare him away quickly. Slow down, pick a time and place where he won't feel threatened, and you both can talk about where your relationship is and where you'd each like it to go. Nothing ventured, nothing gained.

Alice

In Love, but Not in Lust

Dear Alice,
I have been going out with my boyfriend for nearly four years and we are both approaching the engagement decision. We get along great and never lose the ability to have fun and laugh together. The only problem

is that while he wants to engage in intimate activities often (we are still both virgins), I am not that interested. I love him, but I still don't get physically turned on with him as I do while fantasizing about other guys. Is it wrong to marry someone whom you don't feel a total "romance novel" passion for?

IN LOVE, BUT NOT IN LUST

Dear In Love, but Not in Lust,
First of all, it sounds as if you and your partner are in a healthy relation-ship . . . you get along great and have a lot of fun and laughter . . . quali-ties that many sexually passionate relationships are missing. You have been together for four years, so it's likely that you know by now if you're well suited in terms of interests, values, energy levels, lifestyles, temperaments, and personalities. Ask yourself: Does this relationship enhance who I am or diminish who I am? Do I genuinely like my part-ner? Do I respect my partner? Do I even admire my partner? When happily married couples have been asked to describe their relationships, it's not love or sex that they mention, but companionship and respect. Think about the qualities and characteristics that are: (1) essential; (2) reasonably important; and, (3) luxuries in your ideal relationship. In your situation, ask how you would feel after ten years of marriage and great sex but devoid of laughter, fun, or other shared intimacies.

Loving someone and being happy have more to do with you than the other person. When the time for commitment draws near, many people's fears begin to surface and demand attention. Talking with someone may help. Often an older, wiser friend, family members, or counselors can help you sort out your feelings.

Alice

Interfaith Couple

Dear Alice,
I'm upset because I am dating this Jewish guy who I love very much and who loves me. The problem is that in his parents' eyes, I am not the "perfect" woman for him because I am not Jewish. I understand their concern that Judaism is passed through the mother, but I have made it known that I would be more than willing to convert. Yet I don't think that they are completely satisfied. They often ask my boyfriend how this and that Jewish woman is doing and it really upsets me.

I don't know what to do because we are both family-oriented and this just isn't going to work out unless things get resolved. It would be a real shame too. It's upsetting me so much that I'm beginning to see my boyfriend in a different way.

THE SHIKSA

Dear Shiksa,

If you haven't already, you need to have a frank, nondefensive talk with your boyfriend about your thoughts and beliefs about religion, what it means to you now, and what it might mean in your future together. You also need to listen to his feelings, thoughts, beliefs, and expectations about his religion, and separate what each of you wants and believes as individuals and as a couple. Only then can you begin to discuss how his parents act toward you.

If, and when, you get some clarity on the religion issue, you can have a more rational discussion of how you feel his parents treat you because you're not Jewish. Rabbis who assist in the conversion process have experience with these sorts of issues, and you'll be able to benefit from their wisdom and experience. Keep in mind that your primary bond is with your boyfriend and not with his parents.

Alice

Can't Make a Commitment

Hi, Alice—

I just discovered this service, and hope you can help me. I'm a grad student (mid-twenties) and was very deeply involved with a man several years older than me. Although it was a monogamous relationship—we had a wonderful and very fulfilling sex life, and were generally very happy in each other's company—he was unwilling to make a firm promise not to date other people if he found someone he liked. I broke up with him because I didn't like what this ambiguity was doing to me—making me extremely possessive, jealous, etc. We have both been hurting a great deal since then and were planning on getting back together . . . but he backed out because he doesn't feel able to make a commitment. Part of this is cultural (he's Indian, I'm American), and part of it is probably developmental, as he didn't start dating until quite late by American standards.

In any case, we were considering marriage at one point last summer, and I am still deeply in love with him. He still has very strong feelings for me as well, but I get the sense that the fear of commitment is paralyzing him. I'm at the point where trying to let go and get on with my life seems to be the only viable option, but I'd love to hear your suggestions and comments.

HEARTBROKEN

Dear Heartbroken,

Take a step back and take care of yourself. Stop worrying about whether this guy will make a commitment and acting as if you're afraid to take your next step for fear that he will or he won't commit. Live your life and rearrange your expectations concerning him. Don't spend all your time with him talking about and belaboring the commitment issue—spend your time with him developing a relationship, having fun, and enjoying each other. Be honest with yourself and with each other. Be real—commitment or not. Maybe someone else will come along, or maybe he'll come around. It will only happen while you're pursuing your own hopes and dreams, not while you're anxiously awaiting an answer from him.

You said you've considered marriage to each other . . . have you discussed the cultural differences? Do you know if he'd like children? How he'd like to bring up children (i.e., religion, schooling, etc.)? Have you met his family? Has he met yours? Again, work on developing a relationship with him, learning more about him, while at the same time pursuing your own interests and leaving all possibilities open. The actual words—commitment, marriage—are not what's important with this guy. It's important that neither of you feels trapped, and that both of you have the time to know each other and yourselves well enough to make good decisions for your future.

Alice

Why Did She Break Up with Me?

Dear Alice,
I don't know what I did wrong. My girlfriend of one and a half years broke up with me out of the blue. We never fought or argued. I asked her why; she said, "I don't know." I asked her what did I do wrong, and she said, "Nothing." She was my first ever girlfriend and I was planning to ask her to marry me. I don't understand what I did wrong. There has to be a reason. Why won't she tell me?

Dear Reader,
This must be a terribly tough time for you, especially considering that you were planning on proposing to this woman. It's hard to start over when you thought you had your life all squared away. But start over you must! Have faith and believe in yourself—it will become easier with time.

Alice remembers a college friend who had been happily going out with someone for a while, and then she abruptly left him. Her reasons had nothing to do with him, but with her desire to explore herself and the world a little more before settling down (which is where she thought the relationship was heading). Something similar could have happened with your girlfriend. Or maybe there is something else that she's not telling you.

What really matters is that you realize you did nothing wrong and that you couldn't have prevented this. In order to heal, you need to have a sense of closure. Why it ended needs to be clear to you; otherwise, you are likely to have doubts about the relationship and yourself for a long time. Let your ex-girlfriend know that an explanation, or one reason, for breaking up with you will help you to go on with your life, just as she has been able to go on with hers. She didn't do this without any reason at all. Even if it has nothing to do with you, you deserve to know at least part of the reason why. She still may not tell you. In fact, she may not even know, but at least you will have asked.

Although you need to grieve for this loss, make sure that it doesn't consume you. Talk with friends and family about how you feel. Knowing that people in your life love, support, and care about you can be comforting. Know that you are a good person, that you will be okay on your own, and that someday, you may meet that special someone who will feel the same way as you do about sharing your lives together.

Alice

Disappointing First Time

Dear Alice,
I recently had sex with my girlfriend. It was the first time for both of us. Her hymen broke and she bled a little and even cried but she said she *loved* it. I, on the other hand, felt no pain, but, at the same time, I did not have a lot of pleasure. I expected the first time to be much better, but her vagina seemed to be too relaxed and I did not feel a lot of pressure on my penis. Virgins are supposed to have tight vaginas to make sex more enjoyable. My girlfriend used to go to ballet for ten years and she always does the splits and squats. Do you think that made her vaginal muscles relaxed, or is it just that she did not know how to please me? I am really frustrated and lied to her, telling her I loved it, too. Please help me out.

DISAPPOINTED

Dear Disappointed,
It is not uncommon for people to be disappointed when they have their first sexual intercourse. The experience is filled with expectation, hope, anxiety, excitement, and fear. For some, it is important to get "this virginity thing" over with. Often, pressure is a greater factor than pleasure.

Since women are all different, the tightness of the vagina, or of the vaginal "grip," varies. If you place your finger just inside her vagina and ask her to squeeze, you will probably feel her vaginal muscles tighten.

It is not clear to Alice if her vagina could be tighter, or if you have an unrealistic expectation. For example, how do you masturbate? Few vaginas are able to grab onto a penis as strongly as one's own hand. If that might be the case, you can teach yourself to masturbate using a looser grip. Use a water-based lube or your other hand. Changing your pattern could help you learn to respond to different stimuli so that you increase your own opportunities for pleasure.

Being a good lover takes time, patience, trust, talking, listening, and practice. Truthfulness and authenticity also play an important part, since sexuality and intimacy involve more than gymnastics. Along these lines, Alice suggests that you do not tell someone that you love the sex if you do not. It is not fair to her/him, and it is not fair to you. Furthermore, it interferes with "continuous improvement"! Relax a bit; build confidence in yourself, in your body, in hers; and bask in the challenge and opportunity to learn together.

Alice

He's a Virgin, She's Not

Dear Alice,
I recently got back in a relationship with my old girlfriend from about a year and a half ago. We are in a long-distance relationship, which makes it very hard. She has lost her virginity since the last time we were together and she seems to have enjoyed sex a whole lot. I am a virgin, and I think that when she comes into town in a couple weeks she will want to have sex. I do love her, and she loves me. I want to have sex with her, but I am not familiar with the vagina, and I don't particularly know how to please her. I figure that since she talks about sex, she really likes it, so I don't want to disappoint her, especially since it's my first time. Please help me.

SIGNED, LOST VIRGIN

Dear Lost Virgin,
Alice is confident that you will learn to be a good lover with and for your girlfriend by talking with her, kissing, and touching her, and that she may be happy to teach you. Remember that you are learning to please not every woman, but one woman. In addition, do not think about her pleasure at the expense of yourself. If you are too much "in your head," you'll miss out on your own pleasure as well.

Alice

Practice Sex with Best Friend

Dear Alice,
I was a virgin until about five months ago, and after three hours of foreplay, I finally penetrated and came right then. Since then, my girlfriend and I have broken up, but are best friends now. I have a strange

uncontrollable urge to go down on every girl I see (I think because I enjoy a turned-on girl more than I enjoy anything).

Neither I nor my best friend are seeing anyone, and "friends" have sex all the time, so what is the best way to ask her to let me "practice"? After my first "real" sexual experience, I feel incredibly inadequate, especially since we broke up not long after that. I really want to get better. Christ, I'm nineteen and not getting any younger.

ACTIVE TONGUE

Dear Active Tongue,

Alice is delighted to know that you are eager to give women pleasure, since giving and receiving go hand in glove. It's no wonder you're eager to have sex. You're nineteen; your hormones are flowing; and, it's fun, pleasurable, and exciting. In some ways, like a pump being primed, once you have had sex, you have even more sexual energy.

You say you're eager to have oral sex with your best friend. Alice assumes you mean your ex-girlfriend. Casually speak with her. Say something like: "I feel a bit awkward asking you this. Remember when we were seeing each other and fooling around [or having sex, or making out, or whatever words you are comfortable with]? I really enjoyed making love with you, and wonder if you might consider the possibility of continuing the sexual part of our relationship.... I'd really like to give you pleasure. I trust your judgment and value our communication. Perhaps you could help me become a better lover? What do you think?"

You need to be prepared for her answer. She may say "yes," "maybe," "tell me more about it," "let me think about it," or "no way!" It takes courage to ask, and asking is the only way to increase the likelihood of getting what you want.

If the best friend with whom you'd like to practice is not your ex-girlfriend, you can use the same kind of casual but self-revealing approach. "You know, there is something I'd like to talk with you about that makes me feel kind of awkward, and I hope you will hear me out before you react." Then tell her what you were thinking about. Friends usually respect and depend upon gentle honesty. You can skip the potential pitfalls of sex with friends by looking for a brand-new partner who's not a current friend.

Alice agrees with you. Becoming a tender lover takes time and practice; however, you do have your entire life to learn. If your best friend is unwilling, too uncomfortable, or fearful that it might jeopardize your friendship, then Alice suggests finding another partner with whom you can "practice." By the way, on TV, "friends" seem to have sex all the time, but Alice thinks reality has a different script.

Alice

Too Much Sex, Too Little Relating

Dear Alice,

I'm a twenty-five-year-old guy, average looking, and I think I have a normal personality. I met this very nice and pretty girl a little more than a month ago. Almost since the beginning, all she wants to do is go to bed and make love. This was great in the beginning, but, you and some guys out there may think I am crazy, I am starting to get worn out. I like her very much and we get along great in bed, but I want to date her just like my friends date their girlfriends, although my friends tell me they wish they had my problem. Anyway, when I suggest going out, she shrugs her shoulders and says that she likes to be in bed with me. I'm sure that you get a lot of inquiries about how to move a friendship over to bed. Can you give me some advice about how to move the bed over to a friendship?

SEXED OUT

Dear Sexed Out,

It sounds like you and your girlfriend have different expectations of this relationship. You would like to nurture it and give it time to grow and develop. Your girlfriend is into the physical pleasure, without the emotional obligation. In bed, your girlfriend feels powerful and in control; she may not want any further investment.

Talk with her about your wants and desires. Tell her you'd like to develop a friendship with her, both in and out of bed. Mention things you like to do—go to the movies, take long walks, play chess, whatever. Approach it in a general way, rather than asking her specifically. Find out what her expectations are for the relationship, and what she likes to do, etc. If she sticks to her first response, that she likes being in bed with you and nothing more, you need to make some decisions. Is it worth staying in this relationship for the sex? Would continuing to have sex with her keep you from finding someone else with whom you might be more compatible? Can you stay in this relationship for what it's worth without getting emotionally involved (as it might not be reciprocated)?

Yes, your problem may be different from many other men's, but it is not unusual. It's good that you're starting to think about what qualities would fulfill your needs in a relationship.

Alice

Girlfriend Won't Swallow

Dear Alice,

My girlfriend and I have been dating for a year, and I love her very much. We have a mutually fulfilling sexual relationship, and we communicate well. Recently, I told her of my fantasy of her performing oral sex on me and swallowing my sperm. She said that would be "gross," and has never brought me to climax during oral sex because she does not want me to come in her mouth. I perform oral sex for her, and I enjoy having her sexual fluids on my face and tasting them. We have discussed sexual fantasies before and have pleased each other very much. But she will still not accept my sperm in her mouth, and I feel like she does not want to accept a part of me into her body—that she does not have the fullest desire to please me. When I first asked her to do it, I expected her to want to pleasure me, to have desire for my penis. Now, I feel like she thinks my body is not desirable. My question is: what must I do or say to make her change her mind, to make her understand how much I wish she'd do this?

SIGNED, B.J.

Dear B.J.,

Perhaps you could look at your experience in two ways: your girlfriend could agree to go down on you, and you can agree not to ejaculate in her mouth; or, if she already goes down on you, accept that this may be enough for her right now.

There are probably many reasons why your girlfriend chooses not to swallow your semen. Some people worry about possibly not liking the taste and/or texture. You could ejaculate, and both of you could do a taste test. Others worry about gagging and vomiting, or getting sexually transmitted diseases (STDs). Ask her about these thoughts with an "I want to learn" attitude. Similarly, think about gently expressing to her not just what you want, but what it means to you. Communicating in this manner will not guarantee a change in her behavior and needs to be done without that expectation; however, it could foster greater understanding, and even intimacy, in your relationship.

In the meantime, you could focus on all the ways your girlfriend shows you that she cares for, accepts, and loves you, rather than on what you are not getting from her. You have probably noticed that the more pressure you place on her (or anyone), the more she will run away from what you would like her to do. Be aware of, and respect, her wants and needs, while still acknowledging your own. Similarly, when you go down on her, do it because you want to, not as a proof of your love, or as a trade-off, or investment, in what she might do for you in return in the future.

Alice

Can Boyfriend Tell about Abortion?

Dear Alice,

Do you think it is possible to have an abortion without my boyfriend knowing? I think I might be pregnant and I do not want to have the baby. If I tell my boyfriend, he will not approve. Is it possible for me to have one and not tell him about it? Do you think that when we do resume sex, he will notice?

I Really Need to KNOW!!

Dear I Really Need to KNOW!!,
Yes, it is possible to have an abortion without your boyfriend knowing. You will be instructed by your medical provider not to have sex (vaginal, oral, or anal), or even orgasm, for two to three weeks after the procedure. This is critical, since you will be bleeding during this time, and microorganisms can get more easily into the reproductive tract under these circumstances, creating risk for infection. Your challenge will be to figure out how to explain avoiding sex with your boyfriend at this time. Of course, this may not be a problem, depending upon how often you spend time together, how close you live to each other, and how frequently you have sex. Perhaps you could arrange the procedure, if you need it, to coincide with a vacation or trip you would take on your own.

Right now, however, you are not sure you are pregnant, so you need to establish that first. You can use an over-the-counter pregnancy test, go to a clinic such as Planned Parenthood, or see your own health care provider.

As for your question concerning whether it is possible for you to have an abortion and not tell your boyfriend about it, it seems to Alice that only you can answer that question. Physically, there would be no way for your boyfriend to know. But only you know whether or not it is possible for you not to tell him. If you are thinking of your boyfriend as a long-term partner or possible husband, Alice suggests you consider this: trust is basic to this kind of relationship. In that case, what would it be like for you to keep this information from him? What if he finds out later? What if there were complications? At what point might you tell him, if at all?

If you would like to explore some of your feelings about this, or if this situation is more complicated than your letter suggests, then it may make sense to talk with a counselor or someone you trust. Talking with someone may help you clarify your motivations, voice your fears, and facilitate potential communication with your boyfriend; however, it is your body and your decision to make.   RES

Alice

First Year—No Boyfriend?

Dear Alice,
I am so lonely. I'm not ugly or a loser or anything; in fact, I'm an attractive, upbeat, and outgoing first-year college student. But no matter what I do, I can't get a guy to be interested in me as anything more than

a friend. Please tell me what I'm doing wrong. There are a lot of guys I'm interested in, but none of them will give me the time of day. There is one guy I really like. He is a senior and president of a fraternity. I see him every now and then and I've been dying to approach him, but I'm not up for rejection. I guess I should just do it, right? I mean, what do I have to lose besides my pride . . . I'm just kidding! But, seriously, what should I do?

Sincerely, Infatuated to the Nth Degree

Dear Infatuated to the Nth Degree,
It sounds like your self-esteem is pretty high, so "just doing it" doesn't sound like a bad idea. If this fraternity president says, "I'm not interested," your pride should ride high because you tried. Again, nothing ventured, nothing gained. On the other hand, your boldness might bowl him over—then you'll be an attractive and upbeat First Lady. Watch out, Hillary!

It's also okay not to try so hard. Remember to take care of yourself first—work on becoming an interesting person, having higher self-esteem and confidence, being a good friend, and adjusting to college life. Being alone, or without a partner, does not necessarily mean being lonely. Learning to be with yourself, discovering your likes and dislikes, understanding your feelings and beliefs, in the long run will make you more attractive to a potential partner. So, if you can stop your chasing for a while and take some time for yourself, when you least expect it, a Mr. Right might come knocking at your door.

Alice

The Up Side of a Long-Distance Relationship

Alice,
My friend and I have been involved in a long-distance relationship for six months now. We keep in touch with each other on a regular basis, calling and visiting each other. I feel that the distance between us will cause our relationship to end. We have been seeing each other for a year and a half. What are our chances of being together in the future?

Miles Away

Dear Miles Away,
As Alice looks into her crystal ball, she sees that there is another way to think about your situation. The future, of course, is unclear, even for Alice, so why not focus on the present? Your distance could be considered a blessing in disguise, allowing you to come to know your friend in many ways that close proximity could stifle. Proximity can breed taking for granted the opportunity to talk at any time. It can also lead to physical intimacy (Alice doesn't know if you are sexually intimate) before

you are both ready. Distance, combined with telephone calls and writing, electronically or through snail mail, can foster an enviable intimacy which results from learning about another's qualities, values, ways of thinking, sensitivities, dreams, and aspirations. This intimacy can make your coming together much more special. Alice knows there are some people, in circumstances similar to your own, who spend more time writing their thoughts and feelings to the recipients of their affections than they spend in face-to-face conversations with people they live with day in and day out. Many day-to-day relationships are characterized by superficial conversation, and few, if any, meaningful heart-to-hearts. So, Alice is suggesting that you not run away from your long-distance relationship, but nurture and savor it.

It is important for you and your partner to talk about what you're feeling, and what your concerns are. S/he may be wondering about the same things. If being together on a daily basis is what both of you want, then you can begin to strategize ways to make this happen. Will you need to wait until you graduate? Can one of you transfer schools? Or change jobs? Leave the possibility open, too, that you may continue in this coupleship for a long time, and that would be okay, too. Alice believes there are many "right" ways to be involved in a loving relationship.

Alice

One-Night Stand or True Love?

Dear Alice,
Recently, I met a beautiful student named "Sarah." As I am a student in the same school, we naturally started talking about our classes and job prospects. We went out to dinner that night and one thing led to another. We slept together. The problem is I *really* like this girl and I don't know how to make her believe it. I've tried calling her several times, and her roommate tells me that she will call me back. Needless to say, she never does! Am I being majorly rejected or what? She is the first girl here who has really interested me. I'm told I'm good looking, but I'm beginning to wonder. I'm six-two, 190 lbs., blond hair, blue eyes, well-built, and work out regularly. I lifeguard at the same beach that she went to this summer, and offered to take her to my parents' house out there for a long weekend. Should I just resign myself to loneliness or should I keep the dinner reservation for that weekend?

SIGNED, SEVERELY SMITTEN FOR SARAH

Dear Severely Smitten for Sarah,
Alice's guess is that, yes, you were "dissed." Passion, along with building trust, getting to know the other person, developing mutual respect, and learning to like your partner beyond the original physical attraction

are all ingredients in lasting relationships. So, don't feel that you must resign yourself to loneliness, for growth comes from *all* of our experiences. Next time, if you think it's for real, take it slow and easy.

Alice

Fantasizing about Another Woman While Having Sex with Your Girlfriend?

Alice,

Is it okay for a male to think about another female when he is having sex with his girlfriend?

SIGNED, FANTASIZING?

Dear Fantasizing?,

Yes, it's common for a man to fantasize about other women, or even other men, during lovemaking. It does not mean that you do not love your girlfriend, or that you are not true to her. Fantasizing is different from acting. Some people readily accept that no matter how much they love and are turned on by their partner(s), they will continue to be turned on and have fantasies about other people. Some folks are troubled by this reality. Alice believes it's one of the joys of life.

Alice

Only Attracted to Asian Women

Dear Alice,

I'm a twenty-three-year-old grad student. I am now, and have always been, sexually attracted only to Asian women. I've had many sexual experiences with many different women from all corners of the globe, but this preference has become fanatical. Why?

· OBSESSED

Dear Obsessed,

Alice can't tell you why your preference has become fanatical, but there are a few questions you can ask yourself that will give a framework for thinking about your preference. First of all, there are many countries that make up Asia. Is your preference for women of any specific Asian ethnicity? Given the diversity both between and within Asian countries, have you noticed any difference in your experiences with individual Asian women? Do you think all Asian women are: petite, shy, passive, naive, deceptive, obedient, aggressive, diligent, studious, sweet, unfriendly, fashionable, nerdy, have an Oriental or sexual mystique, Geisha girls, Dragon ladies, mail-order brides, etc.? These questions can help you examine generalizations you might have about Asian women. With stereotypes—of Asian women, Asian men, and almost every other group you can think of—some people fit them but more do not. If you do have images of how Asian women are, how have your experiences fit these stereotypes? Have you been disappointed? Is the idea of how Asian women are "supposed to be" what turns you on? Or, is it the individual woman you are with who is attractive to you?

Back to your question on why your preference for Asian women has become fanatical: What does "fanatical" mean to you? Do you mean you prefer to date Asian women? Does it mean that you stay home from school or work obsessing and fantasizing about Asian women? What is the problem you have?

There is no conclusive research on why some people are attracted to blacks (or to whites), to redheads (or to blondes), to short people (or to tall people), to heavy people (or to slender people), to breasts (or to buttocks), etc. Alice encourages you to look at your personal values and generalizations, and to work with each relationship or sexual encounter as a new and different one—with each woman as an individual person. Enjoy and appreciate her characteristics for being herself, in addition to her identity as an Asian woman.

Alice

S/M Role-playing

Alice,
Is safe S/M role-playing normal? And where does one draw the line if mutual consent is established?

C.V.

Dear C.V.,
In S/M, or sadomasochistic sex play, the mutually agreed upon play-acting is based on fantasy situations of dominance and submission. One partner will "force" his/her will on the other, *consensually* experimenting with activities that involve physical pain, discomfort, or intensity, until the other gives the signal to stop. S/M pushes the boundaries between pleasure and pain.

Mutual consent is what distinguishes S/M from abuse and assault, just as consent distinguishes sex from rape. S/M can encompass physical and/or psychological interactions, and may cause pain, but not physical or emotional damage. Accidents can happen during S/M, just as in any other physical activity, but this differs from abuse.

For some, S/M play can increase sexual pleasure and open up hidden issues of power, which are always present in human intimacy. Trust plays a large part in S/M activity. Some refer to S/M as sensuality and mutuality. Partners need to talk with one another before they begin a "scene" to learn what each of them likes, would like to try, and would not like to do under any circumstances.

If you're not sure where to draw the line for yourself, try fantasizing about it first before acting. If in your fantasies you go beyond your own limits of behavior, it's okay because that's exactly what fantasy is, a mental testing ground for limits. If your fantasies repel you because you are afraid you might act on them, this is important info about yourself and your limits. Remember, you are in control. If you're not in control, then it's *not* S/M.

Alice

Calling Out Ex's Name

Dear Alice,

My girlfriend and I have been having sex with each other for the last six months. Just before we began seeing each other, she had gotten out of a pretty serious relationship. She insists it is over and that she has no feelings for him. I believed her up until recently, when we were having sex and she cried out his name. I like her very much, but, of course, this incident has made me very insecure about our relationship. I'm not sure whether she needs more time to get over this guy, if I'm getting myself into a position where I'll get hurt, or if I should just ignore the whole thing altogether. What should I do?

Signed, Sleepy or Dopey?

Dear Sleepy or Dopey?,

The only person who can answer your questions is your girlfriend. Because she didn't give herself much time between him and you, she may still have unresolved issues from that relationship. She also may not have broken the habit of calling out his name.

Your best bet is to discuss the incident with her. She probably would welcome the opportunity to talk with you about it. Even though you may be hurt by her reply, isn't it better to know than to remain uninformed and insecure?

Alice

AN ALICE READER RESPONDS TO "CALLING OUT EX'S NAME"

"I have had two serious long-term relationships (several years each), both of which were very wonderful. However, there was only about a month's span between the end of one relationship and the beginning of the other. It did take me a while to sort through my emotions and become certain about my feelings. However, long after this, I had the natural tendency to call out my ex-partner's name. It had absolutely *nothing* to do with my love or commitment to my girlfriend. It was purely a learned reaction that became deeply ingrained in me, like when one says 'ouch' after touching something hot. After having three years of sex with my first girlfriend, it was difficult to break the habit of calling out her name, which was so closely associated with sex. It was not her that I was really calling out, just her name."

Gay, Lesbian, Bisexual, or Questioning

How Do I Know If I'm Gay?

Dear Alice,
I have a problem. I've never considered myself gay, but I have begun to care for my best friend a little more than I think I should. I get jealous when he finds a woman he likes, and begins going out with her, and I have become very protective of him, since he is a few years younger than me. I don't know if I am just a little jealous that he is able to find someone, and I am not, or if I am gay and am beginning to like him in that way. When I think about it, he fits my idea of my perfect mate. And I often wonder what his penis size is. Help me. Do you think I am gay, or just suffering from jealousy and penis envy?

Dear Reader,
Let's just pretend for a minute that there is no such thing as a heterosexual, bisexual, or homosexual man and woman. Instead, there are only "sexual beings." If this were the case, your question might read:

> Dear Alice,
> I have a problem. . . . I have begun to care for my best friend . . . I get jealous when my friend is attracted to another person and spends a lot of time with them. . . . I don't know if I am just a little jealous, or if I am sexually attracted to my friend. . . . I think about my friend's body, and I'm sure we would make a perfect couple. . . . Do you think I'm suffering from jealousy and sexual attraction?

When the social taboos, and the personal "baggage" they inspire, are removed from discussions about gender and nonheterosexuality, your situation sounds pretty darn normal. Your friend is someone with whom you spend lots of enjoyable time. Whether or not you are sexually attracted to him, it stands to reason that his spending lots of time with others, for whatever reason, would generate feelings of jealousy.

The only person who can answer your question, "Am I gay," is you. Alice wonders if you have similar attractions to, and "envious" thoughts about, other men friends, and if you allow yourself social opportunities outside of your best friendship. Sometimes, the only way to find out what really turns you on is to reach for the light switch and explore your feelings in search of inner peace. As you know, Alice believes that your choices lead to self-learning experiences, not prison sentences. If you decide to "branch out," however, your best friend's switch may not be the one to flick. You are the best judge of how your friendship would fare if you communicate your feelings. As frustrating as it may be, you might try to spend some time with other people and activities when your friend's time is otherwise occupied.

You are lucky to be able to articulate these important and powerful feelings. And your friend is lucky to have someone looking out for him. Alice reminds you to always look out for yourself, too: your goals, desires, and right to learn more about who you are.

Alice

Feeling Guilty about "Gay Thoughts"

Dear Alice:
I'm a fifteen-year-old male teen who recently had a mutual masturbation experience with a male friend of the same age. Although I have always been interested in girls, now when I masturbate, I fantasize of having sex with another boy—like my friend. But, when I finish masturbating, I feel guilty about my gay thoughts. I don't know what is going on, am I gay or bi? Should I have sex with another man? What can I do?

SINCERELY, GUILTY TEEN

Dear Guilty Teen,
First, Alice offers you these thoughts about guilt from British psychiatrist R. D. Laing:

> True guilt is guilt at the obligation one owes to oneself to be oneself. False guilt is guilt felt at not being what other people feel one ought to be or assume that one is.

You might take some comfort in knowing that both your same-sex mutual masturbation experience, and your "gay thoughts" when masturbating, are shared by many. Some of these guys get happily married to women, have kids, raise cocker spaniels, and so on. Others have relationships with guys, live together, and sometimes marry and have children. Still others deny and hide their feelings—whatever those feelings might be—and often become unhappy because they are not true to themselves and others. Some younger and older men feel strongly about publicly identifying themselves, in some way, as gay, straight, or bi, while others are content with living their happy lives in private.

All of this is to say that your interest in girls may continue. You may still fantasize about guys, and maybe you'll even have sex with other men. It's all up to you—from the people you have sex with, to those with whom you share your feelings, to who and what you decide to call yourself. Your confusion and desire for answers about your sexual feelings are certainly understandable, but your willingness and ability to express yourself, as you have to Alice, will undoubtedly help you sort out your feelings now and in the future.

Alice

Should I Explore My Sexuality?

Dear Alice,
I'm a senior in high school, and, just recently, I've been attracted to a few girls at my school. I also get aroused when I see two women having sex or kissing. I've had three boyfriends in high school, and I think I am still attracted to men. I would really like to experiment with girls to see if I am a lesbian or a bisexual. What should I do?

Dear Reader,
Alice is confident that your willingness to contemplate, and possibly explore, your sexual feelings will only add to your future well-being and peace of mind. Safe sexual "experimentation" provides a wonderful opportunity to learn about oneself: likes and dislikes, passions, and goals. If you like sex with women, fantastic. If you don't like it, don't continue to do it. If you enjoy sex with both guys and gals, lucky you. If you're confused, keep exploring the issue by talking with peer support hotlines, mental health counselors, or friends and relatives (if you are fortunate enough to have such open and caring personal contacts). There are other women your age with similar interests. Keep your eyes and ears open for opportunities to meet them, if you make the decision to explore your desires. **RES**

Alice

Interested in Lesbian Sex

Dear Alice,
We are two straight sophomores who are considering lesbian activity. This is not a joke. We have always been intrigued by lesbians and have

been asking the question, "How do they do it?" Obviously, a great deal of the enterprise must involve oral activity, but what else can we do?

SINCERELY, INTERESTED IN LESBIAN SEX

Dear Interested in Lesbian Sex,
What two women do in bed is as varied as the many women we know. Two women may kiss and hug, caress each other's bodies for hours, or have quick sex. They may kiss, suck, and caress each other's nipples and/or clitorises, touch their vulvas with fingers and tongues, press and rub their bodies and their vulvas, or masturbate together. One person, both, or neither may orgasm once or several times. They may look at erotic pictures, tell and/or read sexy stories, share fantasies, or sleep together without sex. As you see, much of this is similar to heterosexual sex.

Often, there is an incorrect expectation that a woman would know how to be a perfect lover to another woman, since she knows what pleases her. However, all women are different. Communication is key, as in all types of sexual relationships. Remember that having sex with a woman for the first time, or at any time, involves a lot more than what happens just sexually.

Alice

Lesbian Oral Sex: Is It Better to Give Than to Receive?

Dear Alice,
As a lesbian who has recently "come out," I've noticed some women get into giving oral sex more than receiving it. Why is that?

THANKS,
NEED ANSWERS!

Dear Need Answers!,
No one knows for sure why some women like to give oral sex rather than receive it. However, Alice has some hunches for you:

- Giving feels powerful to some women, and receiving makes others feel vulnerable.
- Some women are more aroused by the act of giving, enjoying the smells, tastes, and sounds of their partners as they pleasure them.
- Women in many cultures are taught to give rather than to receive.
- Some women think their vulvas are "dirty," and are uncomfortable with someone kissing them "down there."

The point is not to dwell on "why," but rather to give and receive pleasure, acknowledging and celebrating the wonderful differences in people. Other than consent, there are no rules or "shoulds" in sexual behaviors or patterns. Enjoy.

Alice

Coming Out to Mom

Dear Alice,

How do you think I should go about coming out of the closet to my mother?

Dear Reader,

One of the goals of National Coming Out Day (October 11) is to motivate people to say, "I am proud of who I am." Whether or not your decision to talk with your mom about your sexual orientation is inspired by this annual celebration, bravo for your desire to be honest, to grow, and to be more true to yourself.

The direct approach would be, "Hi Mom, I'm gay . . . this is important to me, and I would like to talk with you about it." Or, "I'm a lesbian . . . if you'd like, we can discuss what this means." This "cut-to-the-chase" method can get you right to the "where will we go from here" stage, cutting out much of the agony that commonly precedes publicly saying, "I'm gay, lesbian, or bisexual." Another approach is: "Mom and Dad, there's something important I'd like to talk with you about. You know how much your love and support mean to me. I'm depending on your strength when I talk with you about this. I'm gay [or a lesbian or bisexual], and it's important to me that you know this." Or, "Do you remember when we watched *Ellen* together? Well . . ." However, Alice certainly realizes that being direct can be painfully difficult for both parent and child.

In lieu of a litany of suggestions for direct and indirect coming out strategies, Alice suggests reading some of the many books on the subject. You might know of teachers, counselors, health care providers, clergy, friends, or role models who can provide you with advice and support. Doing so will likely boost your confidence and generate a variety of ideas during this important process. **RES**

GOOD LUCK AND CONGRATS,
Alice

Nonconsensual Relationships

Please Hold While I Masturbate

Dear Alice,
Recently, during a phone conversation with my boyfriend, he told me that he turned the volume up on his phone. Soon after, he began to masturbate, while he was talking. I am well aware of phone sex, but the conversation never came up. I had no idea what to say to him. It was very loud and there was no mistaking those sounds. Should I confront him or let it go? Do many men find this satisfying? He complains about not being able to sleep. Could this have something to do with this?

Dear Reader,
Not only did your boyfriend not give you his undivided attention during that phone conversation, but his behavior was not consensual. Alice believes that your relationship calls for your partner to indicate his "phone sex" intent and to get your permission to "let his fingers do the talking." Sure, many men and women, couples and singles, find consensual phone sex satisfying—even relationship-saving when two partners are geographically separated. Is he pulling his cord in the name of sleep-improvement? Alice encourages you to ask him about his masturbatory behaviors—such a conversation might make for a clearer connection for both of you.

THANKS FOR CALLING,
Alice

Former Abusive Relationship

Dear Alice,
My current girlfriend is still getting over an abusive relationship that she was involved in two years ago. The abuse included repeated rape

throughout the two-and-a-half-year-long relationship. She has never been able to enjoy sex and cannot bring herself to do it again. Despite her feelings for me, she cannot relax enough during sex for it not to hurt her. I have not forced her into having sex she cannot enjoy. We have been together for nearly a year now and the problem does not seem to be getting better for her. She has nightmares and is uncomfortable and afraid in many day-to-day situations. She is worried that going to a counselor will mean she will be in counseling for the rest of her life to get over this. This has become such a hindrance to us being happy that I sometimes wonder if it is best to stay with her to try to help her through this, or whether I am out of my league.

Dear Reader,
Your girlfriend can go to a counselor for a while and learn to manage her feelings. Many, many survivors of abusive relationships have been able to put their past behind them enough to open doors to new (and healthy) relationships.

She can do some research to find a counselor or group that specializes in treating people who have been abused. In that safe, supportive space, your girlfriend can talk, learn, and set her own agenda. With help, the strong, fearful feelings do not have to last a lifetime.

Healing takes time and requires courage to face the beast. If your girlfriend does not take the opportunity at this time to make some of the important changes in her life, then it may be that she is not ready. You, in that case, have some choices to consider, including cutting your own losses and moving on.   **RES**

Alice

Relationship—Abusive?

Dear Alice,
What is the criteria for determining if a relationship is abusive? My husband has never struck me in anger or injured me, but he is constantly poking, tickling, flicking me, etc. When I tell him to stop, he usually says, "Why should I?" and continues a little bit more. It's like a kid tormenting a little sister. He gets right in my face and sometimes pokes me in the chest while he's telling me something. There's never any anger until I get mad at him for doing it, and then he tells me he's just playing. The other night when I told him to stop poking me, he said, "I'll do whatever I want." That really bothered me. When he does get angry, he usually just ignores me, but occasionally he'll throw something (but not at me). What do you think? How can I make him understand that his "playing" is upsetting? Is this type of behavior a precursor of actual violence?

Dear Reader,

Has your husband been treating you in this manner for a long while? Or has this behavior occurred more recently? What caused you to speak about it now? Did it start before or after your marriage? Has he ever acted this way to other people? **Your husband's behavior toward you, which apparently he considers playful and harmless, is harassment.** He bullies and teases you to a point that provokes anger and torment in you, and Alice strongly encourages you to deal with it as soon as possible.

Your husband is exhibiting immature and inappropriate behavior—that's not your fault. He may want more attention from you (because he may feel neglected in the relationship); it could be related to something outside of your relationship, such as problems with his job, other family members, friends, etc., and he is transferring his anxiety over these matters to his relationship with you, possibly in order to establish some control or power; if this behavior started recently, then it could reflect a medical or psychological condition that did not occur before; or this may be his "funny" (but unhealthy) way of showing you affection.

Obviously, you have made several attempts to talk with him about his behavior, but to no avail. He will probably continue to "play" and torment you unless you become more assertive in your response (beyond just telling him to stop). Tell him about what is going on, find out why he is treating you in this way, and let him know how it makes you feel—that it is disrespectful of your feelings and hurts you. This may be hard, but try to remain as calm as possible, especially when he ignores your requests for him to stop. His tuning you out makes communication difficult, if not impossible, at that time. If this is his typical reaction, then gently ask him about his behavior at another time, when he has regained composure.

If there *never* seems to be a good time to approach him about the situation, then consider seeking professional help for yourself, for him, and/or for the two of you as a couple. To encourage him to go, tell him how much you love him and how much the marriage means to you (if this is how you feel), and that if he also values the relationship, then the two of you need to seek help together to resolve the problems that could strain and eventually break up your relationship. Alice urges you to *prioritize your needs* over his, especially if he seems uncooperative or unwilling to seek help. If he will not go, and you want to make a change, by all means, contact a counselor, psychologist, or social worker in your area as soon as possible.

Your husband needs to realize that he can't do "whatever he wants" to you because he doesn't own you, and that being married to you does not serve as justification for his behavior. You need not tolerate such behavior from him. He needs to respect you and treat you as your own person, not as an underling or object. If he values your marriage and relationship, and if he wants it to grow and solidify, he needs to realize that a successful and healthy relationship relies on equality, mutual respect, and hard work on his part, too.

It is very difficult to say whether or not this type of behavior is a precursor to physical violence. However, it seems that emotional violence/abuse/harm already exists in your relationship. Get the help you need and deserve in dealing with him. Getting help now may prevent possible physical violence in the future. Domestic violence hotlines are another resource—even in advance of actual physical violence. **RES**

Alice

Men Pressured to Have Sex

Hi Alice,
Why is it that, in all the movies and stuff about sex, it is always the woman who feels pressured? I felt pressured my first time and no one would believe me if I told them. Any comments would be helpful.

SENSITIVE GUY

Dear Sensitive Guy,
You bring up the beginnings of a huge debate about gender stereotypes and societal norms in the United States and other countries. Alice has heard from, and knows, men who feel similar to the way you do about your first sexual experience, and often about subsequent sexual experiences. Contrary to commonly held beliefs that men are "too big," "too strong," "too much in control," or "too much into sex" to be pressured or forced into sex, it happens. Exact numbers are difficult to determine because of a lack of research and official records, and men's unwillingness to disclose it.

Alice would encourage both men and women to choose when or whether to have sex. Pressure from others can, and does, unfairly influence us in this decision. Also, once a person has chosen to have sex, this does *not* take away his/her right to say "no" at other times during his/her life. Saying "no" to sex often is a way of saying "yes" to ourselves.

Your question alone helps a great deal in dispelling myths about men's sexuality. Thank you for writing.

Alice

Sex with Four Friends—Mutual?

Dear Alice:
You have an excellent service and give great advice. That is why I feel comfortable asking you this question. About three weeks ago, a group

of my friends and I went out to a movie and then a club where we each had some alcohol. After the club, we went back to a friend's room, where the group gradually dispersed until there was only myself, two male friends, and one female friend. We began to play sex games. Eventually, we all were naked, on my friend's bed. The female of the group was the center of our activity. She seemed to want it and even encouraged what the three of us started doing to her.

Although we all were tipsy, it was a great sexual experience for all of us, or so I thought. My two male friends have no problem with what happened. The only thing is that my female friend won't speak to us or return any of our calls. I saw her walking down the street the other day and tried to talk to her, but she wouldn't even raise her head to look me in the eye. Do you have any idea what is wrong? Could my friend feel that she was raped? I want to apologize, but I'm not sure what to do.

WHAT'S GOING ON????

Dear What's Going On????,

Although your woman friend did not say "no," either verbally or nonverbally, this does not mean that she said "yes." Alcohol is a disinhibitor, meaning that people do things when they're buzzed and drunk that they may not otherwise do when they're sober. Your question mentioned that she "even encouraged what the three of us started doing to her." It wasn't doing something *with* her, but *to* her, implying, to Alice, a one-sided situation, without mutual consent or mutual participation, and clearly, she doesn't want to talk about it with any of you, and that, too, needs to be respected.

Yes, your woman friend could have felt that she was raped. This incident also could have been a trigger for other things, possibly bringing up a painful experience from her past.

If she *were* willing to talk with you, make sure it's private and "safe" for her and you. Let her know that you want to hear her interpretation of that night's events, how she feels now, and what she'd need to feel more resolved. Listen carefully. Do not interrupt, criticize her, or tell her your interpretation. See how she's feeling about the incident, and then explain what happened for you, if she would like to hear it.

Alice suggests you reevaluate what happened to avoid getting involved in a similar situation in the future. Consider the power dynamics—in this case, the ratio of men to women was three to one, and there was drinking involved, so clear judgment was impaired. Finally, considering all that was going on, was it even possible to use good judgment? Or was, or is, your good judgment telling you this was not okay? These are things for you and your men friends to think about in order to protect other women, as well as yourselves.

Alice

Girlfriend Broke It Off—Am I Stalking?

Dear Alice,

My girlfriend just broke up with me after one year of relationship. She didn't give me any reason. She says she has no time to give a reason. Last night, I called her every half hour, but she didn't want to pick up the phone. This morning, she told me that if I keep calling her, or I am around her or her place, or trying to follow her, then she would call the police and sue me. My question is: is it against the law if I am trying to get in touch with her by being at the same place as she is? Is it against the law if I wait for her in front of her door?

HOME ALONE

Dear Home Alone,

It seems clear that your ex-girlfriend doesn't want to see you, talk to you, or have anything to do with you right now. She has been definite and clear about her wishes. You absolutely need to back off and stay away from her.

By calling her every half hour, you are *harassing* her. Yes, this is against the law in most places; and it is more than an annoyance everywhere. Waiting in front of your ex-girlfriend's door, or frequently being in the same area she is, is classified as stalking, and is illegal in many places. In other locales, it would be up to your ex-girlfriend to notify the police and get an order of protection that would not allow you to have contact with her, be on her property, or come within a certain distance of her. The order would be served to you, and once you have seen it, if you violate the terms, you could be arrested.

What you are describing is serious. You need to leave your ex-girlfriend alone for a while, or maybe forever. Whatever her reasons for breaking up with you, it is clear that she is not willing to discuss them with you right now. Don't try to figure your girlfriend out; spend your time nursing your hurt and trying to get on with your life. See a counselor or a therapist to cope with your pain, and discuss alternatives to "haunting" your ex. Be calm, stay away, and move on with your life.
RES

Alice

Sister in Battered Relationship

Dear Alice,

I am having a problem with somebody else's relationship. It's my sister. I love her dearly and I know that she is being beaten by her boyfriend. She is tied to him by the fact that she has a child of six months by him. She doesn't want to come to her family for help. I think that this is largely because she is ashamed of herself and his behavior toward her. I simply cannot "mind my own business" because I am genuinely worried for her safety and the safety of my niece.

Part of me wants her to sort the problem out for herself, but she is immature and is used to having men do things for her. This has been going on for some time now. What can I do to stop him?

YOURS, CONCERNED SIBLING

Dear Concerned Sibling,

Talk with your sister. Let her know that you know what's going on—that her boyfriend is beating her. She may have an incredible sense of relief to know that someone else knows about it and is willing to approach her. Many battered women ask for help first from their friends and families, and sometimes receive answers like, "It's your duty to stay with him," or "You have to do it for the child." Your response that she's not a terrible person, that she has the power to change the situation, might give her courage to face her situation.

She also may be in denial about the beatings and react defensively toward your overtures to acknowledge and help. That's okay and normal. It's still important to let her know that you know what's going on and that she can depend on you for help and support. You might also want to get in touch with a domestic violence hotline. They can help you with your conflicting feelings about your sister's situation, as well as give you referrals and information about the nature of domestic violence.

When you speak with your sister, it is unrealistic to expect that she will immediately change her entire life. As outside observers, that's what we might think will happen; however, there are many more factors at play in a domestic violence situation than meet the eye. Support her and tell her that you care and think she's important. Also, let her know that when she's ready, help is available—give her places she can call for assistance. **RES**

Alice

Talking with Parents

Curfews on Break

Alice,

I just went home for my first Thanksgiving break, and my mother had the nerve to try to give me a curfew! I told her that I am safe, don't drink, and have tame friends, but that we like to hang out until late because we haven't seen each other for so long. I was out until about 3 A.M. each of the first three nights, and my mom knew where I was going each time I went out (usually to a friend's house to hang out with people she knows and likes). I told her what I was doing and with whom, even though I really don't think it's her business anymore, just because I wanted to put her mind at ease, because I know she gets nervous about me being out late.

Well, on my last night home, I fell asleep hanging out at my boyfriend's house, and I just really wanted to stay with him all night because he goes to college far away and so I rarely see him. Plus, I hate how usually after we have sex, I have to just leave—I'd prefer to stay and cuddle/sleep with him all night. I woke up at 3:30 A.M. and even though I wanted to stay, I went home because of my mother. She was awake when I arrived, and furious! I'm not exaggerating: she was pacing back and forth and almost hyperventilating in fury! She says that even though she knows I'm safe, she is very uncomfortable with me being out so late and that I will have a 12:30 curfew during Christmas break! She said that she's a single parent who worries a lot, and I'm very unfair by not accommodating her. I said that I was being fair by constantly reassuring her that I'm a safe driver and telling her where I am, even though it's none of her business and my tiny hick town is a million times safer than the city, where I usually am. She says that I'm not being fair enough, that I'm not using good judgment by staying up until 3:30 every night (isn't that *my* decision?), and that I should be less selfish by coming in a few hours earlier. Those hours with my boyfriend and friends are precious, and I hate having to feel guilt, worry, or dread about going home when all my other friends are relaxed and having fun. What can I do? Am I being unreasonable?

TIME WARPED BY MOM

Dear Time Warped by Mom,

You have gained some independence at school, and, from the sound of your e-mail, you are doing a good job of managing your new life as an adult. However, you have run into this snag. You may be so angry and hurt that you are unable to see things through your mother's eyes.

Your mother has told you what she feels comfortable with—she needs you to be home by 12:30 A.M. so she can feel secure that you are safe. When you do not come home until 3:30 A.M., she feels frightened and anxious. She is a single mom, and you may be the only child she has. Of course, this is a lot of responsibility for you; however, this is how she feels.

Focus on having an adult-to-adult conversation with your mother. Talk with her over coffee or tea, when you are both relaxed. No one likes to negotiate when s/he is tired, afraid, anxious, angry, or hurt. Tell her what you have noticed about her behavior, and how it makes you feel—that her anger makes you feel as though you cannot be trusted to make good decisions for yourself. Perhaps you can also let her know how much it means to you to see your friends, what you like about being with your boyfriend, and how much you miss him. Listen to her feelings and observations as well.

Then, use your problem-solving skills. Figure out ways to meet both of your needs. Come up with and evaluate the solutions together. Maybe your friends could meet you at your house, so that your mother, who seems to like your friends, knows that you are all together and safe. She could be in another room, or have a friend over for her to be with. Maybe you and she could work it out that your boyfriend could visit you at your mother's place, or even stay the night . . . stranger things have happened.

The most important thing is to talk with each other as you let the caring come through. Your mother loves you, and, under your annoyance or anger, Alice is confident that you love her, too. Love, some rational ideas, sharing feelings, having an adult-to-adult conversation, and coming up with creative solutions together may be your next steps to adulthood.

Alice

How Do I Tell My Parents I'm Pregnant?

Dear Alice,

I am pregnant and my ex-boyfriend is the father. He broke up with me before I found out I was pregnant. He's going out with another girl now and acts like he doesn't want anything to do with me or our baby! Neither my parents nor his parents know yet. How do I tell them? I don't want to go through this as a single parent. What should I do?

WORRIED, IN

Dear Worried, IN,

If you have decided to keep the pregnancy, you need to tell your parents. Many parents, perhaps most, will be more supportive than you imagine. Maybe mom and dad, or people close to them, have gone through similar experiences. They may be upset at first, and disappointed; but, trust that they will help you decide about your next steps. However, if you are afraid they would be so upset that they might harm you, Alice suggests that you share your situation first with a favorite teacher or coach at school, a school counselor or nurse, or a health care provider.

Your ex-boyfriend and his parents may or may not be involved in your present or future decisions. Alice suggests that as hard as it will be, that you face the inevitable, and sit down with one or both of your parents, soon.

Alice

Living Room Littered with Roommate's Rubbers

Alice,

I have a problem. The problem is my new roommate. We didn't know that he was gay when we asked him to be our roommate because he went out with girls before he moved in. After a month of living with us he started going to gay night at the local clubs and then found this guy. It is a week later and when my other roommate came home from seeing his girlfriend he found condoms all over the place, he didn't even clean up his mess! What should we do? We still have to live with him for another year.

Help Us

Dear Help Us,

Alice agrees. Sloppiness stinks, whether it's leaving around opened, used condoms (assuming that's what we're talking about), dirty socks, magazines, or dishes. Inconsiderate slobs come in all shapes, sizes . . . and sexualities. If you and your other roommate are bugged solely by the mess of rubber rubbish in your common living space, then initiating a nonconfrontational, nonjudgmental face-to-face with the litterbug about your mutual needs for cohabiting in peace would likely be the best strategy for dealing with this issue.

On the other hand, if the two of you are uncomfortable with your new roommate's sexuality (and Alice suspects that you might be, based on the tone of your question: "We didn't know that he was gay when we asked him to be our roommate" and ". . . and then found this guy"), then the latex litter "problem" could be a minor symptom of a more serious issue: your discomfort with your roommate's desire to have sex with men. Or the roommate in question could be scattering his "scum bags" in response to unspoken hostility that he's picking up from the two of you. Or maybe he's "showing off" because he's getting messages that he's inferior to you. Or perhaps this is his way of telling you who he is, and a roundabout way of getting to know you. These are a few thoughts to consider. If this homophobia theory holds water, then solving this problem resides primarily with you.

GOOD LUCK,
Alice

Help—My Roommate's a Lesbian!

Dear Alice,
I need advice. I think that my roommate is a lesbian. Help!!!!!!!!!!!!!!!!!!

Dear Reader,
Lucky you. What an opportunity, and a chance, to learn about someone (presumably) different from you! This is one of the most significant benefits of college—the chance to expand your horizons.

If your roommate were a lesbian, the question to ask yourself is "So what?" What does it mean to you? How is it significant? Remember that she is the same person she was before you had the hint that she may be a lesbian. If she had likable traits before, then she will continue to have these likable traits. If she were unpleasant before, she will probably continue to be unpleasant. Her possible lesbianism does not change your roommate at all. It just gives her another dimension.

Alice wonders what makes you think your roommate is gay? Make a mental list of the signs that indicate to you that she is a lesbian. Keep in mind that your assessment may be incorrect. She may be bisexual, in a phase, experimenting, or woman-identified without the sexual component. Her behavior, or the behavior of any lesbian, does not have the power to change or influence your behavior.

Think of what you would like to say to your roommate. Perhaps write your thoughts in a letter that you would not send. This letter is for you to examine your feelings and fears. You may then want to talk with her about some of your feelings, not by asking her to justify or explain herself, but by explaining your observations, your concerns, and your eagerness to learn. Then let her respond. She may not tell you directly because she may need your support and friendship, and could be afraid of losing it. Even if she denies her lesbianism, at least you have opened the door. (Alice wonders if your roommate suspects that you are heterosexual, and how she feels about that.)

There is a great deal that we can learn from lesbians, and that they (and we) can learn from bisexual, questioning, unlabeled, and nongay women, if we just keep an open mind, open communication, and an open heart.

Alice

HOMOPHOBIA

Often, heterosexual people who don't have a lot of experience with gay men or lesbians have some degree of homophobia. Homophobia is an irrational fear, and sometimes loathing, of homosexuals or homosexuality (or of bisexuality, too). Ask yourself what you are afraid of. Some are afraid that gay people may try to seduce or "convert them" to homosexuality. Some fear losing the friendship of their roommate. Some lose trust. Some worry that it's a reflection of their own sexual feelings. Some worry about the assumptions and disapproval of others. Homophobia, like racism, limits the potential for great friendships. By dealing with homophobia, you can learn about yourself and expand your world.

Roommate Masturbates Every Night

Alice,

I'm a freshman with a problem. I have a roommate who masturbates every night and it makes me sick. She waits until she thinks I'm asleep and then really goes at it. One night she even woke me up after I was asleep. I find it disgusting to hear her moans of passion as she plays with herself. Should I tell her to stop or should I just find another roommate?

DISGUSTED

Dear Disgusted,

A good rule when someone is doing something that bothers, annoys, or irritates you is to let her/him know of your irritation and give her/him a chance to change. You can always take more drastic measures later. (This is a really helpful tip in any type of relationship—how many times have you heard someone say, "I didn't realize that bothered you!"?)

Of course, sex can be much harder to talk about because it's personal and private. To her credit, your roommate *does* wait until she thinks you're asleep before she goes at it. People sometimes masturbate as a way to release tension or fall asleep. Maybe you could first try a simple face-saving tactic like rolling over and asking, "Are you okay?" when she starts to moan.

If dropping hints doesn't work, you could be more direct with her. When approaching this potentially awkward conversation, think about what you want to change: Do you want her to wait until you *are* asleep before she masturbates? Do you need her to be quieter?

Do you want her to masturbate in the hall (just kidding) or bathroom before she comes to bed? Maybe you'd prefer she masturbate at another time when you're not around. Perhaps you feel that *your* privacy is being invaded. Or if you are disgusted by masturbation, you might want to read about female sexuality and the functions of masturbation.

Also consider sexual words that you're comfortable using, or any metaphors that will let her know that you're awake and offended. Practice a few different lines beforehand so you're comfortable when you start the conversation. If you decide to talk with her about her masturbatory habits, make sure you include these three things:

- What's been going on—specifically, what you hear at night.
- How it affects you; how you feel (i.e., offended, uncomfortable, etc.).
- What needs to change; ideas for changing the situation—what options you see for her.

If you can't come to an agreement, earplugs (available at drugstores) or asking for a room change will likely do the trick.

Alice

Floormate Leads Reckless Life

Dear Alice:
There is a woman living on my floor who I think is living a reckless life. Within the first couple of weeks at school, she has already had two one-night stands with two different men—one of whom she met at a fraternity party and who was ten years older than she is and who has children. Now you ask how I know all of this? Well, she told me along with all my other floormates. The disturbing thing is that she brags about these sexual encounters and acts so nonchalant about them. In fact, she had to use PCC (post-coital contraception or emergency contraception) when she had sex last time because the condom broke on her and "her friend." I'm beginning to think that she is insecure with herself and that she uses sex as a means to overcome her insecurities. The sad thing is that my floor is disgusted with her and her behavior. She is not only putting herself in danger, but also all the other unsuspecting people who have sex with her or her partners. Somebody needs to speak with this woman and tell her that she is being stupid and reckless with her health. By the way, if she is reading this, I want her to know that our floor doesn't consider her more mature than us just because she's had more sex than us. Rather, we consider her stupid, insecure, and whorelike.

AFFECTED

Dear Affected,

You may have more insight into this woman's situation than she does, and you definitely have a better idea of how her behavior is looked upon by others. If you choose to approach her, be aware of your motivations. If you can do it, approach her clean and clear of your own judgments, and solely with concern for her. You cannot speak for everyone, and getting a group together to talk with her about her behavior might put her too much on the defensive. You can only speak for yourself and your concern for how she is treating herself.

What can you say? Be honest and sensitive. If she is so insecure, she doesn't need the extra paranoia of thinking everyone on the floor is talking behind her back. Confront her gently and voice your concern. "I'm concerned because you seem to be reckless about your sexual health." "I'm concerned about your liaisons with guys because of the threat of HIV and AIDS these days. Do you feel like you're being safe?" "Hey, have you gotten any of the new information about sexual communication and STDs? It's really helpful if you're sexually active." Or, "If you're being selective and safe, I think it's better if you keep your sex life private because it shows more respect for yourself and to others."

Talk with your resident adviser (RA) about having some educational programs on your floor about sexual communication and safer sex. Your RA can mention to the speaker that the floor is concerned about one person's behavior, so that the program can be tailored appropriately. That way, you wouldn't have to confront her directly and make it a personal thing between the two of you. This might be the wisest approach to avoid alienating her from the rest of the floor, and to give her a chance to get some good information about her sexual health.

Alice

Go to Alice at www.goaskalice.columbia.edu for more Relationship Q & A's, including these:

- "A" Is for Affair with Professor?
- Bisexual or Bicurious?
- Brother Gets All the Girls
- Dinner = Sex?
- Don't Love Him Anymore?
- Falling in Love with an HIV+ Person
- First Sexual Relationship
- Flirting
- How Do I Let Someone Know S/he's Special?
- Incest
- Looking for Love on the Information Superhighway
- Male Rape Possible?
- Ménage à Trois?

- Not Getting IT Enough
- Obsessing about Fellow Student?
- Rape Survivor Needs Help with Intimate Relationships
- Selfish Lover?
- To Be or Not to Be . . . Single?

SEXUALITY

Since all Alice queries are anonymous, she has become an especially popular advisor on sexuality. A lot of people feel too embarrassed to discuss sexuality with their health care providers, parents, and even partners. Alice hopes that her question-and-answer format not only provides information, but also sets an example for clear communication, which is a key element in a healthy sex life.

Ads, movies, television shows, novels, and music videos certainly muddy the picture. Sex looks so simple: flawless, beautiful couples exchange knowing glances, "hookup," and, without a word, begin thrashing around the bed in mutual ecstasy—no zipper fumbles, diaphragms, condoms, or discomfort.

So, of course, Alice readers are curious, and frustrated. Sex looks so easy—why is it painful sometimes? And what if one partner doesn't feel like having sex right now—there must be something wrong with *that*. What's the "correct" size for a penis, anyway? What, technically, is a virgin? Alice hears panicky questions, too: "Have I done something that seriously jeopardizes my health, my relationship, my reputation, my future, or my life?"

Body parts are mysterious, too. Private parts are incredibly complicated: they're packed with highly sensitive nerve endings, hidden muscles, and miraculous body fluids. Combine this with tidal waves of hormones telling us when to cry, get angry, attack, run, have sex, or just go back to sleep. Then there's the equally volatile brew of conflicting psychological needs for love, commitment, freedom, independence, stability, security, and variety. Human sexual response changes at different points in life, too. But, being aware of your preferences and dislikes, from moment to moment, is the essential starting point. If that includes finding a partner, discovering her/his sexual needs is the next step. A pleasurable sex life may begin one night by yourself with your dominant hand or one very special vibrator, or it may evolve over decades of experiences with many lovers, or with one longtime companion.

In this chapter, Alice will replace myths with a wide-ranging battery of facts: the physiology of orgasm; how to lead the mysterious clitoris to its full potential; where exactly the scrotum hangs out; along with even more specific concerns, including genital odor, vaginal noises, and erections (or the lack of them).

For couples—straight, lesbian, gay, bisexual, or questioning—Alice will address issues related to timing, sexual fantasies, menstruation during sex, slippery intercourse, anal intercourse, and the gamut of sexual appetites, just to name a few. Alice explores solo sex with just as much frankness and verve while acknowledging that masturbation, for some, still carries guilt and fear. She'll discuss commonly held beliefs, like whether or not it stunts growth (it doesn't) or leads to psychological harm (pretty unlikely); and, for men, she'll contemplate the ins and outs of finding something safe to penetrate (glass flasks from the chemistry lab may not be the best choice).

Alice readers prove that everyone has a unique sexual self. Each Alice reader possesses his or her own set of expectations, moral beliefs, physical differences, and experiences—some possibly traumatic, some deeply romantic. The smallest, almost invisible traits can determine what feels pleasurable and what turns us off. Hopefully, after reading this chapter, you'll not only feel inspired to go ask Alice for more advice and information, but you'll also feel more comfortable asking your partner, your proctologist, your gynecologist, your urologist, or (with the help of a mirror) even asking your own body what's going on down there.

Genital Wonderings

Virgin Is Eager to Use Tampons, but Worried about Hymen

Hi Alice,
I am a virgin but I want to use tampons. Can I even though I am not broken???? Please answer quickly. I start going to the Y in a few weeks!!!!!!!! I have no one else to ask. I heard about your Web site on a news station. Thank you so much!!!!!!

Dear Reader,
Hymens come in various shapes and designs. If your hymen is still intact and shaped like a person-hole cover, or a septum (a thin line of skin which divides the center of the vaginal opening, as does the septum of our nose), then this thin membrane of skin may stretch or break. On the other hand, if you have a hymen shaped like a crescent moon around the bottom or side of the vaginal opening, then tampons may not interfere at all. Interestingly, not all women are born with hymens, and hymens can break or stretch without women knowing it. Strenuous activities, such as bicycle riding, horseback riding, stretching, or dancing, can also cause the hymen to break. Lastly, a woman's hymen could have already been broken or stretched by sexual activity, even if she has not had a penis inside of her.

So, for all these reasons, Alice encourages you in your tampon adventure. It is a rite of passage, and think of the stories you will tell your friends or write in your journal!

Alice

Clitoris—Where Is It? Why Doesn't It Work?

Dear Alice,

I really don't know where the clitoris is. I have tried many times to touch my girlfriend's clitoris, but she can't feel anything. Of course, she can't get any feeling from intercourse. What can I do now?

SEARCHING FOR THE WILD CLITORIS

Dear Searching for the Wild Clitoris,

Alice is delighted that you are searching for your girlfriend's clitoris, since that is her pleasure center, or "joy button." The clitoris is a hooded body part at the top of the genitals, above the urethra and below the pubic bone and hairline. Human sexuality and human anatomy texts often have photographs or diagrams of the vulva and its parts which you can both use as a map to find her clitoris (what a treasure hunt!). A health care provider can also show your girlfriend where her clitoris is.

Female anatomy can be pretty confusing since there is a lot going on "down there." Women, unfortunately, are not encouraged to look at their vulva and identify their many intricate, delicate, and powerful parts.

Your girlfriend needs to learn how to make her clitoris respond to stimulation, and, thus, spring to life. Then she can teach you what works for her. Perhaps a referral to sex therapy would be your next step, especially if this is something that your girlfriend would like to change.

The other thing to think about is what *is* happening when you are with your girlfriend, rather than what *isn't* happening. Are you both feeling pleasure, valuing being together, and each feeling cherished and special? Do you enjoy each other's caresses? Perhaps these are the things to focus on, not the orgasmic response. Men tend to measure their success as lovers based upon the strength, kind, and number of orgasms they produce in their partners. How about redefining sexuality in terms of pleasure? It may even expand your own. **RES**

Alice

Women's Urine Exits From?

Dear Alice,

Does urine exit the female body from the vagina or the clitoris?

Dear Reader,

Neither.

Urine exits from a separate body part called the urethra (the "pee hole"), which is below the clitoris and above the vaginal opening. Refer to diagrams in human sexuality and anatomy text books to help make this more clear, or read the directions for using tampons since they have illustrations and information that you might find useful.

If you are talking about your own body, Alice suggests that you take a mirror, a flashlight, and some time and privacy to explore your "down under." If this is about a partner, or when (and if) you have a woman partner, you can explore and unravel this mystery together.

Alice

GETTING TO KNOW YOUR GENITALS

Getting to know one's own genitals is really important, much in the way regular breast and testicular self-exams help folks understand what is normal for them. That way, they have a reference point so that when, and if, there are any changes, they can identify them. **Body knowledge is body power!**

Genital Odor

Dear Alice,

For like several years I have been afflicted with a really smelly crotch. It's like I sweat a lot down there and it just has a really sweaty vaginal odor. I bathe regularly but nothing really helps; by the end of the day I always smell funky. This wouldn't gross me out if it was just an occasional problem, but it happens every day. What can I do?

THANKS, STINKY

Dear Stinky,

It is really important for women to recognize their own scent so they know what is normal for them and can recognize any change(s) in their bodies (similar to doing breast self-exams). Perhaps you may perceive that your normal vaginal scent is a problem—but it may just be your normal scent. However, having a sweaty or strong vaginal odor is another issue.

Vaginal odor can be caused by several factors. The most common cause is vaginal bacterial overgrowth known as bacterial vaginosis, which has a "fishy" or "musty" smell. "Fishy" smells can also result from vaginal infections, such as trichomonas vaginalis, and, in some women, from semen in the vagina. The vagina could also smell "yeasty" because of vaginal yeast overgrowths.

Synthetic underwear, pantyhose, tights, and Spandex exercise clothes do not allow air to circulate around the vulva (the outer lips of the vagina). A moist environment promotes overgrowth of normal skin bacteria that could cause vaginal odor.

A physical exam by a health care provider can determine whether or not the odor is being caused by something that is treatable with a medication, such as for bacterial vaginosis, trichomonas, and yeast. In these cases, the unpleasant smell usually goes away after the treatment. The physical exam can also detect other health problems that might cause unusual body odors.

Vaginal odor could also be caused by excessive sweating because it produces a moist environment. Applying cornstarch can help control moisture and odor, temporarily, as you have already discovered. You may just be one of the women who needs to bathe twice a day, similar to men who have to shave twice a day.

Alice

TO CHANGE VAGINAL ODOR, TRY THE FOLLOWING:

- Wash your vulva with warm water and unscented, gentle soap with mild antibacterial action (this will help keep the skin intact and make it less likely for microscopic cracks to develop, where bacteria like to grow).
- Wear underwear and exercise clothes made from materials that "breathe," such as cotton.
- Wear loose pajama bottoms or a nightgown—or nothing at all—to let your vulva "breathe."
- Keep your vulva as dry and aired as possible because bacteria love moist, dark, and trapped environments.
- Don't use antiperspirants, deodorant tampons, and powders with talc or perfumes or other feminine hygiene ingredients, because they can be irritating.
- Douche no more, since it has been linked to Pelvic Inflammatory Disease (PID). [See "Symptoms of Pelvic Inflammatory Disease (PID)" on page 113.]

Changes in Vaginal Scent

Dear Alice,

Over the past several months, I've noticed a distinct change in my vaginal odor or "scent." It has taken on a more sweet, pungent aroma, which is very different from the musky odor to which I was accustomed. This has me somewhat concerned because I no longer smell like myself! I liken this dilemma to that of an identity crisis!

Is this a natural change in my body—something that will continue to evolve and change as I grow older (I am twenty-five), or could there be a health- or medical-related explanation? A possible dietary deficiency? An illness? Could a change in sexual partners play a part?

WANTS TO KNOW!

Dear Wants to Know!,

Alice would like to commend you on your awareness of your scent, your own unique signature.

Think back on your recent life. When your scent changed, was there anything else in your life that changed at the same time? Many of the factors you mentioned could explain your change in scent. Diet changes, hormones (such as when women are pregnant), and vaginal infections could all affect vaginal scent. A change in partners could as well, since semen (if the partner is male) mingling with your own fluids during intercourse alters what smells like you. Of course, if it is an unpleasant, or even a foul, odor, that is usually indicative of an infection, such as yeast or trichomonas. These are treated with either over-the-counter or prescription medications; however, neither sounds like the scent you are describing.

It may be nothing, but check it out for peace of mind.

Alice

Whom Should I Thank for My Penis?

Dear Alice,

Okay, I have looked in just about every place possible. I was just curious about the genetics of genitalia. Is the size of a penis inherited from the father's or mother's side? I have found more than enough info on the size, etc. I just want to know what side of the family my penis came from (no pun intended). Thanks.

Dear Reader,

After doing some genital gymnastics herself, Alice wound up in Washington, D.C., before finding an answer to your penile pondering. According to the National Center for Genome Research at the National Institutes of Health, penis size, like height, weight, and general build, probably comes from both mom and pop. Research on size-related genital genetics is scarce because funds and brain power are, understandably, spent on finding treatments and cures for genetic disorders, like human growth hormone deficiency, which can cause stunted penile development. Alice hopes that this information doesn't cause you to lose a bet, or, worse yet, start a family feud.

Alice

Tremendous Testicles

Dear Alice,

I'm on my school's track team and I don't know if I'm doing something wrong. When I run, my testicles seem to get in the way and are sore afterward. They seem too big. Is that possible? The jocks I've tried don't help much and we are issued stretch shorts that don't hide them well at all! It's embarrassing and sometimes it hurts to ride my bike, too. They have always been that size but is there something else I can do?

WONDERING

Dear Wondering,

So, your cup runneth over. Like penises, breasts, vaginas, hands, feet, noses, and almost every other endowment, testicles and the sack (scrotum) that they sit in vary in size, shape, and texture. The degree to which this hormone- and sperm-producing hardware descends differs from man to man, too. Temperature sometimes plays a role as well: "your boys" (thank you, Kramer) pull closer to your body when you are cold, and "hang out" when your thermometer is in the comfort zone. This automatic action keeps sperm at their required temperature. (Don't worry, Alice isn't going to suggest that you pack your privates in ice before your next track meet.)

Have you tried wearing underwear or a jock strap one size smaller than the ones you usually sport? If it doesn't cut off your circulation when you're moving about, briefer briefs might give you that extra support you need to both reduce your pain and reduce your anxiety about how you look in shorts. Staying with sporting goods, do you have proper shock-absorbers? Do you wear shoe cushions and sneakers that help buffer the violent pounding of many athletic endeavors that rattle even the tiniest of testicles? The same goes for your bike seat: additional padding is often essential for a smoother ride.

Even if you're really strolling around in shame over your bountiful basket, Alice and her male friends wouldn't be a bit surprised to learn that you are actually the envy of your teammates, some of whom have no doubt contemplated stuffing their stockings with a sock or potato to boost their profiles.

Alice

Testicle Hurts

Alice,

This is a serious query about a health problem I'm having. My left testicle HURTS! I am quite concerned. It's not sharp pain but a gradual aching pain, but it's damn tender when I touch it. Is this testicular cancer, testicular torsion, a hernia, the consequence of an active sex life, or simply the result of two successive bouts of masturbation? Please help me resolve this.

SWOLLEN BALLS

Dear Swollen Balls,

Make an appointment for a full health exam, and discuss this problem in the context of the rest of your life, including any recent changes before your testicle started to hurt.

Testicular cancer most commonly appears as a firm, painless swelling of one testicle. Cancerous lumps in the testis are generally not tender when they are touched. Testicular cancer is a relatively rare form of cancer, usually occurring in men between the ages of fifteen and twenty-five years, especially if they have an undescended testicle.

Other causes of swelling of the testis, which are harmless: hydrocele, a collection of fluid in the scrotum; epididymal cyst, a fluid-filled swelling of the epididymis (the structure behind the testis where sperm mature), which may also cause fever and discharge from the penis; and varicocele, varicose veins in the scrotum, which is described as feeling like "a bag of worms." Inflammation of the testis can also be related to bacterial infections.

Torsion of the testis occurs when a testicle rotates, and the spermatic cord becomes obstructed and the blood supply is cut off. This most commonly occurs around puberty and causes acute severe pain and

HOW TO DO A TESTICULAR SELF-EXAM

Men are encouraged to do a monthly testicular self-exam to become familiar with their anatomy, and to note if any changes occur. Do a testicular self-exam during a shower, when the heat of the water relaxes the scrotum. Rotate each testicle between your thumb and forefinger, making sure you feel a round, firm surface. Look at the rest of your scrotum's contents for any changes. If you have questions about this, ask your health care provider.

swelling of the testis. The first symptoms of a hernia usually include a bulge in the abdominal wall and abdominal discomfort.

If during sex you are engaging in S & M (sadism and masochism), with twisting, pulling, or squeezing of your testicles, this may be a cause of pain. Otherwise, average masturbatory or sexual techniques do not cause your testicles to swell. It may be simply coincidence that you had more sex than usual before your testicle swelled.

Alice

Boyfriend's Uncircumcised Penis Smells

Alice,
Maybe this is a weird question, but my boyfriend is uncircumcised. If he hasn't taken a shower right before we make love, his penis smells. I assume it is the secretions getting stuck under the foreskin. Have you had any other questions about this? I'm really very curious to know if this is a problem.

FORESKIN CURIOUS

Dear Foreskin Curious,
The foreskin is a fold of skin that covers the glans of the penis (a.k.a., the head). Circumcision removes the foreskin from the penis. Men with uncircumcised penises need to pull back their foreskin and wash the area underneath at least once a day.

Smegma, a cheesy substance that can have a "particular" scent, is secreted from tiny subcutaneous glands beneath the foreskin. This is probably what you are noticing on your boyfriend's penis. The area under the foreskin is also ripe for bacterial growth. Infections can easily develop under the foreskin if isn't pulled back and washed. A yeast infection, which has symptoms that include redness, swelling, and a pasty discharge, is also a possible occurrence when the uncircumcised penis is not cleaned properly.

Shower or bathe together before sex. Wash his penis, pulling the foreskin back. Or tell him that you're concerned about getting a vaginal infection, and ask that he please wash before having sex. As a last resort, take the super-direct route: "Your penis stinks—let's give him a bath." Choose which approach you think will work best. Alice bets one of these will work.

Alice

Shave Your Pubic Hair?

Dear Alice,

I'm wondering about what happens to a man's pubic hair after you shave it off completely. Would the pubic hair be permanently shaven off or would it grow back? If it does grow back, would it become hairier than before, like beard growth?

Curious

Dear Curious,

Shaving your pubic hair is by no means permanent. As the hair starts to grow back, however, it can be very itchy and uncomfortable. If you only shave once, your hair usually grows similarly as before. While shaving any body part may seem to increase hair growth, which may appear more coarse, the number of hair follicles stays the same. What may have appeared to be increased hair growth when someone was maturing and beginning to shave was not due to shaving, but to normal growth and development. By the way, this applies to women as well.

Alice

Sexual Questions

Where Does the Penis Go for Intercourse?

Dear Alice,

My new girlfriend and I had sex for the first time this weekend. Later in the evening, she was curious about something . . . "Where is that thing going???" she asked. She mentioned that full insertion was painful and she wanted to know what I was hitting, and "how far does it go?" Being admittedly a bit rusty on my knowledge of the anatomy of the female body, I told her that I *thought* it went no further than the "uvula" (whatever that is), but that I would do a little research, maybe see what I could get off the Net and get back to her.

NEED DIRECTIONS

Dear Need Directions,

A penis goes into a vagina. Inside the vaginal opening are walls made up of soft tissue. This tissue tends to mold around a penis, fingers, tampons, or any other object that may be placed inside the vagina. The length of the vagina varies from woman to woman, and extends with arousal.

When you mentioned the uvula, perhaps you meant the vulva, or outer genitals, which consists of the visible sexual organs: the tip of the clitoris, the clitoral hood, and the inner and outer lips. As for what you're "hitting," it could be your girlfriend's cervix, which hasn't yet changed position. When she's aroused enough, her cervix will have moved out of the way, and her wetness will make sex more comfortable. For more information about the anatomy and physiology of sexual and reproductive organs, look at a basic human sexuality text in your local bookstore. The graphics may make it more clear.

Alice

Conservative Considers Coitus

Dear Alice,

I'm a Christian, very conservative in upbringing, and I'm having difficulties in discussing sex in an open and casual manner. I told my male friends that sex should be done within the parameters of marriage. But they told me that I should have a first sexual experience so as to satisfy my wife or maybe a girlfriend (I don't have one yet). Should I follow their opinion regarding this? Should I first know the dynamics of sexual intercourse before doing it with her? I would appreciate your kind response. Thank you.

GENTLEKID

Dear GentleKid,

Conservative or liberal, talking about sex can be awkward and confusing, as well as exciting and fun. As you know, Alice believes that considering, and communicating about sex can be just as important as "doing it," so thanks for the reminder.

The right answer for you is the one that satisfies your beliefs. The choices that make you feel most comfortable are the ones that are right for you. Of course, sometimes you can't know what's best for you until you sample your options. Sure, what you learn from past sexual experiences can add to the pleasure of future ones; but, for many, the energy and excitement of the "first time" is unrivaled by all the sex that follows. And when it comes down to it, your partner at the time is the best teacher of all, as each of your partners will be turned on (and will turn you on) in different ways.

Sex is just one part of the picture—your future partners will want you for so many other reasons, not the least of which is your "gentle-kid"ness.

Alice

Deciding to Devirginize

Dear Alice,

I am an eighteen-year-old virgin, but my boyfriend wants to have sex with me. We have been dating now for eight months, and he says he has been waiting long enough. I have this fear of having sex because of the consequences, but I try to tell myself that as long as I use protection, things like that shouldn't happen.

I'm not sure what I'm asking for; I'm not sure it's advice either. Right now I'm reasonably sure that I don't want to have sex, but this little voice (probably his) keeps asking "What's the big deal?"

I know it's not a big deal, but it's something I really believe in, and I want to wait. I only have one life to live and I want to do it right. I did a lot of things I ended up regretting, but this is really important to me. The only thing is, I have no problems fantasizing about making love to him. I just have trouble with carrying out the actual act. I really need to ask if you think my fear of sex is unnatural or just a product of the way I've been raised?

Is there any way I can get over all the horror stories of regret and painful first times and just give myself to the guy of my dreams?

Confused

Dear Confused,

It sounds to Alice as though you are choosing not to have sex right now, and she supports you in that decision. Your letter says clearly that this is something you really believe in and that you want to wait. It doesn't matter if you are making this choice out of personal conviction or fear; it is your personal choice at this time and it deserves to be heard and respected. If your boyfriend chooses not to be with you because you choose not to have sex with him, or anyone at this point, then where is his respect for your opinion and your convictions? And for you? Would you want to be with someone who is so impatient and who seems to have more respect for his own needs and desires than for yours?

Alice is delighted that in your fantasies you have pleasure when you think about being sexual with him. This is important when you finally do choose to become sexually active. It also is a way to give yourself pleasure now.

You will "give yourself to" or choose to become sexual with the guy of your dreams when you are ready, and only you can decide when that is. Alice asks you, if you feel so strongly about waiting, then what's the rush? You will be sexually active for many years. This is an important decision, and no one should tell you to have sex when you are not ready. It *is* a pretty big deal.

Continue to explore your feelings of closeness with your boyfriend. Keep talking with him about the things you are willing to do with him—socially, romantically, sexually—as well as the things you are not willing to do with him. Perhaps there are ways that both of you can get your needs met—while you still remain a virgin—and you won't have to think about contraception or sexually transmitted diseases (STDs). In the meantime, you can learn the facts about contraception and STDs by yourself and together. Both of you can read some related Alice questions, for example. That way, when you do choose to have sex, you will be more prepared.

Have courage, girlfriend. Sex can be wonderful—the first, fifteenth, and fiftieth time—when *you* choose to have it. The when, where, and with whom, are up to you.

Alice

Am I Still a Virgin?

Question #1:

Dear Alice,

Me and my boyfriend had sex the other day. But he didn't fully insert . . . so he just went in a bit. I didn't want sex so we stopped. So am I still a virgin? Thank you!

Question #2:

Alice,

How about if I am a virgin and I use the condom in my first experience. Am I going to keep being a virgin???

THE BOY

Dear Reader and The Boy,

It sounds like keeping your virginity is important to both of you.

In the first scenario, Alice would say that it's not entirely unreasonable for you to still consider yourself a virgin. If you want to be completely literal about it, you could say that you're one-half or three-quarters a virgin, depending on how far his penis went in. Just joking! The main point is that you decided you weren't ready to have sex. You wanted to keep your virginity, and you did just that.

As for "The Boy," Alice cannot say the same. Sex with a condom is still sex. If you use a condom the first time you have sex, it's still considered your "first time." Loosely translated, that means the time you "lost your virginity" (although Alice thinks we may need to rethink this phrase and think about what we are gaining). Naturally, Alice applauds your decision to use a condom and hopes you will continue. Even though it won't protect you from a loss of virginity, it will help protect you against numerous sexually transmitted diseases (STDs) and fatherhood.

Much goes into the decision to have sex for the first time. Often peer pressure, strong emotions, uncertainty, curiosity, guilt, fear, exploding hormones, and _____ (you fill in the blank) are involved in this big life event. It sounds like both of you have given some thought to what your virginity means to you. And Alice hopes that when, and if, you do decide to have full insertion sex for the first time, you'll be happy with that decision.

Alice

Male Virgin Wants to Be Normal

Dear Alice,

I am a twenty-one-year-old male student and still a virgin. I am very shy and do not have any girlfriends. I masturbate almost every day, but desperately want to have real sex. I have thought about paying a prostitute, but I am not sure. Are there any groups for people in my situation, i.e., people who want to lose their virginity and be normal?

VIRGIN

Dear Virgin,

Normal by whose criteria? Everyone wants to be normal. Of course you are normal if you are a virgin at twenty-one, but peer pressure may try to force you to feel you're not. At what point does being a virgin seem abnormal? There are plenty of twenty-one-year-old male virgins around; however, you will never know since they will not tell you. To them, it remains a private matter. It is not considered acceptable for men to be virgins since, with socialization, they believe it is their job and responsibility to be sexually knowledgeable and experienced.

Try thinking about your virginity in another way. How would your life change if you were no longer a virgin? What would be different? From your letter, it seems more important to you to no longer be a virgin than it is to have a girlfriend. Is that true for you? What is it about being a virgin that is a burden to you?

Think about the possibility of finding someone you want to get to know better, someone that you might like to spend time with, and someone you think you could feel comfortable with, so that a relationship may grow. This path of rethinking your goal and plan will help you connect with another person rather than focus on the isolation. As Alice sees it, it is not your virginity that is the problem, but your sense of isolation and loneliness.

Alice is glad you asked about a group. When you think of joining a group, however, Alice would suggest finding one where you are interested in being involved, rather than focusing on your "problem." If you find a social, political, or community service organization where you feel committed to the issues, you will be more likely to meet others who feel the way you do. You can build on this and cultivate quality relationships.

Alice's hunch is that the more time you spend with others, involved with issues you want to learn more about or are committed to, your need to "devirginize" will subside.

In the meantime, rethink your ideas about masturbation. Masturbation *is* real sex. What it isn't, at this point, is partner sex. Masturbation can relieve the tension of sexual energy, and even loneliness, temporarily. Clearly, you can still masturbate as you go on your search for a larger social network, and, ultimately, a partner with whom to share your feelings, activities, closeness, joy, humor, and sexuality as well. Finally, many people masturbate even when they have a partner. It is a part of their sexuality, not a partner replacement. So, as you search for a partner, enjoy yourself every step of the way.

Alice

Afraid to Have Sex?

Hi, Alice.
My girlfriend and I have been going out for more than two years now. I am a first-year student (eighteen years old) and she is seventeen. We haven't had sex yet, but during the last year and a half we tried pretty much everything there is besides it. I really feel this is the right time, but when I try to talk to her about it, all she says is that she is afraid. She says it is not that she does not believe in losing virginity before marriage, she is just afraid. I don't want to pressure her, but I just feel that maybe I am not the right person for her or something. What should I do? Thanks.

CURIOUS

Dear Curious,
Why not let things lie where they are for the moment? Is there something special that you think will happen the moment you first have intercourse? You can continue to pleasure each other as you have, making each other feel safe and secure in your relationship, and then, at another nonstressful point later on, approach the subject again. What might she be afraid of? Is it pregnancy? HIV? Other STDs? If it's any of these, you both can make an appointment to see a health care provider together and discuss having sex. You can also read books together to learn more about your sexuality.

You need to talk with and trust each other. When, and if, you finally get to it, your lovemaking will be more intimate.

Alice

Painful Sex

Dear Alice,
I have never had sex, but I have tried now twice with my boyfriend, and it has been incredibly painful. It's felt like there is a barrier inside me, and the second time I bled. I feel like I am relaxed, and my boyfriend is very gentle and slow, but it still really hurts—more than I think it should. I am able to use tampons—I'm not that small—but I don't know what the problem is. Is it supposed to hurt this much? Could there be something wrong?

PENETRATION?

Dear Penetration?,
This barrier you describe may or may not be your hymen. An unstretched hymen may cause you some pain or discomfort. However, you mention that there was some blood during your second attempt. This could mean you have partially or fully stretched your hymen by now.

Being relaxed is an important part of having comfortable sex, and so is being sufficiently aroused and well-lubricated before trying to put your partner's penis inside of you. One way to remedy this situation is to spend a long time touching each other, kissing, and caressing before you try to have intercourse. Intercourse then becomes an extension of other touching, and your body may be more physically ready for it. Your partner may place his finger(s) inside your vagina while touching and/or kissing your clitoris till you are comfortable, and even feel pleasure.

If you find that the pain with intercourse, or attempted intercourse, does not diminish at all over time, then seeing a health care provider is your next step. S/he can help determine whether or not you might have a local infection, such as a yeast infection; or a reaction to a birth control product, like foam, spermicidal jelly, or lube; or vaginismus, a strong, involuntary tightening of the vaginal muscles, which does not allow a penis in (or sometimes a finger, or even a tampon). For vaginismus, a referral to a sex therapist is your next step. Call the American Association of Sex Educators, Counselors, and Therapists (AASECT) for the name of a therapist near you.

As you are just becoming sexually active, now would be a good time to have an annual exam and discuss contraceptive options and safer sex, so make an appointment to check in with a health care provider in any case. **RES**

Alice

WHAT IS "LUBE"?

"Lube" is a water-based, nongreasy, gel-like clear substance which allows for safer, more pleasurable sex and protection by increasing the body's own natural lubrication.

Period When Boyfriend Is Visiting

HI Alice,
My boyfriend goes to another school, and will be visiting me soon. Unfortunately, I'll get my period the day before he arrives. Is there any way to make your period shorter?
SIGNED, NOT IN THE MOOD FOR KOTEX

Dear Not in the Mood for Kotex,
It is fine to have sex during your period—in fact, orgasm may help relieve menstrual cramps. Some women find that sex during their

period is more enjoyable as they are less worried about becoming pregnant, and they find that the menstrual blood acts as a lubricant. You and your partner both have to feel comfortable, though, with the sight, feel, smell, and taste of your blood. In order to hold back some of the flow, you may want to take a bath directly before having sex. Throw a towel under the two of you, so that you don't have to change the sheets, clean the table, mop the floor, etc., after sex.

Another possibility is to get fitted for a diaphragm. In addition to being an effective form of birth control when combined with contraceptive jelly, it works well to hold back menstrual blood during your period.

Be creative—two heads are better than one.

Alice

Vaginal "Farts"?

Dear Alice,
Have you ever heard of vaginal farts? Well, most every time I have sex, especially in certain positions, air seems to get pushed inside of me and what happens sounds suspiciously like a fart. It's embarrassing. Any way to prevent this and does this happen to other women?

SIGNED, DESPERATE

Dear Desperate,
Yes, it does happen to other women, and yes, it can be embarrassing! Vaginal "farts," or "varts" as another reader once named them, occur when air gets into your vagina during intercourse. During arousal, the vagina lengthens and the uterus moves, creating more air space. Often, the "fart" occurs when the walls of the vagina and uterus return to their unaroused positions. Extra lube may make the difference. You also may want to stay away from certain positions for a while, to spare yourself the embarrassment. Your other option is to say something like "It's awfully drafty in here," to distract your and your partner's attention from the noise. Or, just say, "Excuse me."

Alice

What Is "Frigidity"?

Dear Alice,
Could you give me some information about frigidity?

Dear Reader,
"Frigidity" is a judgmental term usually used by a man to describe a woman who does not orgasm through penile thrusting, or who is not

open to him sexually, or who does not want to have sex as often as he does. The assumption is that she is cold, unfeeling, unresponsive, unavailable, or that something is wrong with her. It is not a term sex counselors, sex therapists, or health educators use these days, because of its negative connotation and incorrect assumptions.

According to professional lore, Alfred Kinsey, the famous sex researcher, said that there were no frigid women, only inept men. Of course, that reflects a heterosexual model, and it doesn't have much compassion for men. Alice could update that to say, "There are no frigid women, only uneducated men and women." The more information women have about their bodies, the more pleasure they can receive.

From now on, Alice recommends that "frigid" be used as a term to describe a bitter winter, an unheated swimming pool, or a butcher's meat locker.   RES

Alice

Girlfriend Gets Too Wet

Alice,
When making love with my girlfriend, she says she gets too wet, doesn't like it, and would like to know if there is anything she can do to lessen the wetness just a bit.

CARING

Dear Caring,
Your girlfriend may have cervicitis, a disease that is known to cause lots of discharge. Also, if you have oral sex, the germs of your own mouth and throat might be causing her discharge. Does she use an IUD? Any type of foreign body in the uterus can increase vaginal fluids.

There are women who expel large amounts of fluid upon orgasm; there are people of both sexes who pee a bit when highly aroused; and then there are people who are quite regularly wet when sexually aroused. However, for most individuals, hot and juicy are synonymous! You and she may be making a problem over what is, at worst, an inconvenience, and what would be for many people a blessing. If she has an examination and there is no medical cause for concern, you can try the "terry cloth approach." Keep a towel near the bed and use it sensuously to dry off your girlfriend and yourself during sex.

Alice

Dry Up My Wet Dreams!

Alice,
I have a normal sex life with my wife (once or twice a week), but I have been having a problem lately. I have had about four wet dreams last

year. I don't know why but I feel really bad about this. Is there something wrong with me? How can I stop this???

FEELING HELPLESS

Dear Feeling Helpless,
Lucky you! You're getting sexual satisfaction when you're awake and
when you're asleep. If your wet dreams aren't diminishing your desire
to have sex with your partner, then could your troubled mind be a product of the association of nocturnal emissions with adolescence and limited adult sexual activity? True, wet dreams are more prevalent among
these groups, but they should be thought of as "normal" for all other
males, too. Okay, so maybe you'll have to do the laundry a little more
frequently, but isn't that worth the pleasure, as long as you can free
yourself from anxiety common to this natural occurrence?

SWEET DREAMS,
Alice

Girlfriend Gags During Oral Sex

Alice,
My girlfriend enjoys performing oral sex on me, but can't seem to get
much more than the head in her mouth without gagging. How can she
learn to take more in? Oh, incidentally, I'm just of ordinary penis size.

FELLATIO

Dear Fellatio,
This is an area where the two of you will need to negotiate and work on
it together. Ask her specific questions about the point at which she starts
to gag: Does her mouth feel too full? Is your penis touching the back of
her throat, or the sides? Or, more important, is this something she even
wants to do?

Once you and your girlfriend find out more about what happens
when she starts to gag, together you can try to solve the problem. If it's
purely a physical thing, have her try using her hand to guide your penis
into her mouth. That way, she can control when, how far, and how fast
your penis will move. Try different positions, with you on your knees,
lying down, with her on top, standing up, etc., to see if there is one position or another where she feels more comfortable and in control. See
what works, being willing to delay or give up your oral pleasure for
other pleasures if she is unable to do it.

Alice

Need More Information on Cunnilingus

Dear Alice,

I enjoy performing cunnilingus on my partner and she enjoys receiving it as well. Are there any techniques that can help me increase the pleasure she receives from oral sex?

ORAL MAN

Dear Oral Man,

Your partner is the best resource available to answer your question. Ask her what she likes and what turns her lights on before you go down on her and while you are doing it. Pay attention to her signals (moans and cries of delight or discomfort) as you try variations of your own style, or ask her about her fantasies. Many women would be thrilled to have you as their partner!

Alice

Cunnilingus and Menstruation?

Dear Alice,

If one has a long-term partner and neither AIDS nor any other STD is a concern, is there any medical reason not to perform cunnilingus on a menstruating woman? My significant other is particularly horny during her period and would love cunnilingus at this time. I am willing but curious.

SAFE

Dear Safe,

If there is no history of STDs for you and your partner, then go for it. Orgasms can help relieve menstrual cramps, so sexual activity during menstruation can be a bonus.

For those of you who don't like the idea of oral sex during a woman's period, know that on some days she has a lighter flow than others; and, when a woman takes a bath, often her period stops for a while.

For those of you who are unsure of your partner's STD status, you can use a dam or an opened-up rectangular piece of nonlubed condom to protect both of you during her period. (Plastic wrap also works in a pinch.) (See "What's a dam?" on page 106.)

Alice

Can't Stay Erect

Dear Alice:

It seems that I can't maintain an erection for more than a couple of minutes during intercourse. In fact, sometimes it doesn't seem to want to get up and play at all. The girlfriend is really starting to take this personally, but I know it's not her fault. Help! Are there any vitamins, diets, etc., that may help?

SIGNED, HERE AND GONE

Dear Here and Gone,
Erection problems can be mainly physical, mainly psychological, or a mambo combo. You say that you are unable to maintain an erection during intercourse. Can you keep an erection when she touches your penis with her hands or mouth, or when you masturbate?

Some men have problems keeping erections at the beginning of a relationship. Then, after they become more comfortable with their new partners, their erections become more reliable. Pay attention to your erection patterns to help you decide if you need to see a urologist or a sex therapist. If you have erections when you wake up or through masturbation, but not with a partner, that's important information that says your body is working correctly, physically. For the time being, why not receive pleasure and not worry about erections? These kinds of difficulties are common and transient. You can view them as part of life rather than as problems. Or, if it *is* a problem for you, sex therapy may make a difference. **RES**

Alice

PENIS SIZE

Unaroused penis size varies greatly among men. There is less variation in size, however, among erect penises since smaller penises enlarge more during erection. The average length of an aroused penis is 5 3/4 inches. *Men tend to underestimate the size of their penis* since, when they look down at it, a portion of it is covered by their pubic hair. Remember, size may be important to both men and women, but what you do with it is the larger issue.

Objects in Anus During Sex?

Alice:
I think this web site is fantastic and incredibly healthy for everyone. Maybe, with the help of things like this, we'll actually get to the point someday when people can ask about things like this without having to need anonymity.

Anyhow, the reason I'm writing is that I would like a little info. Are there medical risks associated with anal penetration? What if the object is larger than a finger? Should penetration occur only so far?

EXPERIMENTING

Dear Experimenting,
Hooray for the idea of openly talking about sexuality! Forget the future, start now—with your partners and friends.

As to your questions, the anus can be stimulated with fingers, tongue, penis, or any slender object. It is a highly sensitive area for many people. Your body will tell you when something is in too far, and then you need to tell your partner. Objects may be sucked up into the rectum past the sphincter. So, hold on tight. The anus is less elastic than the vagina, so ask your partner to be gentle. Make sure objects are inserted slowly, the person receiving is relaxed, and use a lube. Lube is especially important since the anus is *not* self-lubricating. Since moving objects from one person's anus to another's vagina or anus can cause infections, wash the penis, finger, or object first before inserting. Men inserting their penis into someone's anus can use a condom with extra lube. Rimming, or using your tongue to stimulate another's anus, is made safer by using a dam or an opened-up rectangular piece of nonlubed condom (see "What's a dam?" on page 106), kissing and licking through the thin latex.

Some people have said that they like having something in their anus during sex, with no pressure or movement, just presence. Other folks are really turned on by objects—a finger, penis, or dildo—moving in a rhythmic motion in their anus (they like the sensations deep inside). Whatever you like, have fun and be safe.

Alice

Receiving Anal Sex: What Does It Mean?

Dear Alice,
I am a well-adjusted late twenties male with a steady girlfriend. Lately, I have been increasingly fantasizing about various types of anal penetration. I have discovered that during masturbation, this brings me very intense pain/pleasure. Even though I think it may be satisfying to experiment with a vibrator or other objects inserted by my girlfriend, I find myself drawn toward trying the real thing (i.e., having anal sex with a penis). The problem is, I definitely do not consider myself homosexual and, in fact, the thought of the actual act with another man actually repulses me. Am I trying to have the real thing without going through a bisexual experiment or what?

Dear Reader,
One beauty of human sexuality is its freedom of expression through a range of pleasure possibilities. We can satisfy ourselves with fantasies and masturbation. We can give and receive pleasure through touching, holding, kissing, and intercourse. We can involve just one or two areas of the body, or turn on everything from head to toe. We can be ourselves, and we can play games. We can let our fingers do the walking, perhaps picking up a few sex toys along the way. We can communicate our passions, or we can "take the Fifth."

We can also chip away at this "sexual constitution" by hanging labels on our thoughts and actions—labels that act like a ball and chain around our desires. Your enjoyment of anal penetration, from whatever source, and for whatever reason, does not in and of itself mean that you are bi-, hetero-, or homosexual. Throughout our lives, we all live on a dynamic continuum of sexual desires. It is often socially and culturally influenced discomfort with sexuality in general—let alone private behaviors not defined as "normal"—that push us to pigeonhole our sexual thoughts and actions into comfortable and manageable boxes.

Alice applauds you for getting in touch with what flies your flag. You might share your fantasies with your girlfriend, if you think they would enhance your relationship. You can also pursue anal sex satisfaction now, later, or never, remembering that sexual experimentation of any kind does not mean a lifelong commitment. The choice is yours.

Alice

G-Spot

Alice,
What is the "G-spot" on a woman and where is it?

VAGINAL

Dear Vaginal,
The G-spot has been identified as a sensitive area right behind the front wall of the vagina, between the back of the pubic bone and the cervix. (A man's "G-spot" is his prostate.) When this spot is stimulated during touching or sex, some women's orgasms are accompanied by "ejaculate" from the urethra. Ernst Grafenberg, who first wrote about female ejaculatory fluid in 1950, stated that fluid expelled by women during orgasm was not urine, as was the common belief, but instead, secretions which are similar to a man's ejaculate minus sperm.

There is an ongoing debate over whether such an anatomical feature actually exists. Erogenous zones vary from woman to woman. The term G-spot is often used generically by both women and men as a label for a woman's most sensitive spot within the genital area. For some women, there doesn't seem to be any specific spot in their vaginas that is sensitive to stimulation. For others, the G-spot is quite real, with evidence to prove it.   **RES**

Alice

Kegel Technique

Hi Alice!
Could you describe the male and female versions of the Kegel technique in detail, including mention of how often it should be practiced for the maximum benefit in the least amount of time?

KT?

Dear KT?,
Kegel exercises were developed by Dr. Arnold Kegel to help women, especially after childbirth, regain bladder control by strengthening their pelvic muscles. Dr. Kegel later discovered that his exercises also increased orgasm intensity. There are many variations, but the exercises are similar.

For women and men:

• Locate your pelvic muscles by stopping the flow of urine midstream.
• Contract the pelvic muscles hard for one second and then release them, ten times in a row, three times a day. Gradually increase the number of contractions so that by the end of one month, you are doing ten contractions, twenty times a day.
• Vary the exercise by holding the contraction for a count of three and then releasing it. You can mix the exercises up, some short and some long.
• Kegel during commercials, every time the phone rings, at each stoplight when you are driving or riding, while you are waiting for your Web search results—find your own regular pattern.
• Kegel when having sex for extra pleasure for you and your partner.
• Do the Kegels for a minimum of six weeks. Results will not be immediate, but eventually you will be able to notice a difference.

Note: Some practitioners recommend that pregnant women do up to one hundred extra Kegels per day to strengthen their pelvic muscles for the work they're about to do.

Alice

Sex and Disabilities

Dear Alice,

What can you tell me, a caregiver, about male quadriplegics and sexual intercourse? I take care of a young gunshot victim who is dealing with his sexuality. I would like to better understand what he is dealing with.

THANK YOU, A CONCERNED CAREGIVER

Dear A Concerned Caregiver,

Begin to learn about sex and disability by talking with the person you care for. The reason for this is that you already have established trust with this person, and, hopefully, he with you.

If his disability is one that has developed recently, one of the challenges is encouraging him to get to know his new body, to see what feels good where, and to know how he responds, so that he can know what to expect when he is with a partner. It is important to know that even people with exactly the same kind of injury can differ in their perceptions and sensations.

Perhaps Christopher and Dana Reeve are our most recent inspirations. Not only have they talked about Mr. Reeve's rehabilitation after his horse riding accident, but Reeve shared feelings and facts about their "new" sex lives during an ABC news interview. People with seemingly overwhelming disabilities often can meet others, develop relationships, marry, and have children. Of course, it may take some time, encouragement, work, and support for people with disabilities to adjust before becoming more positive about themselves and their outlook on life.

One way of approaching this subject with him is to rent movies, such as *Coming Home* and *The Waterdance*. Also, contact the Sexuality Information Education Council of the United States (SIECUS) for a current bibliography on sexuality and disabilities. **RES**

Alice

Masturbation

Masturbation: It's Still Okay

Hey Alice,
I heard a lot of people saying masturbation is the best way to relieve oneself, but doesn't it cause harm?

Dear Reader,
Assuming that by, "relieving oneself," you mean answering sexual urges, then, of course, masturbation is one great way to experience self-pleasure. As long as you're not stimulating yourself in public, or refusing food, friends, and gainful employment because you can't keep your hands off your privates, then the only masturbation-related harm will remain with those who poo-poo it, and the effect that their ignorance or moral beliefs have on people seeking to satisfy a most natural desire.

Go WILD,
Alice

Masturbation Inhibits Growth?

Dear Alice,
Does masturbation affect your growth if you are not yet fully grown?

Dear Reader,
NO, masturbation does not stunt growth. Neither your penis, nor any other part of your body, including your height, is affected. Masturbation also does not cause blindness, hairy palms, or insanity, as some people have heard. Furthermore, masturbation does not cause men to lose their precious body fluids because more are being continually produced.

Masturbation causes pleasurable, soothing, exciting, orgasmic, and, ultimately, relaxing sensations (and guilt, at times, for some).

If your question is more about being short in stature, there are many other possible causes, including heredity. You can check with your pediatrician, if you are concerned, but be confident that masturbation is *not* responsible.

Alice

Holy Hand Job!

Dear Alice,
I started masturbating when I was nine. Recently, I have discovered that sticking my penis into every hole that I see, whether it be a hole in the wall or into a flask in chem lab, is the most incredible experience that I have ever felt. The last time I did this, my best friend walked in on me. Now he thinks that I am totally crazy and I don't know what to do. Alice, PLEASE HELP ME!

HOLE FETISH

Dear Hole Fetish,
If your friend had never plunged his penis into an opening designed for something other than masturbation—prior to walking in on your latest round of creative self-stimulation—he probably ran home in ecstasy to discover a wonderful new world of pleasurable monkey-spanking possibilities. If Alice were you, she'd wait for a big thank-you, not a strait-jacket. Now, without any intent to dampen your crusade for that perfect "hole-in-one," although it may be exciting to masturbate in a "forbidden" place, Alice encourages you to use good judgment, discretion, and privacy. Also, be careful not to throw all caution to the wind: Was chem class in session when you performed that experiment? Did you clean out every last drop of hydrochloric acid from that flask? Did you use lube to prevent getting stuck? And was the Bunsen burner turned off and safely put away? Other sharp and breakable objects, electrical wiring, and matter used by others, such as the main course for tonight's dinner, should also send up red flags. Just ask Alexander, the hero of Philip Roth's *Portnoy's Complaint*, with whose desire and ingenuity you will no doubt identify.

Alice

Surprise! It's Masturbation!

Dear Alice,
As young girls, my friend and I discovered that the simple activity of shimmying up the pole at the playground would produce a wonderful tingling feeling! Later, we realized that this was probably sexual in nature! Is this type of activity a common occurrence among youngsters? Could the simple muscular tension involved cause orgasms?

Dear Reader,

Is it common? Yes. Movements that give pleasurable sensations are common for youngsters (as well as for oldsters). For years, sexual arousal and orgasm have been observed and recorded in young children. Similarly, sex play, such as "doctor," is also common since children are naturally curious about their bodies.

Can it cause orgasm? Yes, yes, yes! If the sensations are intense enough, muscle tension and/or clitoral pressure can and does cause arousal, pleasure, and orgasm.

Alice

Wants Girlfriend to Masturbate

Dear Alice,

I have a rather strange question.

My girlfriend does not masturbate. We've talked about it a few times, and she has basically said that she would like to be able to masturbate, but can't get the feeling that it's "dirty" or "wrong" out of her head. She has no problem with me masturbating (she enjoys it, actually)—but she simply can't get herself to do it. Any suggestions to help her feel more comfortable with herself and her body?

ARGH

Dear Argh,

Research shows that women learn to masturbate later than men, often during or after college rather than during puberty. This process includes two parts: learning to orgasm and learning to feel good about it. In the 1970s, women would meet in women's groups with safety, humor, and support to talk about many things, including orgasm—having them, not having them; how to have them, how to have them more frequently; what works, what doesn't work; how to have them with partners; and their feelings about orgasm. Ironically, this is not happening today. So for similar information, she can check out some of the materials and videos available at woman-sensitive, sex-positive bookstores.

Your girlfriend is not alone. There is plenty that she can do to learn (you can learn, too!), *if* this is truly a path your girlfriend wants to take! She may need *privacy* and time alone to explore her own body and to experiment, learning for herself what sensations are pleasurable. Sometimes, a nonallergenic lotion, a lube, or a vibrator can make a difference. Practice, information, and pleasure go a long way in minimizing feelings of "dirtiness" and guilt.

Alice noticed that you signed your letter "argh" and wondered about that. What is causing your frustration? Why is it so important to you that your girlfriend learn to feel comfortable masturbating?

What would change in your relationship if she were to masturbate? What would change for you? What would change for her? (These are questions to ask yourself, and the answers may prove interesting.)

Alice

Masturbation Fantasies?

Dear Alice,
I am curious about men's masturbation fantasies. Specifically, I am wondering what men think about when they are looking at an adult magazine or videotape and masturbating. Are they thinking about being with the woman they are looking at, or what?

WANNA UNDERSTAND

Dear Wanna Understand,
The following sentiments are possibly among those silently spoken by men (and women) pornography viewers everywhere—and let's start off with your entry:

- "Oooh, I'd love to do it with her/him."
- "Look at those (fill in the blank)!"
- "Those breasts can't be real."
- "I wish they'd show more of him/her."
- "Where's the damn rewind button!"
- "That's not a bad idea . . . maybe we could try that this weekend."
- "Why aren't these people using condoms?"
- "If only I could come eight times in ten minutes."
- "I didn't know toe-sucking could be a turn-on."
- "Do you think they're paid well?"
- "My grandmother could write a better script than this."

If your man likes to peruse the pages of adult magazines, or occasionally pop in a copy of "Forrest Hump," you could ask him your question directly. Who knows—his answer might pique your own interests.

Alice

Horny All the Time?

Dear Alice,
I masturbate about two or three times a week, but I still feel horny all the time. I think about sex during class and other situations. I think this is also affecting my life. I can't help it when I get an erection during class, and it seems so obvious that I'm afraid other people may find out. What should I do? Is this natural? I especially think about this one girl, who I've had a crush on for a few years. I always think about her during

class, but then I feel like a dirty scum when I'm around her. Am I just sexually repressed?

SIGNED, HORNY

Dear Horny,

Masturbating two or three times per week is well within the normal range. It's also normal for men, including young men, to feel horny all the time, and to have sexual fantasies. Horniness can increase or decrease when under stress, and also when inundated by stimuli, including memories or desires.

When you get erections in class, there are ways of remaining discreet. Alice is sure that you already have a few tricks. Erections are a reaction to a sexual signal. Often, if you think about something asexual, or something that is a total turn-off, like your next exam, you can lose your erection.

Think about specific ways of discharging some of your sexual energy, such as masturbating more frequently. In terms of the woman you have a crush on, try talking with her. Sometimes, by acting on your feelings, you can put this looming sexual energy into perspective.

Alice

No Privacy to Masturbate

Dear Alice,

I used to always masturbate at least once a day before I came here to school. However, now that I have a roommate, I can never find time alone to masturbate. I feel a need to masturbate at least once a day, but now I can't go through with my urge every day. Thus I start thinking about masturbation during class, and it's really affecting my mind. I need to masturbate or else I can't function correctly. Please help me out. Maybe there is another means to get out my sexual urges.

ALWAYS AROUSED

Dear Always Aroused,

You clearly know what you need to function effectively. The issues seem to be logistical. You need to develop either creative ways to find privacy or creative ways to masturbate with the privacy you have.

For example, since this is such a priority, you need to find some kind of private time and private space. Some people masturbate in the shower, since that was the only place they had privacy growing up. Men sometimes soap up their penis and go to town. Some women use a mild soap on their clitoris to make it slippery, or press with their fingers without extra soap; some use the spray of the shower. Of course, if you have never masturbated standing up, this may take some adjustment, but it does add to your options.

What about going to the bathroom and closing the door for privacy? What about when you or your roommate is in the shower? It is hard for Alice to believe that there is absolutely never a time when you are in your room and your roommate isn't and you're sure s/he isn't going to come home. Did you ever have time in your room alone for private phone calls? How do you arrange them? You might say, "I need to make a private phone call tonight from 9 to 9:30 (or from 3 to 3:30 P.M.)." This gives your roommate time to plan to be invisible, and you a block of time to do your thing, although Alice is not suggesting that you try this tactic every day.

Perhaps you could run home for a "lunch break" when your roommate is away from the room. If you are worried about starting to masturbate and then hearing the key in the door, try a code, like placing something prearranged on the doorknob, i.e., a tie or a ribbon, to signal that you don't want to be disturbed. It could also be a note that says, "Do not enter till 2:30 P.M. Studying (or napping)." Your roommate may be relieved since this would give him/her permission to take time alone in the room as well.

Realistically, how much time are you actually talking about? Many men can, and do, come within two minutes of beginning to masturbate. Similarly, Alfred Kinsey found that many women orgasmed through masturbation within five minutes, a brief amount of time. Alice is not advocating fast orgasms, since they tend to minimize pleasure; however, what is wrong with a quickie in a pinch? You do deserve at least one orgasm a day, and, if you're creative, Alice is sure you can come up with a way to find the privacy to give it to yourself.

Alice

Decades of Masturbation Enthusiasm

Dear Alice,
I have a comment, rather than a question. I see many questions from young folks who are concerned about masturbation and wonder if it is harmful. I am seventy years old and have masturbated at least once, sometimes two or three times a day, for most of my life, since I was about ten years old. I still do it. I am healthy, happy, have several grown children and grandchildren. Masturbation has been a constant, welcome, warm, and healthful companion. My advice? Enjoy it, and let your body be your guide.

AVID READER

Dear Avid Reader,
Alice couldn't have said it better!

Alice

Orgasms

Am I Having an Orgasm?

Alice,

How do you know when you've reached orgasm?

UNSURE

Dear Unsure,

Orgasm is a reflex, usually accompanied by pleasurable feelings, that occurs when the body has had sufficient, effective sexual stimulation. Orgasm reverses the bodily processes of increased blood flow into the genitals and muscular tension that occur during sexual arousal, allowing the body to return to its unaroused state.

Orgasm is a full body response. For men, rhythmical contractions occur along the penis, urethra, prostate gland, seminal vesicles, pelvic muscles, and anus, and are usually accompanied by ejaculation. For women, contractions occur in the lower part of the vagina, in the uterus, and in the anus.

However, where the contractions occur and what sensations you experience are two different things. Each person has different sensations each time orgasm occurs—for example, changes in breathing, a feeling of warmth, sweating, body vibrations, altered consciousness, or need/desire to moan or cry out are common experiences for women. Many women would say about orgasm, "I don't know how to describe it, but I know it when I feel it."

Some women orgasm, but do not know it. They think that what is happening to them is too tame to be considered an orgasm. It is important to concentrate on what you *do* feel, rather than discount your experience by comparing it to an imagined sensation. Women can teach themselves to orgasm by touching their clitoris in pleasurable ways until the intensity turns into sexual release. If you are not sure if you are experiencing an orgasm, read Lonnie G. Barbach's *For Yourself: The Fulfillment of Female Sexuality* (one of the orgasm bibles). Orgasm is not a magical gift someone gives you—it's a physiological response that is learned with practice.   RES

Alice

Multiple Orgasms—Possible?

Dear Alice,
Is it true that a woman can have multiple orgasms?

Dear Reader,
Oh . . . Yes . . . Yes . . . Yes . . . Yes . . . !

THANK GODDESS!
Alice

Girlfriend Fakes Orgasms

Dear Alice,
My last girlfriend was really sex-hungry. We were having sex for a long time, then, I started wondering if she fakes her orgasms or was really having a good time. After hearing that most women (not all) have vaginal contractions, I found out she might be faking. When I spoke to her about it, she started faking the contractions as well. This made me real sad, I couldn't make her come. I couldn't imagine what the problem was. I entered a circle of confusion and self-accusations for something that I'm doing wrong.

The girlfriend never cared for not coming because she said she loved me the way I was. It's important, but sex life is important as well. Now I have a new girlfriend, and since I'm afraid I can't please her, I can't get an erection. I think I have a psychological problem with that. By myself, when I think about girls, I *do* have intense erections, and I can masturbate, no problems at all when I'm alone, but with girls, I just can't have erections. What do I do to fix this problem?

THANKS IN ADVANCE, MR. ERECTION-LESS

Dear Mr. Erection-less,
It seems like your trust has been compromised, since your ex-girlfriend was not having orgasms and you thought she was. Having an orgasm is an intensely personal experience, and a *learned* response. Men have orgasms easily because they have been practicing for years, usually since puberty. Many women do not start masturbating until college, or later, when they learn about orgasm and masturbating from books, or by finally trying it themselves. This means that as adults, they simply have

less practice than men. Similarly, it is easy for men to orgasm during intercourse since the way they masturbate is similar to the kind of sensations and stimulation they receive during intercourse. A woman's pleasure center is her clitoris. During intercourse, the clitoris often gets ignored. So what seems to be a fairly easy response for men is not as easy for women. To save face, or to "protect" their partner's ego, some women fake orgasm.

It's not your *job* to make a woman come. Her orgasm is hers, and she may or may not choose to have one. She also may or may not be able to share it with you. This is not about being a good lover. It is about her choices, and the way the two of you communicate. Since you are now with a new partner, you could start off your relationship by telling her how important it is for you to learn how to touch and please her the way she likes. She may be able to show or tell you, or it may be an experience that you learn about together.

Try taking some pressure off yourself and enjoy being with your new partner. Place the emphasis on getting to know her, and, when you do get sexually intimate, think about pleasuring each other without focusing on your erection. If you get one, fine; and, if you don't, it's okay, too. It is possible, and often pleasurable, to be sexual without an erection. It can add a whole new dimension of creativity and excitement that may not be there when you take your erection for granted. And, you may well find that when you stop worrying and start enjoying yourself and each other, your erections will return naturally. Remember, the key to erections is pleasure, not pressure.   `RES`

Alice

I'm NOT Faking Orgasm

Hey Alice,
How can I convince my boyfriend that I do not fake my orgasms? When he asked me if I have started faking them, I got really hurt. We have been dating for about five years and he questions this now?
SOMEWHAT INSECURE ABOUT SEXUALITY

Dear Somewhat Insecure about Sexuality,
Perhaps you might pretend to doubt the authenticity of *his* orgasms just to see how he responds. Alice bets that something has probably happened to make him question his skill as a lover, or his belief in your honesty. Maybe he is getting older and feels less secure, or perhaps he has read something in a magazine that has made him question you. There is no way of knowing unless you ask.

You might begin with, "What is making this an issue for you now?" Subsequently, talking with him about how you feel may make it safe for him to talk about what is going on for him.

Bottom line, however, is that your own sexual response is fine, especially if it's fine with you. His uncertainty seems to be the more central issue.

Alice

No Orgasm with Intercourse

Dear Alice,
Well, okay. This is my problem. My boyfriend and I have been sexually active for about three months. I enjoy making love to him very much, but intercourse doesn't give me any pleasure. He can easily bring me to orgasm through oral sex, but I don't feel any pleasure from regular sex. NONE! Sometimes I can't even tell if he's inside of me or not. I feel so bad about it, and we've been trying to find some information that might help us, but there isn't any. Why is this happening? It isn't like I don't know how to have an orgasm; I do, I've masturbated so I know what to do, but nothing works for intercourse. Can you help me?

Dear Reader,
The vagina, or birth canal, understandably has very few nerve endings. The clitoris, or joy button, has as many as a man's penis. In order to orgasm, you need to touch what works. During intercourse, the clitoris rarely gets touched. Some women learn to orgasm through intercourse with practice. Since your clitoris—the most sensitive body part on a woman—is not located inside your vagina, reaching an orgasm through intercourse is difficult. While you are making love with your partner inside you, touch, press, and rub your clitoris with your fingers. You may have to move your body so that you can do this, and that can be part of the fun. It really is okay, too, if you have your orgasms before or after intercourse. Don't drive yourself crazy . . . it's a matter of anatomy and variety.

Alice

Easing Orgasms for Women

Alice,
What about women who find it hard to orgasm? Can you advise?
SIGNED, LOOKING FOR PLEASURE

Dear Looking for Pleasure,
Pressing and rubbing the clitoris cause pelvic fullness and body tension to build up to a peak. Orgasm is the point at which all the tension is suddenly released in a series of involuntary and pleasurable muscular contractions. The contractions can be felt in the vagina, uterus, and/or rectum. Orgasms can be mild, intense, ecstatic, or sensuous, depending on the women, the environment, the moment . . .

Many women have difficulty orgasming, either by themselves or with a lover. Lack of information and/or shame about touching one's own body, and unknown fears, keeps some women from learning how to orgasm.

The following interferes with orgasming:

- Not noticing or misunderstanding what's happening to your body as you get aroused. It's easy to think about abstractions—how to do it right, why it isn't going well, getting bored with yourself, wondering what your lover is thinking, whether or not your lover is impatient, whether or not your lover can last—when you might be better off concentrating on sensations, not thoughts.
- Fear that you won't have an orgasm, even though you are aroused, and so you don't want to get into the hassle of trying, repressing your sexual response.
- Fear of asking too much and seeming demanding of your partner.
- Fear that if your lover concentrates on your pleasure, you will feel such pressure to come that you won't be able to—and then you don't.
- Trying to orgasm simultaneously.
- Conflict about, or anger at, your partner.
- Guilt about having sex, so you can't let yourself really enjoy it.
- Rushing into sex—being swept off your feet, just like in the movies, and being swept under the rug when it comes to climaxes.

Lonnie G. Barbach's *For Yourself: The Fulfillment of Female Sexuality*, and Betty Dodson's *Sex for One: The Joy of Self-Loving*, are the orgasm bibles. Some hints about relaxation and effective techniques for achieving fulfilling orgasms, whenever you want them, can be found in these books.

Alice

Boyfriend Takes a Long Time to Ejaculate

Hi Alice!

My boyfriend has trouble ejaculating, usually taking a long time. I was wondering if it could have to do with his constant masturbation during most of his young life. Could it be that the problem is me? Is there a possibility that we can improve the situation?

ELLE

Dear Elle,

There is no standard for how long it takes a man to reach orgasm, so the fact that it takes your partner a long time may just be how his body works. Your boyfriend may be more familiar with orgasming by himself than he is with you. He may be used to the grip of his own hand, which is different from the sensation of vaginal muscles. For others, it takes time to build trust with a partner, to feel like you can really "let go."

Drugs, prescription or otherwise, can also inhibit orgasm for both men and women.

Some women would pay big money to exchange situations with you. They are the ones whose partners come too quickly. Ask him if there's anything you could do sexually that would make him feel more aroused—ways he would like to be touched, held, or talked to. It's important that you don't take his lack of orgasm as a personal affront— thinking that you are not arousing him. On the other hand, if this is a problem for him, he may choose to see a sex therapist. Focus on your sex life as a unique experience, rather than fall back on preconceived notions or expectations of what *should* be occurring sexually. **RES**

Alice

Prolonging Arousal/Lasting Longer

Dear Alice,

What is the best way to learn how to prolong male orgasm when having intercourse? It seems that I might get thirty seconds of penetration before I blow my top. I'd like it if I could enjoy the situation and add to my partner's pleasure by helping her orgasm.

HELP!!

Dear Help!!,

It seems to Alice that you are describing two issues: one is lasting longer than you do, and the other is helping your partner orgasm. Orgasm is a learned response. People learn what kind of stimulation and touching effectively brings them to orgasm.

Many men often learned to have a rapid response pattern because they had no privacy when they were young and needed to finish masturbating quickly, before someone walked in. If you want to learn to last longer, your challenge is to increase the amount of time you spend in arousal.

You might try the "Stop-Start" method. For example, when you feel you are approaching the point of no return, stop what you are doing with and to your partner, and just do nothing, or hold each other, until the urge to ejaculate subsides. Then start again and stop again when you feel you are approaching orgasm. It may take a few tries to identify the point of no return, and to stop *before* then, but you do have the rest of your life to practice and "get it right." (Alice doesn't think it will take you a lifetime to learn this.) Tell your partner when you need her to slow down or stop her movements for the moment, have sex with her on top, and relax. Well, not too much, if you know what Alice means.

The second issue that you raise is the pressure you feel to help your

partner orgasm. Alice suggests looking at the situation differently. Her orgasm is hers, and it is not your "job" to "give" her an orgasm. Alice wonders . . . have you spoken with her about what you want? Have you asked her about what she wants? Her answers may surprise you.
RES

Alice

WHY SOME MEN COME QUICKLY

In nature, male animals need to orgasm quickly before they are attacked and eaten by predators. It is humans who have considered it desirable to extend their pleasure and the pleasure of their partners(s).

Go to Alice at www.goaskalice.columbia.edu for more Sexuality Q & A's, including these:
- A Penis, Not a Ramrod
- Briefs or Boxers?
- Curved Penis
- Erection Comes and Goes
- Hey Penis, You're So Vein(y)
- Hymen Stretching
- I Thought She Was a Woman: My Real-life Crying Game
- Increase Penis Size?
- Interval Training for Multiple Orgasms
- Light Period = Pregnant?
- Masturbating Friends
- Pregnant from Pre-cum?
- Responsible Erotica?
- Semen Changed Consistency
- Soapy Sex in Shower
- Spice up Sex Life?
- The Small Penis Club
- To Come or Not to Come?
- Transgenderist

SEXUAL HEALTH

Y ou don't have to be sexually active with many partners to have a sexual health concern. Single people with few partners, people with partners in long-term monogamous relationships, or even those who have never had sex can find themselves scratching an itch in a place they've never seen, or feeling a lump they didn't notice until it had grown to an alarming size.

Alice covers these maladies as well as birth control issues in this chapter. Until recently, for some people, birth control was a taboo subject, and still today, it is discussed with hesitation and discomfort, even between partners. Yet it's now a booming industry, offering a variety of methods and even over-the-counter pregnancy tests. Modern science has delivered the goods, but human emotion is still a main ingredient in this intimate kind of decision-making ("Maybe he doesn't need to wear a condom—I don't want him to think I'm hassling him," or "Birth control pills seem so unnatural—shouldn't she take a break from them every once in a while?").

Whether you want to start a family or are responding to an unintended pregnancy, Alice is here to help you make informed and better decisions. She also includes a section for specific health concerns of women—breast implants, breast lumps, skipped menstrual periods, endometriosis, PMS (premenstrual syndrome), and the case of the disappearing tampon.

Alice will then explore a range of sexually transmitted diseases (STDs). Although researchers now know more than ever before about the causes and treatments of STDs, the emotional aspects of navigating a healthy sex life remain as challenging as human nature can make it. Things get even more interesting if you consider the fact that one of the most common symptoms of an STD is NO SYMPTOM AT ALL. With chlamydia, for example, it can take a long time to realize there's a problem because there may be NO SYMPTOMS; so, chlamydia is often untreated because it has not been diagnosed. Untreated, chlamydia can cause pelvic inflammatory disease (PID); and, if chlamydia is not treated in time, it could lead to infertility in women and men. Women who delay or postpone getting diagnosed or then treated, or who don't have regular gynecological checkups, are at greater risk.

Sexual health problems can raise issues of shame and embarrassment: "What if those bumps are herpes? How could I have gotten it? What does the doctor think of me? What if I run into someone I know in the waiting room? I don't want to tell my partner. Do I have to tell my partner? What if s/he finds out? What if s/he leaves me? Will anyone ever love me?"

And, after nearly two decades of headlines about AIDS (acquired immunodeficiency syndrome), the thought of HIV (human immuno-deficiency virus) infection crosses many people's minds, too. For others, it's a stressful, constant fear ("I seem to be losing weight—do I need to get tested?"). For some, they act as if "it's not going to happen to me." While there is still no known cure for people who have the viruses that cause AIDS, a number or treatments are now available that enhance and prolong the lives of many who are HIV-positive, particularly when they are diagnosed early.

On one hand, the age of AIDS has opened the door to more frank discussions and awareness about sexual health. But, the misinformation is ever-rampant, much of it spawned by social stigmas associated with homosexuality. ("I'm a man who only has sex with women, so I'm not at risk for HIV, right? Isn't it only the gays who have to worry?" Or, "Lesbians don't need STD education because they don't really have sex.") Alice will clarify the definitions of "safe" and "safer," with questions ranging from kissing to oral sex to intercourse.

Accurate information, and action, are still the best "vaccines" for staying healthy—emotionally and physically. You have the freedom to decide for yourself what you're truly comfortable with, and what you will do, if you know the probable outcomes. Facts are the ultimate pro-phylactics, and resources are the sometimes necessary backups.

Reproduction

Semen Goes Where?

Dear Alice,
I was just wondering what happens to semen after it has been ejaculated into a woman's vagina. Does it just stay there until it dies, or does it seep out? If it stays in, what happens to it once it dies?

THANKS, PRUDE AND WONDERING

Dear Prude and Wondering,
Semen (the fluid that carries sperm), if ejaculated into the vagina, could either travel farther into the vagina, or seep out and eventually dry up, or both. Semen that remains in the body will carry sperm that can survive for approximately three to five days.

When semen evaporates in the open air, the sperm it contains die. Some women use minipads advertised for "light day periods" when they are out, and about, to help absorb the semen that seeps from the vagina.

Alice

Life of Sperm

Dear Alice,
How long do sperm live if they do not fertilize an egg?

Dear Reader,
Sperm live inside a vagina for about three to five days. The important thing about your question is that if you have sex without using contraception up to five days before an egg bursts from the ovary (ovulation), the egg could be fertilized. For example, you could have sex on Monday and fertilize an egg that is not released until Friday. The egg, on the other hand, has a much shorter lifespan—about twenty-four hours. So,

having sex right before ovulation—and up to one day afterward—would be prime for fertilization. Whether or not you want that to happen is another story. . . .

Alice

Fertile Times?

Alice,

When can a woman, during her menstrual cycle, be at high risk for pregnancy? I've heard two answers: fourteen days before or after your period. Which is it?

CONCEIVING ONLY IDEAS

Dear Conceiving Only Ideas,

The simple answer to your question is that the egg bursts from the ovary (ovulation) approximately two weeks *before* the beginning of your next menstrual period. A common misunderstanding is that the egg bursts from the ovary at midcycle, halfway between menstrual periods. This is only true when the cycle is twenty-eight days long (something that cannot be known for certain until that particular cycle is over and menstruation begins).

A woman can become pregnant from unprotected intercourse up to five days before ovulation. Sperm can survive in a woman's body for three to five days, waiting to fertilize that egg during ovulation. Therefore, guessing how long your period usually is and counting backward fourteen days is not an effective method of birth control.

The fertility awareness method of birth control (a studied, standardized monthly procedure), however, can be quite effective if used diligently and properly. Being aware of your fertile times involves counting days, observing cervical mucus, taking your body temperature with a basal thermometer daily, and charting your own observations. This method also requires a highly motivated person. **RES**

Alice

Pregnant?

Dear Alice:

Yesterday, while standing in front of a terminal, I suddenly was hit with a feeling of intense weakness. It wasn't a stomachache, but a wave of weakness and nausea (perhaps? I'm not sure what nausea is). I quickly left the terminal and went to a bathroom and used it appropriately (no diarrhea). Afterward, I felt fine, but there was still a feeling of something moving around in my lower stomach (intestines?).

My immediate thought was that it was "morning sickness," a symptom of pregnancy. However, I had thought that this occurred during the end of the first trimester. This seems impossible because I haven't been missing my period. If I did conceive, it could have happened only during last week. Wouldn't it be too early to tell? Do you recommend the store-bought home tests? When would those become effective (i.e., how many days/weeks after conception would the testing be accurate?)

THANKS A LOT, ANXIOUS

Dear Anxious,
Throughout your letter, there is an assumption being made that you have had unprotected sexual intercourse. Going on this assumption, the usual early signs of pregnancy (one to two weeks after conception) are: a missed period; a period with less bleeding or fewer days than usual; swelling, tenderness, or tingling in your breasts; frequent urination; nausea or vomiting; feeling bloated or crampy; increased or decreased appetite; changes in digestion (constipation or heartburn); and mood changes. Keep in mind that signs of pregnancy vary from woman to woman and pregnancy to pregnancy. Also, since you suspect pregnancy but haven't had a test yet, you don't have to assume that you are definitely pregnant. However, you need to find out.

You can test for pregnancy days after unprotected sex. Home pregnancy tests are accurate if the instructions are followed exactly.

Alice

BASAL BODY TEMPERATURE

Basal body temperature is the temperature of the body **when you first wake up**. This needs to be measured using a basal thermometer (a basal thermometer is a special thermometer used to track ovulation that measures temperature in tenths of a degree, like the standard oral thermometer, but its numbers are magnified to make it easier for you to read your basal body temperature more clearly) immediately after waking in the morning to be most accurate. Women need to have a basal thermometer ready by the bed because any movement (even getting up from bed to get the thermometer) can cause the temperature to fluctuate.

Basal body temperature needs to be measured and recorded every day for several months; after a rise and a plateau, there will be a sharp drop in temperature followed by menstruation, which would indicate that the woman is ovulating.

HOME PREGNANCY TESTS

Using a home pregnancy test is getting easier all the time. You used to need an early morning urine sample, but now you can do it at any time of the day, at almost any time in the cycle. A home pregnancy test is accurate seven to ten days after unprotected intercourse. This is because the test cannot detect the human pregnancy hormone until about one to two weeks after conception.

Masturbation before Intercourse: Pregnant?

Dear Alice,
If a man masturbates shortly before having intercourse, will the likelihood of the woman becoming pregnant be diminished?

JUST WONDERING

Dear Just Wondering,
While it may seem that a man depletes his semen supply in the first ejaculation through masturbation, he does not. For the second ejaculation, sperm are not only replenished, but also remain in the entire urethra (the tube inside of his penis which also transmits urine), increasing the likelihood that sperm will also be present in his pre-ejaculate. From puberty, men continually produce sperm, unlike women, who are born with all of their eggs and release one, or perhaps two, per month.

Keeping this in mind, masturbation before intercourse can relax you, for example, before a date; can remove some pressure; or can help some men last longer when they do have intercourse; however, it is not an effective form of contraception.

Alice

Pregnant without Intercourse?

Dear Alice,
My girlfriend and I masturbate and have oral sex every day and we really enjoy it. One thing that concerns me is that although we have not had sex yet, we have frequent genital touching; we use our genitals to rub each other to get excitement. Will this cause some possibility of getting pregnant? Both of us have never had sex before.

DON'T KNOW

Dear Don't Know,
There is a small chance that your girlfriend could get pregnant without intercourse. If the sperm from your ejaculate or pre-ejaculate gets near the lips around her vagina when she is fertile, the sperm can move into the vagina, hook up with an egg, and fertilize it (a.k.a., conception). If you want to make sure that your girlfriend doesn't get pregnant, either use a condom, or make sure both ejaculate and pre-ejaculatory fluids are far from her vagina. Also, if you touch your own semen and then touch your girlfriend's vagina with your hands, these highly motivated swimmers could travel to the egg.

Alice

Can You Get Pregnant the First Time?

Dear Alice,
Can you get pregnant the first time?

Dear Reader,
Is the Pope Catholic?

Alice

Contraception

Condom Breakage and Slippage

Dear Alice,
I recently started having sex, and we are committed to using condoms. What is the "right" way to use a condom? I know how to put them on and take them off. But I'm petrified about having it break or come off. Also, someone told me that I should pull out immediately after I ejaculate. Is this true? This has happened before, but I have "stayed in" because I wanted my partner to have an orgasm. Is it really important to withdraw immediately after ejaculation?

Thanks for all your help, Having Fun and Being Safe

Dear Having Fun and Being Safe,
Condoms need to be removed while the penis is still hard. Once the penis begins to lose its erection, the ejaculate can leak out. To be safest, pull out after ejaculation, simply because once the ejaculate is present, if it leaks or there is breakage, your risk of transmitting infection or viable sperm is greatly increased. However, if you would like to continue to thrust after you ejaculate, hold the rim of the condom against the base of your penis. Another possibility is for your partner to orgasm before you. When withdrawing, hold on to the rim of the condom with your fingers (or with your partner's fingers). This can prevent the condom from coming off.

Alice

CONDOM USE GUIDELINES

Always use a new condom each time you have sex, and put it on the erect penis before you have any genital contact. When placing the condom on the penis, leave space at the tip for ejaculate (pinch an inch), and gently squeeze this tip as you unroll the condom all the way down the shaft. This air-free space at the end will leave room for the ejaculate, keeping the condom from breaking due to extra pressure. Water-based lubes, or lubricated condoms themselves, also help to prevent tearing of the condom. Spermicidal foam, cream, or jelly increases the effectiveness of condoms in preventing disease transmission and pregnancy.

Condoms—Porous?

Alice,
I have a friend who is very religious and has been telling his children that since the AIDS virus is so much smaller than the pores in a condom, it affords no protection, thereby making abstinence the only option that makes sense. Is there any truth to this story whatsoever, or is he just using this as an excuse to scare his kids? (Not that I would go around his wishes with his family—just curious.)

ATHEIST

Dear Atheist,
Latex condoms, which are the least expensive, most accessible type of condoms at the moment, are designed so as not to allow transmission of the HIV virus, or any virus for that matter. The HIV virus is larger than the pores in condoms.

Lambskin condoms, on the other hand, are made from sheep intestines, and are now advertised as a contraceptive, but not as effective against STD transmission.

Because both user error and manufacturer error exist, condom use constitutes "safer" sex, as opposed to 100 percent safe sex. The only 100 percent safe sex is no oral, anal, or vaginal sex, or abstinence. Tips for using condoms to insure greatest effectiveness in protecting against both pregnancy and HIV (and other sexually transmitted diseases) include storing condoms in a cool, dry place and out of direct sunlight, and using them before their expiration date. If using a lube with your condom, make sure that it is water-based, as oil-based lube causes the latex in condoms to deteriorate.

Good communication and accurate information between parents and children are more effective against risk-taking than scare tactics.

Alice

Spermicidal Tablets?

Dear Alice:

When my girlfriend and I have intercourse, we use condoms and an insertable spermicide tablet. I don't remember the brand name, but it is a white capsule and she inserts it ten minutes before intercourse and it is effective for one hour. Can you tell me how effective this is?

CONCERNED

Dear Concerned,

Spermicides come in several forms of foam, jelly, film, suppository, or insertable tablet. Spermicides are most effective when used with another method of birth control, as you and your girlfriend do. When combining condoms with spermicidal foam, cream, or tablet, you get as close as you can to 100 percent protection.

Alice

HOW TO USE SPERMICIDES

- Read the package directions THOROUGHLY. Each type of spermicide has its own instructions.
- Plan ahead for when to insert your spermicide.
- Check to be sure you have all the supplies (spermicides, diaphragm, inserter, tissues) you need on hand.
- Wash your hands before inserting spermicide.
- Use a new application of spermicide each time you have intercourse.
- Leave spermicide in place at least six to eight hours after intercourse—do not rinse your vagina or douche. (Douching, in general, is also not recommended.)
- Wash your spermicide applicator or inserter after each use with mild soap and warm water.
- Store your spermicide in a cool, clean, and dark place.

CONDOMS AS CONTRACEPTIVE BACKUP

Condoms, when used with other methods such as the diaphragm, cervical cap, spermicidal foam or jelly, and even Depo-provera and birth control pills, serve as a backup method of contraception.

Diaphragm Effectiveness

Dear Alice,
How effective is the diaphragm? I was on the pill, but it made me ill and depressed. However, I miss the spontaneity and reliability of it. What about the cervical cap?

JUST SAY NO TO HORMONES

Dear Just Say No to Hormones,
Both the diaphragm and cervical cap are barrier methods of contraception. They work by physically blocking the sperm from entering the cervical opening. Both are made of rubber: the diaphragm is in the shape of a shallow cup, and the cap is more like a thimble. When a diaphragm or cervical cap is fitted correctly and used properly, the success rate is high. Both of these methods are used with spermicidal jelly or cream, creating a double form of contraception: physical and chemical.

You can insert a diaphragm before intercourse. It needs to be left in for at least six hours after intercourse. If you have intercourse a second time, add more cream or jelly without removing the diaphragm.

A cervical cap is smaller than a diaphragm. It's not absolutely necessary to use a spermicidal cream or jelly with a cap, but it's certainly recommended. The cap is designed to provide an almost airtight seal around the cervical opening. An advantage of the cervical cap is that it can be put in on a Friday night and left in for the weekend. The cervical cap only comes in limited sizes which do not fit all women.

In order to get fitted for either a diaphragm or cervical cap, make an appointment with your regular gynecologist or woman's health care provider.

Switching to a lower dose pill may help with depression. Discuss this with your health care provider to decide what form of contraception will work best for you.

Alice

How Do Birth Control Pills Work?

Alice,
How do birth control pills work?

WOMAN

Dear Woman,
Birth control pills fool the body into acting as if it's pregnant. Birth control pills, also called oral contraceptives (OCs), come in two forms: the combined OC, a combination of two synthetic hormones, estrogen and progestin; and the minipill, which consists solely of progestin. Combined OCs are more commonly used, though both kinds are available through health care providers. The combination pill prevents ovulation by suppressing the natural hormones in the body that would stimulate the ovary to release an egg. By taking this estrogen throughout the month, you insure that no egg will be developed or released for that cycle. Progestin thickens the cervical mucus, hindering the movement of sperm. Progestin also prevents the uterus's lining from developing normally; so, if an egg were fertilized, implantation is unlikely.

The minipills, which contain no estrogen, inhibit the egg's ability to travel through the fallopian tubes, alter the cervical mucus to block sperm, partially suppress the sperm's ability to unite with an egg, and partially inhibit implantation in the uterine wall. For maximum effectiveness, you need to take the pills as prescribed.

Alice

On and Off the Pill

Dear Alice,
I have been on the pill for over a year now. Recently, I broke up with my boyfriend of two years. We still see each other, but I have not had sex since we broke up. I don't plan on having sex with anybody except my ex. My question is if I don't plan on having sex for a long while, should I stop the pill? I am afraid that if I decide to get back on the pill, I will have an increased risk of cancer or something like that. Is this true? Please tell me.

FEELING ASEXUAL

Dear Feeling Asexual,
There is no time limit for using the birth control pill. A woman can use birth control pills safely from the time she becomes sexually active until she reaches menopause, as long as she does not have any of the risk factors (which your health care provider can assess) for taking the pill, and does not develop a major side effect from its use. A rest period is actu-

ally not recommended for a woman wishing to continue using pills in the future, as her system has to adjust hormonally to changes that accompany going on and off the pill, as opposed to the consistency of staying on it. If you do decide to go off the pill, you will still need to think about which other form of birth control you might use in the interim—one that may be used on an as-needed basis (i.e., condoms and foam, diaphragm, etc.). If in the future you restart the pill again, you will not have an increased risk of contracting cancer. You may find it more helpful to talk with your health care provider about your situation and contraceptive choices.

Alice

RISK FACTORS FOR TAKING BIRTH CONTROL PILLS

DO NOT USE THE PILL WHEN YOUR HEALTH HISTORY INCLUDES:
- Cardiovascular disease
- Abnormal blood clotting
- High blood pressure
- Gall bladder disease
- Sickle cell anemia
- Current smoking
- Current liver disease

Birth Control Pills and Weight Gain

Alice,
I have been taking birth control pills for about a year now, and I think they have caused me to gain almost fifteen pounds in that time. Since I work out aerobically at least five times a week and eat a very healthy diet, the exact same as I have been doing for the past three years, I don't know what else could be causing the weight gain. I'm only twenty, so it shouldn't be weight gain associated with aging. Is it possible that the pills are the cause? If so, what can I do about it, short of ceasing to take them?

SIGNED, FEELING CHUBBY

Dear Feeling Chubby,
Birth control pills can alter your water metabolism. Both the estrogen and progestin in the pills can cause fluid retention, a temporary and

usually cyclic effect that often begins in the first month as a result of an increase in sodium. The estrogen in the pill can cause weight gain due to increased breast, hip, or thigh tissue, usually after several months on the pill. This causes swollen ankles, breast tenderness, discomfort with contact lenses, or a weight gain of up to five pounds. Reducing your salt intake moderately can help control this type of water retention.

Some progestin-dominant pills can cause appetite increase and permanent weight gain. Pill-related depression may also lead to increased appetite and weight gain. There are hundreds of reasons why women gain weight that are not pill-related. Talk with your provider about the extra weight you've gained, and together you may be able to find the cause. If your weight gain is determined to be pill-related, your provider can change your prescription to minimize any weight gain.

Remember that exercise, especially weight training, can cause some weight gain in the form of increased muscle mass.

Alice

The Pill and Infertility?

Alice,
I was wondering if there is a relationship between taking the pill and infertility. I have heard stories of women who have been on the pill for five or more years experiencing difficulty or no luck conceiving. Some tell me the birth control pill from several decades ago contained overly high dosages of hormones, and it was these high levels which led to infertility or conception problems. I was wondering if it is true that the older pills contained higher levels, and if so, what are the levels of the pills today? Also, what are the fertility risks associated with the pills available today?

CAUTIOUS KATE

Dear Cautious Kate,
Most reasons why women, even those who've been on the pill, have trouble conceiving are not related to pill use. For example, on the average, it takes couples about eight months to become pregnant once they start trying. Infertility and conception are based on many factors, such as age of partners, sperm count, frequency of intercourse, etc. While a woman is taking birth control pills, any fertility problem is masked.

Many women take the pill to regulate irregular menstrual cycles. Irregular periods are often due to hormonal imbalances. Presumably, the hormone imbalance will remain after a woman goes off the pill because the cause of the imbalance has still not been addressed. In addition, couples in their childbearing years can have infertility problems which do not become obvious until after the woman stops taking the pill and they begin to try to get pregnant, regardless of birth control method.

Yes, pills prescribed today have much lower doses of hormones than those prescribed twenty, and even ten, years ago, but they are just as effective.

Alice

Depo-provera

Alice,

I was interested in using Depo-provera as a birth control method, but I don't know that much about it. I was wondering if you could tell me about the risks and effectiveness of it. I am currently on the birth control pill, so would this cause any complications? Thank you for your help.

NEEDLES

Dear Needles,

Depo-provera is an effective contraceptive method. A woman is given a Depo injection every three months. It is a hormonal (progestin-only) form of contraception, acting by suppressing Follicle Stimulating Hormone (FSH) and Luteinizing Hormone (LH) levels and disrupting the menstrual cycle. Depo is used by more than fifteen million women in more than ninety countries.

If you miss your shot, your chances of pregnancy increase the longer you wait to get another shot. How long this "forgiveness" period lasts depends primarily on how long a woman has been on Depo-provera, so call your provider if you miss your shot.

Your provider will also help you switch from birth control pills to Depo-provera, if that's what you choose.

Alice

Norplant Information

Dear Alice,

I've heard of the Norplant System for birth control. Where can I have it done? Does insurance pay for any of it? Where can I get it at low cost? Thanks!

NEEDS NORPLANT

Dear Needs Norplant,

Norplant is a progestin-only contraceptive method in the form of implants inserted into your arm at your health care provider's office or at a clinic. A single implant can provide up to five years of effective birth

BASIC DEPO INFO

- Continue to use condoms for safer sex in addition to Depo, because you are not protected against STDs.
- Make sure you have a shot every three months (twelve weeks) for Depo to be effective.
- Depo tends to make a woman's periods less regular, and spotting between periods is fairly likely. Some women stop having periods completely. If your pattern of menstruation after being on Depo concerns you, discuss it with your provider.
- Weight gain is common with Depo use.

(Material adapted from *Contraceptive Technology*)

control. Many women find that Norplant works for them, and they especially like the long-term protection.

Norplant failures are rare. Some advantages of Norplant include lighter periods, less severe menstrual cramps and pain, lower risk of cervical and endometrial cancer, and effective long-term birth control.

Some drawbacks are weight gain, breast tenderness, decreased bone density, possible difficult removal, and high initial cost.

Removal takes more time and usually costs more than insertion. Most insurance covers the cost of the implants, and some will also cover insertion and/or removal.

Alice

Emergency Contraception?

Dear Alice,

My girlfriend and I had sex twice one night—the second time we had to change condoms because she was dry and the lubricant had run out. Before I put the second condom on, she asked me to "put it in" without it on for a few seconds; which I did—not entirely all the way though. I instantly realized the mistake and withdrew. Naturally, as I expect, there is a small chance this could have gotten her pregnant. However, this was four days after her period ended, and the condoms we were using had nonoxynol-9 on the inside and outside. I had not ejaculated yet, as a matter of fact I never did ... and I had wiped the tip of my penis prior to doing this to avoid any pre-cum. My question is this: I'm hoping I'm right in assuming the chance of pregnancy is minimal—however, we are considering emergency contraception. What could you suggest? Thanks!

Dear Reader,

There's a minimal chance for your girlfriend to become pregnant from what seems to be you and your girlfriend's understandable curiosity about what unprotected sex feels like and your desire to be as close to each other as possible. Regardless, Alice could tell from the details you have provided that you were very careful—you wiped off any pre-cum on the tip of your penis, used nonoxynol-9 spermicide on the inside and outside of the condom, and considered the time of her menstrual cycle. However, these "precautionary" measures don't guarantee 100 percent contraceptive effectiveness, as you later realized, even if you were inside her ever so briefly.

If you and your girlfriend are concerned about the possibility of conception, then emergency contraception (the "morning after" or "911" pill) is an option the two of you can choose. Emergency contraception needs to be taken within seventy-two hours from the unprotected sexual intercourse. You can call the Emergency Contraception Hotline for more information and nearby referrals anywhere in the United States.

If more than seventy-two hours have passed since unprotected sexual intercourse, emergency contraception may no longer be an option for you, but call the hotline anyway. Otherwise, wait and see if your girlfriend misses her period (Alice knows this can be nerve-wracking). If she does, she needs to see a health care provider for pregnancy testing, or use a home pregnancy test. You and your girlfriend may also consider talking with a provider, if she, or you, needs it for any next steps, about a backup birth control method. **RES**

Alice

RU 486

Alice,

I remember reading about RU 486. Could you explain how it works and what, if any, side effects are linked to it? Thank you.

OPTIONS

Dear Options,

RU 486, or mifepristone, is a drug that causes early abortion in pregnant women. Combining RU 486 with a low-dose prostaglandin (a chemical substance found in the body that can also be manufactured artificially, with a number of different effects on bodily processes, such as uterine stimulation) appears to increase effectiveness without increasing side effects. According to a 1995 World Health Organization (WHO) study looking at the use of the RU 486–prostaglandin regimen since 1982, when this combination is given within seven to eight weeks from the first day of the last menstrual period, a complete abortion occurs in 64 to 85 percent of women. Side effects of this drug combination include bleeding, cramping, nausea, vomiting, short-term fatigue or weakness, and occasional diarrhea.

Mifepristone is administered under a health care provider's supervision. In a small percentage of women for whom the combination of medical drugs is not effective to produce complete abortion, a follow-up surgical procedure is sometimes required. Because of this, close follow-up by a health care provider is necessary.

In the United States, methotrexate (a drug widely in use for the past forty years to treat illnesses, including cancer) is being used to induce abortion, and its action is similar to RU 486. RU 486 has been approved by the U.S. Food and Drug Administration (FDA), but because it is not manufactured and distributed in the United States, it is not generally available.

Alice

Sexually Transmitted Diseases (STDs)

SAFER SEX GUIDELINES

Safer sex means having sex, orgasms, or intercourse without sharing blood, semen, or vaginal fluids.

Safer sex includes ways of minimizing risks of passing HIV and other STDs. Some of these techniques include:

- Using a condom correctly and consistently each time a person has sex
- Using a latex barrier for oral sex—such as an oral dam
- Mutual masturbation
- Sex with clothes on

Use a condom for vaginal, anal, and oral sex. For cunnilingus (oral sex on a female), use a dam; a nonlubed condom that has its ring removed, is cut down the length, and is opened up to form a rectangle; or plastic wrap. (Read "What's a dam?" on page 106 for instructions).

UNSAFE SEX

Unsafe sex puts an individual at risk for HIV and other STDs. This is sex that allows semen, blood, or vaginal lubrication (body fluids) to be passed from one person to another. These body fluids can spread viruses or bacteria.

What's an STD?

Dear Alice,
Sorry to ask and sound stupid, but, what are STDs?

THANKS, STD

Dear STD,
No need to apologize, your question indicates your interest in learning; and there is nothing wrong with wanting to be an informed individual. Alice is certain other people out there don't know what STDs are either.

STDs is an abbreviation for sexually transmitted diseases. It's the term that has replaced VD, or venereal disease. Sexually transmitted diseases are diseases/infections that are transmitted through sex with a person who already has an STD. *Every* sexually active person is at risk for STDs, if a partner is infected. To help reduce your risk, use safer sex guidelines. If you think you may have an STD, remember that it is not a stigmatizing experience—don't let yourself feel so ashamed, embarrassed, or guilty that you do not see a health care provider for a checkup and, if needed, appropriate treatment.

Call the National STD Hotline for referrals to free and/or low-cost clinics located near you, or for general information about STDs, and remember:

RES

"RESPECT YOURSELF, PROTECT YOURSELF."
Alice

WHOM TO SEE FOR AN STD?

- Primary care physicians
- Nurse practitioners
- Gynecologists
- Urologists
- Dermatologists
- Clinicians at STD clinic of local or state health department
- Clinicians at local Planned Parenthood or women's clinic
- Hospital OB/GYNs

How to Ask Someone You're Going to Have Sex with If They Have Any Diseases

Dear Alice,
I really enjoy reading your answers on these pages, but here's the question that I haven't seen addressed on your Web pages or anywhere else

on the Internet. Can you please suggest some appropriate ways to ask a person with whom you're about to have sex if he or she has any sexually transmitted diseases? A few months ago, I met a girl with whom I had sex . . . and, as I found out later, she had herpes. We did use condoms anyway, but there was still some risk in catching herpes since we didn't use condoms all the time.

SIGNED, GETTING SMARTER

Dear Getting Smarter,
There is no A-B-C method of how to ask a partner if s/he has a sexually transmitted disease (STD). In fact, even if you find a comfortable way to ask, if your partner's been sexually active, s/he may have contracted an STD and not even know it. One of the most common symptoms of an STD is **no symptom**. Alice stresses communication with your sexual partner, ideally before you're already in bed together, because this is not a light discussion and could "ruin the mood." More important, asking this question when you're in bed and aroused, and perhaps not thinking as clearly, could lead your partner to flippantly answer "no." Condoms might then be disregarded in the "heat of the moment," with possible regrets the morning after and for some time to come.

Make a decision yourself about when and how comfortable you are about bringing up the STD discussion. It may be that it's something that's not discussed the first few times you have sex—you both just automatically choose to use condoms, as you described in the case with the woman who had herpes. It may be that you're a more verbal person, and need to talk about STDs early on in a relationship. If you're going to talk, use language you're comfortable with. Be as direct as possible, knowing that it's probably going to be awkward. Be yourself. Pick a time and place where you won't be interrupted or disturbed, and when you're not sexually engaged. Talk freely and openly, and have some suggestions ready for how you can learn more about your sexuality and sexual choices together as a couple. Ideas include going to a bookstore to read up on sexual health books and reviewing pamphlets from a health center. Or make an appointment together to see a health care provider to discuss your safer sex options.

Many couples say that they use condoms regardless of their partner's history, and that's how they avoid the awkwardness of this discussion. However, if you're interested in developing a relationship with increased intimacy over time, it's a good idea to discuss STDs early on. It doesn't *have* to be a trust issue, or a discussion of past relationships and promiscuity or prudence, but more a look at the future and caring for yourselves enough to protect each other.

Alice

WHAT'S A DAM?

Oral, or dental, dams are thin, square pieces of latex that prevent possible transmission of HIV and other STDs when placed over the clitoris, vulva, or anus for oral sex. You may be able to buy dams at your local drugstore; if not, you can try the STD clinic of your health department. You can make your own dams with plastic wrap by folding a piece in half. Or take a nonlubed condom, snip off the elastic ring, cut along one side using scissors, and flatten it into a rectangle. Do this right before using it.

A FEW TIPS ON USING DAMS:
- Use a new dam each time you have sex
- Change to a new dam when you change your spots (i.e., anus, vulva)
- Dab a little water-based lube on the side of the dam that will be touching the clitoris, vulva, or anus
- Place the dam evenly over the clitoris, vulva, or anus while stretching the edges of the dam with your hands—then "pleasure" your partner with your mouth, lips, and tongue!

Ex Has STD

Dear Alice,

I am an undergrad at Columbia. I've been going out with a girl here for the past six months. Last weekend I went home (out of NY) and fooled around with an ex-girlfriend. She called me last night and told me that she might have a venereal disease. She went to the doctor this week and told me she would let me know when she finds out for sure. We didn't use a condom.

My problem is, what should I tell my girlfriend? I really love her and don't want to ruin things because of this stupid fling I had. But I can tell she's annoyed that I've avoided her all weekend. I can't exactly tell her next time we get together that I don't feel like fooling around, but I don't know how long it will be before I know if I'm infected. And what do I do if I am? Help!

DESPERATE

Dear Desperate,

The first thing to do is to make an appointment for a full STD checkup. Explain to your health care provider your recent experience, your reason for concern, and any specific info your ex-girlfriend may have given you—i.e., what venereal disease she may have, what symptoms she has, etc. You can use the opportunity with the provider to get information about the specific disease—symptoms, treatment, and prevention of transmission. Get the info yourself rather than waiting for your ex—it will likely relieve some of your anxiety.

As for how, when, and whether to tell your present girlfriend that you may have an STD—Alice is one for honesty in relationships. It may not be easy, but it is possible and important to be honest with your girlfriend.

It would probably help if you had some more information to give her, because part of her reaction will include fear of transmission of the disease to her. Be prepared for anger, jealousy, incomprehension, and fear for herself. There's also a chance that you may be surprised and she may be understanding and forgiving. Whichever happens, you can deal with it.

Alice

HIV and Heterosexual Intercourse

Dear Alice,

How does a man get infected with HIV through heterosexual vaginal intercourse?

JUST WANNA KNOW

Dear Just Wanna Know,

Men can become infected with HIV when they have unprotected sexual intercourse with a woman carrying the virus, most probably via exposure to secretions or menstrual blood in the vagina. During heterosexual intercourse, the man's urethral lining may be exposed to infected fluid that enters through the urethra (the opening and tube in the penis through which urine and semen flow). Another way that a man may become infected is through an open sore, cut, or minor abrasion on the penis which would facilitate viral transmission. **RES**

Alice

HIV from Kissing?

Hi Alice,

I am sure this question of mine may sound stupid and you have been asked a number of times. However, for me it is a very important question relating to my sexual life. My question is: does kissing, with sucking your partner's tongue and lips, transmit HIV? For me, sex without such kissing is no fun! Lately my girlfriend was told by someone that such kissing is risky, and therefore she refuses to give kisses during sex. Waiting anxiously for your reply.

SIGNED, NO KISS NO FUN

Dear No Kiss No Fun,
There have been no documented cases of HIV transmission through mouth-to-mouth kissing. However, risks exist in people with serious gum diseases, if one is HIV infected or has open sores on the lips or in the mouth, or has other diseases (i.e., mono, herpes). Be as informed as you can be, make your choices, and enjoy them.

Alice

Oral Sex, HIV... and Braces

Alice,
I'm a young gay man, and I'm concerned about oral sex and HIV. What are the risks, statistically and in your opinion, of receiving oral sex without a condom? Also, and this will sound kind of funny, I have braces, so I'm assuming giving head is dangerous.

Dear Reader,
Leading HIV research and care organizations, like the Centers for Disease Control and Prevention (CDC) and Gay Men's Health Crisis (GMHC), say that the risk of being infected with HIV via *receiving* oral sex without a condom is virtually impossible.

Where your braces are concerned, if you are giving oral sex, proceed with caution: be gentle with partners and avoid sudden, erratic movements (both of you). If you decide not to take your partner's penis into your mouth, your lips, tongue, saliva, and breath can be wonderful sources of pleasure. **RES**

Alice

Anal Sex for Ten Seconds—AIDS?

Alice,
What are the possibilities of catching anything after having anal sex with a person (with no condom)—even if they say they don't have AIDS—for only about ten seconds and stopping with no ejaculation occurring?

CURIOUS

Dear Curious

Word of mouth is not a good way to determine whether or not your partner has an STD. Remember that one of the most common symptoms of an STD is **no symptom**. This is also true for AIDS. A person can be HIV-positive, but show absolutely no signs of AIDS for years. A person could also be HIV-positive and show up as HIV-negative on a blood test if it is during the "window" or latent period before the virus can be found in the blood. Your partner may not honestly know that s/he has the virus at the moment when you're going to have sex.

It is possible, but unlikely, that HIV could have been transferred from the inserter to the receptor during the very brief period of anal sex you described through the inserter's pre-cum. It is even less likely that the receptor could have transmitted the virus to the inserter in that short amount of time, unless there was tearing and blood in his/her anus. For the future, if you want to enjoy anal sex with a partner safely, *use a condom* from the *very beginning of your sexual encounter* and use lots of water-based lube.

Alice

HIV Transmission: When Does It Show Up on a Blood Test?

Dear Alice,

My question is about AIDS/HIV: I had a sexual affair that lasted two and a half months, and, unfortunately, I was not using condoms. I happen to know nothing about my partner's previous sex life. I know that, for a test to show something, you must wait for six to nine months. I would like to know whether, provided that I am infected, I will experience any symptoms in this six- to nine-month period?

Is it possible to have the virus and not have any symptoms or indications all this time? Right now, I am a graduate student and I am experiencing anxiety, fatigue, sleepiness, weight loss (three to five pounds in the last two months). Are these related to the disease, or is it just in my mind?

GRATEFUL TO YOU,
THANK YOU IN ADVANCE, WRONGDOER

Dear Wrongdoer (Lessons Learned would be a nicer name),

Three to six months from your last unsafe sexual experience is the amount of time you need to wait to get an HIV test. Depending on the source, you will get differing opinions about this "window" of time between infection and HIV antibody detection in a blood test. For example, the Centers for Disease Control and Prevention (CDC) recommends six months, some city and state health departments advise waiting two months, while the Gay Men's Health Crisis (GMHC) suggests a three-month waiting period. Alice thinks that six months is a long time to wait for HIV test results, and a negative or positive test result three months after possible HIV exposure can be considered reliable, although not 100 percent accurate. Early detection of HIV/ AIDS is critical, in light of all of the promising new treatments available.

As for your weight loss, fatigue, and sleepiness, they could easily be stress-induced (i.e., angst about your health, the grind of graduate school, etc.). Symptoms related to AIDS can take years to manifest, so their absence is not the best indicator of HIV status. You know the safer-sex routine, but here's something for you and other readers to think about: one way to prevent some of these pre- and post-sex worries is to think and talk about HIV and safer sex before you become sexually intimate with someone: what will you do, what won't you do? What might you do more, or less, of? Having a strategy is one more way to ward off post-sex anxiety.

Alice

Scared and Hopeless with Herpes

Dear Alice,
I have been diagnosed with herpes simplex 2. Not fun. I am afraid, now, to consider having sex with anyone who does not have it. From the research I have done so far, I have come to the conclusion that it is unsafe to have sex, even with a condom and with no sores. I really don't look forward to being alone, or sexless, for the rest of my life, but I am unwilling to convey the disease to someone that I care for enough to have sex with. Is anyone doing research on a cure for herpes? Can you recommend reading material? Something technical that describes the viral and immunological aspects of the disease?

HOPELESS IN NY

Dear Hopeless in NY,
Herpes simplex is a common virus that is spread by direct skin-to-skin contact. Symptoms of genital herpes usually develop within two to twenty days after contact with the virus, although it may take far longer. For some people, the first attack is so mild that it goes unnoticed. For others, the first attack causes visible sores and flulike symptoms. In either case, the virus eventually retreats to the nervous system and lies dormant there.

Some people have frequent recurrences, while others rarely do; and for many, this number decreases with time. With each recurrence, your body is more prepared to fight off the infection, so there are usually fewer sores, they heal faster, and the outbreak is less painful. The flulike symptoms of the first outbreak are seldom present during subsequent outbreaks.

Herpes affects each person differently. The following factors could bring on an episode: surgery, illness, stress, fatigue, skin irritation (such as sunburn), diet, menstruation, or excessive friction during intercourse.

Your worries about transmission are understandable. Sexual contact poses a risk for transmitting herpes from the time the first symptoms of itching, tingling, or other skin sensations are noticeable, until the area is completely healed. Sexual contact during times when no symptoms are present (asymptomatic) is less likely to cause infection. However, people tend to have sex more often when they have no sores, which increases the risk of transmission.

The virus can become active and transmitted without any detectable symptoms. During this time, the virus travels along the nerves to skin and mucous membrane sites. The presence of the virus at the surface of the skin is referred to as "viral shedding," or "asymptomatic shedding." Herpes virus can be transmitted during viral shedding. There is really no way to tell when viral shedding is occurring. Your body gives you no warning, such as minor pain, discomfort, or a tingling sensation in the skin where the shedding is going on.

There's good news where prevention is concerned. Laboratory results have shown that the herpes virus does not pass through latex condoms. A recent clinical study of women has shown that herpes simplex 2 infection rates are much lower among condom users.

If you're concerned about the long-term—a lasting relationship and possibly having children—don't despair. Couples come to different kinds of peace with herpes. Alice knows several women and men with herpes who have had several partners, have gotten married, and/or have had healthy children, some by C-section and some by vaginal delivery. Your obstetrician (and midwife, if applicable) can monitor you during pregnancy and labor.

Lastly, give yourself the best possible chance to avoid recurrences by maintaining general good health and keeping your stress levels to a minimum. Eat well, sleep, and try to keep a healthy perspective on life.
RES

Alice

Oral Sex with Canker Sores

Alice,
Is it safe to have oral sex when either partner has a canker sore—not a cold sore, but a canker sore? Does the same virus cause both and can you cause genital herpes with a canker sore?

BLISTER MOUTH

Dear Blister Mouth,

Canker sores have not been proven to be caused by a virus, and they are not contagious, or a sign of any other disease. However, if the person performing oral sex has a canker sore in his/her mouth, and s/he comes into direct contact with his/her partner's semen, vaginal fluids, or blood, s/he may well be increasing his/her risks of contracting HIV from his/her partner if s/he is infected. Any type of lesion or opening in the mucous membrane of the mouth makes transmission of HIV more viable than if the lesion weren't there. You'll need to make decisions about how much risk you want to take with your partner—if you want to be extra safe, avoid oral sex when canker sores are present, or use a condom or dam during oral sex to protect each other.

Alice

CANKER SORES

Canker sores appear more often under the tongue and inside the mouth than cold sores caused by the herpes virus. Canker sores can be sparked by stress, trauma to the area in your mouth, allergies, or by a reaction to a particular bacteria.

Chlamydia?

Dear Alice,

Could you tell me about the symptoms of chlamydia and if one test is enough to detect that disease? Thank you.

CURIOUS

Dear Curious,

Chlamydia is an STD caused by *Chlamydia trachomatis*. As with some other STDs, the most common symptom of chlamydia is **no symptom at all**. Comparatively, more women than men are asymptomatic—up to 80 percent of women and 40 percent of men diagnosed with chlamydia may not experience symptoms.

Semen or cervical secretions transmit chlamydia. It usually takes one to three weeks for symptoms to show up, if at all. If you've given unprotected oral sex to someone with chlamydia, it's possible, but unlikely, to get a sore throat. This is even less likely if you've gone down on a woman—the penis is much more effective in transmitting chlamydia to a partner's throat.

In men, the chlamydiae make their way into the urethra, where they can cause discharge and burning when urinating, especially during that first trip to the bathroom in the morning. Some women will experience itching, vaginal discharge, and burning during urination. More often than not, the infection will manifest as mucopurulent cervicitis, a discharge around the cervix. This symptom often goes unnoticed because it is difficult to detect without an examination by a health care provider.

Unchecked and untreated chlamydia can lead to a number of problems, including sterility for men and women alike. If given free reign to divide and multiply, chlamydiae can infect the epididymis (where sperm mature) in men who do not experience any symptoms at first. These men may eventually experience sensations of heaviness and discomfort in their testicles, and inflammation of their scrotal skin. In women, chlamydiae can cause pelvic inflammatory disease (PID) and scarred fallopian tubes. Women who develop PID are also at higher risk for chronic pelvic pain and ectopic pregnancy (when a fertilized egg implants outside of the uterus). PID and ectopic pregnancies can be life-threatening.

It is extremely important to be tested for chlamydia, as well as for other STDs, even if you don't have any symptoms if you're sexually active with partners. And yes, one test is enough to determine the presence of *Chlamydia trachomatis*. Basically, the test involves collecting material from your urethral or cervical area with a swab, and sending the sample to a lab for analysis.

Alice

SYMPTOMS OF PELVIC INFLAMMATORY DISEASE (PID)

- Sudden low-grade or high fever; chills
- Frequent urination, burning when urinating, or inability to empty bladder
- Abnormal or foul discharge from vagina or urethra
- Irregular bleeding or spotting
- Bleeding or pain during or after intercourse
- Swollen abdomen and/or lymph nodes
- Lack of appetite
- Nausea or vomiting
- Increased menstrual pain and cramps

Women with PID may experience some or none of these symptoms; symptoms range from very mild to painful enough to warrant a visit to the emergency room.

Chlamydia from a Toilet Seat?

Dear Alice,

Recently, someone in my hall told me that another girl who lives in our hall has chlamydia. I do not know if it is simply a rumor, but what she told me got me worried. I know chlamydia is a sexually transmitted disease, but is there any way I can get it from her considering the fact that we share the same bathroom? What are the ways in which I can get it from her? Could I maybe get it through the toilet if I sit on the toilet seat after she sat there?

CONTAGIOUS?

Dear Contagious?,

Chlamydia, an STD, is not spread by sharing the same bathroom or toilet seats. It is transmitted through intercourse or genital touching when one person is infected. Chlamydia affects men and women. Chlamydia is important to detect and treat because it can lead to serious inflammation of the urethra or reproductive organs, resulting in damage and even sterility. Since most STDs are not skin diseases, sharing bathrooms does not put one at significant risk for STD transmission.

Alice

Genital Warts

Dear Alice,

An ex-girlfriend told me recently that she has genital warts. She was a virgin at the time we met so I must have given it to her. I am waiting for my test results but I must be infected. I have learned (too late!) that we can't get rid of the virus. If I get married some time later, would I have to use condoms all my life with my wife so I don't pass the virus to her? What are the complications for women?

NANH

Dear NANH,

Genital warts, also called condyloma, are growths caused by human papillomavirus (HPV). They are usually, but not always, spread sexually. The incubation time (time from exposure to appearance of growths) may range from a few weeks to many months or years. Some people harbor the virus and transmit it to others without ever developing the growths themselves. New information has shown that the virus can be found in some people prior to sexual activity. With a long incubation period and the potential presence of the virus without any sexual activity, it's hard to determine the source of the virus. Diagnosis and treatment are important because some wart viruses can cause cervical cancer.

Available treatments for HPV do not completely eliminate the virus. Instead, treatment is aimed at removing uncomfortable growths, reducing the number of viral particles, and, perhaps, stimulating the immune response to help control the infection. Treatment depends on the areas involved. In most cases, chemical, electrocautery (heat), cryotherapy (freezing), or laser treatment is used. Excision (surgical removal of infected tissue) is used only occasionally. Most treatments are done in a health care provider's office, and are tailored to the needs of the patient.

You may want to use condoms with your future partner(s) to protect yourselves. However, with your future wife, the two of you may be comfortable with a mutual decision not to use condoms.

Alice

HPV and Having Children

Alice,
I was wondering about your response to "GenitalWarts." If someone has genital warts, does that mean that s/he cannot or should not have children? If they take the risk, will the resulting child be born with HPV?

CONCERNED FOR THE FUTURE

Dear Concerned for the Future,
If a woman has HPV (human papillomavirus), the virus that causes genital warts, the warts may appear on the outside of the vagina and/or on the inner walls of the vagina and on the cervix. Genital warts don't interfere with a woman's ability to get pregnant. However, during pregnancy, warts may get larger, probably due to increasing levels of estrogen. Warts along the vaginal wall might make the vagina less flexible and elastic during delivery. It may not be advisable to have the warts removed at this point because of the unknown possibility of birth defects caused by the substances used to remove them. Instead, Cesarean delivery might be recommended when there is a possibility of warts being present toward the end of a woman's pregnancy.

As for your question about a child being born with HPV, it's unlikely. There have been some cases where women with HPV in their vaginal canals during birth have passed the virus on to their babies in the form of laryngeal papilloma, which affects their throat, but this is quite rare.

Alice

Yeast Infection

Alice,
Recently, my girlfriend had a yeast infection. She went to the health service and they gave her something to clear up the matter. But the prob-

lem now is that I am noticing that my skin is extra dry and sometimes the skin develops signs of breakage. What could be the problem?

ALWAYS QUESTIONING

Dear Always Questioning,

Candida albicans, and other forms of yeast, grow in the vagina, rectum, and mouth. In a healthy vagina, the presence of some yeast may not be a problem. When a woman's system is out of balance, yeastlike organisms can grow profusely and cause a thick, white discharge that looks like cottage cheese.

Yeast may be transferred from partner to partner during unprotected sex. If you were having sex without a condom or dam before she was diagnosed, or while she was taking the medication, you may very well have gotten a yeast infection yourself. (This may or may not be yeast. This is something for you to have checked by your health care provider.) If this is the case, you could also pass it back to your partner, and then back to you, etc. To minimize this possibility, don't have intercourse, or use a condom or dam, until both of you complete treatment.

Alice

Yeast Infection Treatments

Alice,

My doctor prescribed antibiotics for me twice over the summer. Soon after taking the antibiotics, I got a yeast infection and have been having problems for several months. My gynecologist indicates that, even though the yeast infection is gone, I have a problem with stabilizing my pH balance. I have been taking acidophilus constantly in an attempt to put the "good bacteria" back into my system. My gynecologist indicates that the "good bacteria" has only recovered by approximately 15 percent. Since I have been fighting this for several months, I just wanted to get a second opinion. Can it possibly take six to eight months to recover from the damaging effects of antibiotics? Thanks!

IRRITATED

Dear Irritated,

Antibiotics, such as penicillin, erythromycin, tetracycline, and amoxicillin, are used to treat and prevent infection by killing and inhibiting the growth of bacteria. Antibiotics can also increase your susceptibility to yeast infections, as you well know, because they change the vagina's natural pH, which is normally slightly acidic, and kill off healthy bacteria. A change in acidity creates or allows for an overgrowth of yeast.

Alice would suggest you go back to your doctor and discuss this situation. Ask your provider why it seems to be taking so long for you to return to your normal bacterial balance. And ask if s/he has other suggestions for you to take care of yourself and regain your health. You may also want to get a second opinion from another provider.

Alice

WAYS TO PREVENT VAGINAL INFECTIONS

- Strengthen your immune system through exercise, a balanced diet, and enough sleep to increase your body's defenses against infections.
- Wash your vulva and anus with mild soap and warm water every day.
- Avoid perfumed soaps, feminine deodorant sprays and cleansers, and tampons and pads with deodorant.
- Do not douche. Douching can wash away the healthy bacteria lining the vagina, as well as alter the vagina's natural pH level.
- Use only plain white unscented toilet paper.
- Keep your sugar and caffeine intake to a minimum (too much can upset your natural pH balance).
- Wear underwear, tights, and pantyhose with cotton crotches. Tight clothing creates warmth and moisture which are favorable for the growth of yeast or bacteria.
- Wipe yourself after urinating from front to back so that bacteria from your anus will not get into your vaginal area.
- Wash your sex toys with mild soap and warm water.
- Use a condom on your sex toy or boy toy during intercourse.
- Change the condom between anal and vaginal penetration, and when sharing sex toys.
- Use a lube for sex.
- Get treated (your partner[s], too!) to prevent passing the infection back and forth, even if you're only having oral sex.

(Adapted from *The College Woman's Handbook*. Copyright © 1995 by Rachel Dobkin and Shana Sippy. Used by permission of Workman Publishing Co., Inc., New York. All Rights Reserved.)

Chronic Yeast Infections?

Alice,

I have chronic yeast infections. My doctor basically said that I have a pH imbalance and to stock up on Mycelex or similar creams. This answer, to me, is unsatisfactory. There must be something I can do to keep my pH level in balance, or at least on the acidic side.

I would very much appreciate any information you could provide pertaining to vaginal pH levels, or refer me to good resources. Thank you.

Dear Reader,

It sounds like there is more to this problem than meets the eye. It is not normal to have chronic yeast infections. Did your doctor say your yeast infections are "chronic," or did s/he use another term, such as "recurrent?" The distinction between chronic and recurrent is subtle, but important. *Chronic* means that a disease or condition will be present most, or all, of the time for a very long period of time, possibly for the rest of your life. *Recurrent* implies that you are able to effectively treat a certain infection or condition, but that it's likely to return.

Why does Alice make this point? Chronic yeast infections are usually indicative of a more serious health problem, usually one involving lowered immune response, or even diabetes. If you do have chronic yeast infections, you may want to have a complete medical checkup, including testing for all sexually transmitted diseases (STDs). This will help determine what, if any, systemic problem is causing these yeast infections. So, that's one thing to think about.

If your yeast infections are recurrent, perhaps the medication you're using is not effective for your particular infection. With recurrent yeast infections, it is a good idea to have a culture of the yeast done to figure out what strain of yeast you have. There are strains of yeast that do not respond to the usual antifungal creams. If that is the case, your doctor will be able to prescribe a more appropriate medication.

Perhaps the most simple solution to your problem is to make sure that this is yeast. There are several diseases and infections that appear to be yeast infections, but are not. This is why it is important to see your doctor and have the problem diagnosed each time. Just because you had a yeast infection two weeks ago doesn't mean that the vaginal itching and discharge you are experiencing now is another yeast infection. Women often treat what they think is a yeast infection when, in reality, they have a different infection that may or may not respond to the antifungal cream, or that may be aggravated by the antifungal. Moreover, using yeast infection medication when you don't have a yeast infection can create new problems.

Schedule an appointment for a complete physical and medical workup. Alice can't emphasize enough the importance of getting a diagnosis each time you have what appears to be a yeast infection.

Alice

Burning When I Pee?

Dear Alice,
I have a burning sensation when I pee. Is this bad?

SIGNED, BURNING

Dear Burning,
It's not bad, any more than a cough or sneeze is bad in and of itself. For men and women, burning when you pee is usually a symptom of an infection, a urinary tract infection (UTI), or an STD that's usually easily treated. Make an appointment to get this checked out, the sooner the better for your own personal health. It needs to be treated soon because if left untreated, it could cause permanent damage.

Symptoms may include:

- Needing to pee every few minutes
- Burning when you try to pee
- Needing to pee with hardly anything coming out
- Some blood in your pee (pink pee)
- Pain just above your pubic bone
- Strong odor to your morning's first pee

Alice

TO PREVENT URINARY TRACT INFECTIONS (UTIs)

- Drink lots of fluids every day.
- Urinate frequently, emptying your bladder completely each time.
- Wipe yourself from front to back after a bowel movement to keep bowel bacteria away from your urethra (for women only).
- Wash your hands before having sex, and after contact with the anus before touching the vagina.
- Make sure you are well-lubed before intercourse.
- Pee before and after sex.
- For women, change sanitary napkins and tampons frequently during your period.
- Cut down on or eliminate caffeine, alcohol, and sweets.
- Eat well and get enough rest.
- Manage your stress.

Crabs and Nit-Picking

Dear Alice,

I think I have pubic lice, a.k.a. "crabs." Do I need to see a doctor about this problem, or is there over-the-counter medication of some kind I can use to expel the little buggers from their new home? Also, I'm curious as to how I got them since I haven't had sex for several months and this is a recent development. Can one contract this problem from sharing clothing, towels, or bedclothes?

THANKS ALICE, ITCHING TO KNOW

Dear Itching to Know,

Lice eggs (nits) are small, gray, teardrop-shaped eggs that fasten themselves onto each individual hair. The crabs actually look like mini-crabs, and cause intense itching. Effective, over-the-counter treatments for pubic lice are available at drugstores even though they are used primarily for head lice (read the label for products gentle enough to use on pubic hair and genitals). Look for medications that are 1 percent permethrin creme rinses since they're milder than prescription medications. Shampoo the product into pubic and surrounding body hair as directed. For men, avoid applying the treatment to the tip of the penis. For women, avoid contact with the exposed mucous membranes of the vagina. Another application, after seven to ten days, may be necessary.

Pubic lice is most commonly spread through sexual contact. However, it can also be transmitted by direct nonsexual contact with someone who has lice, or with that person's clothing, bedding, furniture, and other personal belongings.

To help stop the spread of pubic lice and eggs, wash affected clothes and bedding in water that is at least 140 degrees Fahrenheit (60 degrees Celsius . . . hot water cycle), or put them in a sealed plastic bag for two weeks. Sexual partners, roommates, and family members who have been exposed need to take the same treatment steps. Once you've used the medication, remove the nits with a fine-tooth comb or with your thumb and forefinger, guiding the eggs off each hair and dispensing of them in a tissue.

If you've got crabs, you may also have been exposed to other more serious infections—see a health care provider.

Alice

Hepatitis B

Hi Alice:

Just wondering what you could tell me about Hepatitis B. My mother was just recently diagnosed with it, so I'd like some more information about what it is, what it does, who gets it, and the like.

CURIOUS

Dear Curious,

Hepatitis B is a liver disease characterized by inflammation of the liver and liver cell damage. It is caused by the Hepatitis B virus (HBV), present in the blood and all body fluids of an infected individual. Most hepatitis cases are acute, lasting less than one year. Each year, 6 to 10 percent of Hepatitis B infections in the United States becomes chronic, meaning the person continues to be highly contagious, and risks developing cirrhosis of the liver and liver cancer.

Hepatitis B can be transmitted through any contact of contaminated blood or body fluids with breaks in the skin or mucous membrane of an uninfected person. Hepatitis B is primarily transmitted through sexual contact and needle sharing—much like HIV transmission—or through blood transfusion. In some areas of the world, Hepatitis B is endemic and may be transmitted to offspring who become chronic asymptomatic carriers. If you were born in a high-risk area, you need to be evaluated to determine if you are a Hep B carrier.

At first, a person infected with Hepatitis B will not show any signs of disease—no symptom is one of the most common symptoms. Some people experience mild flulike symptoms (i.e., fever, aches, loss of appetite, fatigue). As the disease progresses, many people develop temporary jaundice (a yellowing of the skin) and dark urine.

Safer sex and avoiding unsterile needles (for drugs and tattoos) help prevent Hepatitis B transmission. As a matter of fact, Hepatitis B is the most preventable sexually transmitted disease (STD), primarily because there is a vaccine for it, which is administered in three injections over a six-month period. Because Hepatitis B is highly contagious, all those who have had close personal contact with someone infected with the virus need to be screened and vaccinated. If you are a college student, Alice strongly urges you to get the Hepatitis B vaccination because college is a common place for coming into contact with STDs, and you need all the protection you can get. See your health care provider to be immunized.

For more information on Hepatitis B, the virus or the disease, you can call the Hepatitis Hotline of the National Liver Foundation.
RES

Alice

A TALE OF THREE HEPS

Hep A: Common in children in developing countries, but frequently seen in adults in western countries; spread through direct and indirect contact with an infected person's feces (i.e., via contaminated food and water prepared with unwashed hands).

Hep B: Most common type of hepatitis worldwide, with an estimated 1.2 million carriers in the United States; spread through sexual contact, contaminated needles, and blood transfusions, and from mother to child during, or shortly before, childbirth. Hep B is common among college students. A vaccine is available and recommended.

Hep C: Most common type of hepatitis in the United States, with approximately 3.9 million carriers; spread directly from one person to another through blood or contaminated needles. It's possible, but uncommon, for Hep C to be spread from mother to child or through sexual contact.

Eating Sperm

Dear Alice,
I'm worried. What happens if you eat your own sperm?

Dear Reader,
Nothing, except you might spoil your dinner.

Kidding aside, if it's semen (the liquid in which sperm exits the penis) that you're worried about, all the safer sex guidelines apply when you eat *someone else's* semen. There's still debate about HIV transmission via semen and oral sex, but there are plenty of other sexually transmitted diseases (STDs) that can be passed along by oral sex, too. Swallowing your own semen (virus-free or not) is safe.

Alice

Men's Sexual Health

White Spots on Penis and Tight Foreskin

Dear Alice,
I am a virgin and I've never had any sexual contacts. I have always had, for as long as I can remember, a lot of little white-headed spots on the underside of my penis. I can only assume they are some form of wart—they are small, few millimeters across, and, if squeezed, sometimes the white head can be removed. I am too embarrassed and worried to see my doctor (she's a woman), but I would like to know what they are before I have sex.

Also, I have a tight foreskin. The reason appears to be a profusion of similar, but much smaller, spots, without heads, on the inside edge of the foreskin that seem to have collected together to form a nonstretchy expanse of skin (almost like scar skin). I should add that none of these symptoms cause any discomfort whatsoever.

CONCERNED VIRGIN

Dear Concerned Virgin,
Your white-headed spots, as you call them, on the underside of your penis are probably pearly white papules, common and harmless. These papules are frequently misdiagnosed as condyloma (genital warts).

A tight foreskin, if it causes pain during erection, masturbation, or any other activity, can be released under local anesthesia in the doctor's office. Your best bet is to go to the doctor, even if you are embarrassed, since peace of mind means a lot. And if you're too uncomfortable with your own doctor because of her gender, then see a male doctor.

Alice

Penis Bump—Wart?

Dear Alice,

I have a single white, hard bump on the shaft of my penis. Could it be a wart?

Dear Reader,

The bump that you describe could be a wart. More likely, however, it is a sebaceous cyst. Alice recommends that you have this checked by a health care provider who can diagnose and determine the appropriate treatment for you, if any.

Alice

WHAT'S A SEBACEOUS CYST?

A sebaceous cyst is a catch-all term for a benign, harmless growth that occurs under the skin and tends to be smooth to the touch. Ranging in size, sebaceous cysts are usually found on the scalp, face, ears, and genitals. They are formed when the release of sebum, a medium-thick fluid produced by sebaceous glands in the skin, is blocked. Unless they become infected and painful, sebaceous cysts do not require medical attention or treatment, and usually go away on their own.

The Spotted Penis Mystery

Dear Alice,

I know that having intercourse at a time when I have a vaginal infection will cause my partner to become infected, i.e., get red spots on his penis. What could cause him to get this when I'm not having any symptoms?

Dear Reader,

Red spots on the penis could be caused by an allergic reaction to spermicidal jelly or cream, or to the nonoxynol-9 or lube on condoms. Red spots can also be caused by an asymptomatic infection. It sounds as if you are already on the case and now have some variables to test as well. There also seems to be sufficient reason to get yourself and your partner checked for STDs. You can go to the nearest city or county health department's STD clinic, or to your own health care provider.

Good luck solving your spotted penis mystery.

Alice

Bumps on Inner Thighs? Warts? Molluscum?

Dear Alice,

Hi there, this is a question that has been on my mind for years now, and one which I've felt too embarrassed to ask even my physician because of personal reasons.

My problem is this. On my thighs there are many raised bumps. Usually, there are between five to ten of them, and some can be quite big or painful. I think they are warts of some kind but I am not sure.

They've been appearing on me randomly for about four years now, I guess, and yet I'm wondering if they are sexual in some way? I didn't lose my virginity until two years ago, yet they only appear on my inner thighs and no creams I have ever tried abate them whatsoever. Could I have been born with an odd form of genital warts? Is there a recommended cure for these annoying things? Can I alleviate this problem without the trauma of asking my physician?

For years, these things have been bugging me, and now that I am sexually active, I fear that these might be contagious. They do have slippery/oily liquid in them when they tear.

What do I do? I'm perplexed, scared. When a problem like this sends a twenty-year-old male to tears, it's definitely a problem. Are there any recorded instances of this problem? Are warts on inner thighs common?

BUMPS ON THE INNER THIGHS

Dear Bumps on the Inner Thighs,

First of all, Alice encourages you to speak with your physician just as you did with her. "Hey, Doc, I'm, like, embarrassed to bring this up, but I, like, have these bumps on my inner thighs. Can you tell me what they are?"

These bumps might be molluscum contagiosum, a common skin condition that matches many of the characteristics you describe. Thigh bumps can also be folliculitis (an inflammation of the hair follicles) or some other chronic inflammation.

Mollusca are firm, dome shaped, flesh-colored bumps that may be umbilicated, which means that they have a little dimple in the center. However, there is room for variety in the description: they could be white, translucent, or yellow, and range in size from very tiny (head of a pin) to large (size of a nickel). They can also become red and swollen. They are usually found around the lower abdomen, genitals, and inner thighs. The cause is a virus different from the wart viruses. The virus can spread to other areas of the body, or to other people, usually by direct contact, such as sexual contact, but possibly nonsexual, too . . . for example, via clothing or towels. Fortunately, there are no hidden or future problems or risks. Just the bumps.

Treatment? Easy, though inconvenient. There are a variety of methods, including a scraping procedure, called curettage, and freezing. Repeated treatments may be necessary. Overall, the outcome is better than with other types of wart-removal treatments. Going through treatment minimizes the risk of transmission to another person.

Even though Alice understands your fear, embarrassment, and perplexity, she recommends that you make an appointment as soon as possible. A diagnosis by a health care provider is the necessary first step.

Alice

Women's Sexual Health

Gynecologist for the First Time

Dear Alice,
How soon after losing my virginity should I see a gynecologist for the first time?

JUST WONDERING

Dear Just Wondering,
Usually, women eighteen years and older see a gynecologist or a nurse practitioner whether or not they're virgins. After a woman has had sex with a partner, it is important for her to get a full gynecological exam each year.

You can use this experience to learn more about your body as well as yourself. Let your provider know that this is your first exam and ask her/him to explain each procedure. Routine pelvic examinations include both an external and an internal exam. The health care provider will examine your vulva (inner and outer lips), clitoris, and vaginal opening. After that, s/he will look inside your vagina using a speculum, which may be the most unfamiliar part of the exam. A speculum is a metal or plastic instrument used to hold your vaginal walls apart. It may be a bit uncomfortable—even though this may seem impossible, relax, it does get easier with practice. The provider will examine your vaginal walls for lesions, inflammation, or unusual discharge, and will also check your cervix for the same. S/he will collect a sample of cells from your cervix using a swab. This part of the internal exam is called a Pap smear. Some women feel a slight cramping when the cells are being gathered. The collected cervical cells are then sent to a lab to check for abnormal cell growth and to screen for cervical cancer. The Pap smear does not test for pregnancy, sexually transmitted diseases (STDs), vaginal infections, or other types of gynecological problems.

It's important for young women to get an annual gynecological exam. They may be vulnerable to cervical infection since the surface of their cervixes contains relatively immature, less resistant cells. Early detection and treatment can reduce future complications.

Alice

AN ANNUAL EXAM INCLUDES A GENERAL EXAMINATION, AS WELL AS SOME OR ALL OF THESE SPECIFIC PROCEDURES:

- Questions about full family and personal medical history
- A breast examination, with instructions on breast self-exam
- Listening to your heart and lungs with a stethoscope
- A blood pressure and pulse check
- A blood test (hemoglobin count and complete blood count)
- A weight check
- An abdominal exam
- A pelvic exam
- A Pap smear and STD screening tests
- Evaluation for contraception, if desired

What Is Dysplasia?

Dear Alice,

Last week I went to my OB-GYN for a checkup. I had not been to the doctor in four years because I had moved and not found the time to look for one. (I know, not a good idea.) Well, the results of my Pap smear came back and my doctor said I had dysplasia. She also said that I did not have any signs of warts when she examined me. After questioning her on the origin of this, since I know little about dysplasia, she told me it was sexually transmitted. Is this true? I have heard that no one really knows where dysplasia comes from. I just want more information before I go in for my checkup before treatment. By the way, this didn't show up on my Pap smear four years ago, and I have had the same partner this whole time. Thank you!

Dear Reader,

Yearly Pap smears allow us to keep tabs on cervical cell growth. We can see if they are growing and replacing themselves in a healthy manner, or if the cell growth has become abnormal.

Dysplasia means abnormal cell growth anywhere in the body. In your case, this abnormal growth has occurred on your cervix. Unchecked and untreated, it can progress, possibly to cancer; or, it can heal on its own. The more severe the dysplasia, the more likely it is to progress to cancer. Mild dysplasia may resolve on its own, without any treatment.

Cervical dysplasia has been associated with the presence of the human papillomavirus (HPV), which causes genital warts and is usually, although not always, sexually transmitted.

If you have an abnormal Pap smear, the result may not always say "abnormal with HPV changes." Although you've been with the same person for the past four years, and your last Pap was normal, HPV could have gone undetected before. It is important to have a Pap smear annually so that abnormalities can be detected early.

Dysplasia is further diagnosed with colposcopy, which looks at the whole cervix, and, sometimes, a tissue biopsy. Through colposcopy (a procedure that magnifies the area with a special microscope—a colposcope), your doctor can directly view your cervix and any abnormalities. If your doctor sees any abnormal cells through the colposcope, she will remove them and send them to a lab. This is the biopsy part of the treatment. Depending on the biopsy results indicating the severity of the dysplasia, further treatment may be suggested, which can be simply observing it to see if it resolves spontaneously, repeating the Pap test more frequently, and probably repeating the colposcopy. Other treatment may be recommended to remove the abnormal tissue. A commonly used treatment is cryosurgery, a freezing technique.

Discuss your options with your doctor, or seek a second opinion, if you want, or both.

Alice

Bled from Pap Smear

Dear Alice,

I bled as a result of my last Pap smear. I've never had that happen before and it was a new gynecologist. She said that it was normal. Is that true?

CONFUSED ABOUT BLOOD

Dear Confused about Blood,

Yes, it is true. Bleeding from a Pap smear is normal. Some women who are on birth control pills bleed from a Pap smear because the effect of the hormones tends to make the cervix more sensitive. If you are not on birth control pills, bleeding from a Pap smear may be a sign of a minor abnormality on your cervix, such as an infection or STD, or a result of the procedure itself. Wait for the results of your Pap. If the bleeding is a sign of another problem, the tests would normally show that.

Alice

PMS!

Dear Alice,

Once a month I get PMS-y. I can deal with the bloating and cramps (usually), but, honestly, I go crazy, loony, wacky. My emotions are completely out of control, from extremely happy to totally miserable and crying, with lots of grumpy behavior in between. I actually don't usually realize when I'm behaving irrationally, so when my boyfriend tries to point out that maybe my bouts of anger and tears are caused by hormones I attack him for telling me I'm just an irrational woman. Basically, is there any way to help these mood swings? I'm on birth control pills, which is supposed to help, but it doesn't really seem to do anything.

THANKS, NUTS

Dear Nuts,

Premenstrual syndrome (PMS) is the development of a wide range of symptoms for several days before, and sometimes during, the first day of most, or all, of your periods. Researchers disagree on a definition of PMS, and all efforts to find a biological basis for it so far have failed. These treatments work for some women: Prozac, birth control pills, some vitamins or minerals, and evening primrose oil. Hormone suppressants have not had clinical trials as a remedy for PMS—although it is known that they can have severe side effects when taken in large doses over long periods of time.

Some women have found that home remedies, or rather preventatives, have been helpful in alleviating some of the symptoms of PMS. Reduce your salt, sugar, caffeine, and alcohol intake at least one week before your period is expected. Or, if that seems like too much to ask, try reducing one item at a time in your diet and see if there's any difference. Exercise helps premenstrually, as well as for cramps during your period. Although it seems as if that's the last thing you'd want to do, it can help. Also, vitamin B_6, or pyridoxine, may help. Good food sources include whole grains, green vegetables, molasses, nuts and seeds, poultry, potatoes, and fish. If you want to try a B_6 supplement, 25–50 mg a day may help. Avoid higher dosages because of toxicity—discontinue use immediately if you get tingling sensations. Taking 400 mg/day of vitamin E along with vitamin B_6 may offer benefits as well. RES

Alice

Missed Periods

Dear Alice,
What is the usual treatment for missed periods? I haven't had my period for half a year (ever since I stopped taking the pill). I have also lost some weight. What are the health effects of missed periods?

PERIODLESS

Dear Periodless,
Amenorrhea ("a" means without and "menorrhea" means menstrual flow) is the medical term for this condition. Since you have missed over three consecutive periods, make an appointment with your health care provider. The assumption, from your letter, is that you have already made sure that you are not pregnant, which is the main reason women stop menstruating. Other common reasons include weight loss, hormonal changes, strenuous exercise, a change in one's environment (this has also been referred to as "boarding school" syndrome), and even the eating disorder anorexia.

After going off the pill, your body may take some time to adjust to secreting its own hormones that regulate ovulation and your period. If it takes more than six months for your period to return, a visit to your health care provider is recommended. If the cause of your amenorrhea is due to low estrogen levels, vaginal dryness and a loss of bone density can result (for example, among highly competitive athletes in physically demanding sports). Athletes, regardless of their excellent diet and exercise programs, have lost significant bone mass when their periods stopped. Amenorrhea can have a negative impact on reproductive, endocrine, and muscular-skeletal systems.

Give your women's health care provider a thorough history of your activities, diet, and workload. Let her/him know about any other symptoms you may be experiencing, even if they seem insignificant. It may be nothing, or it may be just the clue needed to determine the cause.

Alice

Endometriosis

Dear Alice,
My girlfriend has endometriosis and I want to know more about it. Thanks.

Dear Reader,
Endometriosis occurs when some of the tissue which lines the uterus begins to grow in another part of the body. In most cases, this growth develops in the pelvic area—on the ovaries, the lining of the pelvic cavity, ligaments, or the fallopian tubes.

Because these growths are made of endometrial tissue, they usually behave like the endometrium, responding to the hormones of the menstrual cycle. Each month, they build up tissue and slough it off. As a result, internal bleeding, inflammation, cysts, and scar tissue can develop in the affected areas.

Common symptoms of endometriosis include: extreme pelvic pain during menstruation, ovulation, and/or sexual intercourse; excessive menstrual flow; fatigue; lower back pain; infertility; or no symptoms at all. Endometriosis can also cause other serious problems, such as ruptured ovarian cysts and an increased risk of ectopic pregnancy. The disease can be debilitating, even interfering with normal daily activities, for days, weeks, and even months at a time. Fortunately for you and your girlfriend, diagnosis and treatment will make a difference. RES

Alice

Breast Implants

Dear Alice,
I always had small breasts until I became overweight. I am now going on a medically supervised diet. I know that I am ready to really lose the weight and keep it off. The only trouble is that I am only a size "B" cup now. When I lose the weight, I am sure to be an "A," or even an "AA." So, I have been considering the possibility of breast implants. Can you tell me some of the repercussions of breast implants? Can you breast-feed later? What happens during pregnancy? What are the health risks? Well, any information you have about the topic would be helpful. Thanks!

FLATTY BUT NOT A FATTY!

Dear Flatty but Not a Fatty!,
Alice wonders what factors have influenced your desire to increase your breast size. Are you worried that you will not be sexy and attractive if your breasts are "too small"? People find themselves attracted to another person because of that individual's personality, attitude, intelligence, athletic interests, and other attributes besides looks.

As you explore breast implant surgery, read information pamphlets and ask a doctor or surgeon for information. Known risks of implant surgery include a painful tightening of the scar tissue around the implant, known as capsular contracture; implant rupture; the formation of calcium deposits around the implant (this makes reading mammograms difficult); temporary or permanent changes in nipple or breast sensation; and, shifting of the implant. Other possible risks still under investigation include immune-related disorders, cancer, and possible effects on pregnancy and breast-feeding.

In the meantime lose the weight, look at your body, and ask for second opinions before going ahead with this surgery. You may find that you are more attractive and in proportion than you think.

Alice

Breast Lump

Dear Alice,
My doctor found a lump in my breast recently. She told me not to worry, but have it checked out soon, by another doctor. She said that it did not feel cancerous, but may be a cyst or fibroadenoma. Can you tell me about what these are exactly, and does this mean a greater chance for breast cancer later in life? What should I expect? Thanks for your help.

CONCERNED

Dear Concerned,
When a lump is found in a young woman, the doctor usually assumes that it is a fibroadenoma and not cancer. A fibroadenoma is a benign, fibrous tumor found commonly in the breast which does not fluctuate with your period. Fibroadenomas are painless, firm, round lumps, usually one-half to two inches in diameter and movable. Multiple fibroadenomas may develop in one or both breasts. The cause of these growths is unknown. They are not linked to increased risk of breast cancer. If removal is necessary, it can be done with either a local or a general anesthetic. After removal, the lump is examined by a pathologist to rule out the small chance of breast cancer. Fibroadenomas occur most often in women under thirty, and are more common in black women.

A cyst develops in the breast when small sacs fill with fluid or semi-fluid material. The size of the cyst may fluctuate during the course of your menstrual cycle. During ovulation and before menstruation, your hormone levels change, causing breast cells to retain fluid. If you examine your breasts during these times, you may find a series of lumps in one or both breasts—especially in the areas near your underarms. These lumps may be present from your very first period, or may develop in your twenties or thirties. Sometimes, the lumps feel a little sore, but they are harmless.

Alice

BREAST SELF-EXAM (BSE)

To effectively monitor any changes in your breasts, the American Cancer Society (ACS) recommends that BSE be done once a month, preferably a few days after your period, when your breasts are not swollen or tender.

TO DO A BSE:

- First, lie on your back with a pillow under your right shoulder, and your right arm behind your head. For your right breast, use the top one-third of the three middle fingers of your left hand and press firmly to feel for any lumps. Move your fingers in a circular motion. Switch pillow and arm position to check your left breast. Squeeze each nipple to check for any discharge.
- Then, in the shower, raise your right arm and carefully examine your right breast using your left hand. Start at the top, outer edge of your breast and press your fingers firmly in a circular motion, feeling for any abnormal lumps in the underlying tissue. Once you've finished with the outer edge, move in an inch toward the nipple and repeat. Repeat this with your left breast. Also, check the area above your breasts and your armpits for any lumps or knots.
- Lastly, stand in front of a mirror with your arms at your sides. Check your breasts for any color, size, and/or shape changes. Also, check for any dimpling or scaling on the skin. Do this check again with your hands on your hips, flexing your chest muscles (by pressing your shoulders and elbows forward). Then, do the check one last time with your hands raised above your head.

The Pill and Breast Cancer

Dear Alice,

I was hoping you could answer a question for me about birth control pills. There is a history of breast cancer in my family (my mother). Is it true that because of this, it is unsafe for me to use birth control pills? A few friends have recently had condoms break during sex, and I am looking for a type of "backup" contraception system.

CONCERNED

Dear Concerned,

At this time, there is no evidence that pill use increases the risk of breast cancer if a woman has a female relative with breast cancer. However, there is some concern that since estrogen can promote some breast cancers, a woman with a strong family history of breast cancer may be at higher risk and wish to choose another method. But, since the pill *may* protect against breast cancer by stabilizing hormones within the breast tissue, the pill is recommended for daughters of mothers with breast or ovarian cancer as long as they are carefully monitored and have regular breast exams as advised by their health care providers. If you smoke, definitely choose another method of contraception because of the increased chance of stroke or other cardiovascular problems.

Make an appointment with a provider to discuss your other contraceptive options.   *Alice*

WITH ONE IN NINE WOMEN GETTING BREAST CANCER AND MANY HAVING NO RISK FACTORS, EVERY WOMAN NEEDS TO DO THE FOLLOWING:

- Carefully examine your breasts each month for unusual lumps (breast self-exam).
- Have an annual breast exam by a health care provider.
- Cut down on fatty foods (i.e., soft cheese, whole milk, red meat, sour cream, etc.) and eat more vegetables and fruits.
- Talk with your health care provider about current drug research findings that may apply to you.

BREAST CANCER AND EXERCISE

F.Y.I.: *Science News* reported the results of a study from the University of Southern California School of Medicine in Los Angeles regarding reducing a woman's risk of breast cancer. It states that women who exercise three or more hours a week in the decade following menarche—the onset of their menstrual cycle—can lower their risk of breast cancer by 30 percent by age forty, compared to their more sedentary peers. Continuing that moderately active lifestyle until at least age forty can cut your risk by almost 60 percent. This is one of the only risk factors for breast cancer that women themselves can have control over. So get out there and get moving.

Tampons or Pads?

Alice,
I am a twenty-year-old foreign student and I am new to the States. One of the first things I learned about the American way of life for women is that tampons seem to be used by my sister students more often than pads. I was not familiar with them before I arrived here and am rather worried about trying to use tampons myself, despite the advantages claimed for them. Maybe you can help by answering a few of my questions, as I find it embarrassing to talk about this as frankly as some American girls do.

(1) Should one use pads or tampons?
(2) What kind of pads or tampons are recommended (I am not familiar with the brands in the stores here)?
(3) What particular advantages do these types have over others?
(4) I have seen some pads described as "overnight." Does that mean very absorbent? Is it possible to wear a pad and a tampon at the same time?
(5) What are panty liners? Do you also use them with pads and with tampons?
(6) I have heard that tampons are sold to girls as young as thirteen. How is it possible that they can use them?
(7) Are there any risks or dangers in using tampons?

NEW TO PLAYTEX

Dear New to Playtex,
You ask some great questions that many American women have as well. Here are some answers: wearing pads or tampons is a matter of personal preference. Pads, or sanitary napkins, come in a variety of shapes, sizes, and absorbencies. Overnight types are usually the bulkiest and the most absorbent, and panty liners are the smallest and the least absorbent. Women use different products depending on the heaviness of their flow.

Tampons are made of soft absorbent material and are inserted into the vaginal opening, like a battery into a flashlight, resting in the vaginal canal to absorb menstrual fluid. Tampons also come in various sizes and absorbencies, with or without deodorant, and with or without applicators. Brands also differ in size, effectiveness, and comfort. Tampons need to be changed frequently to prevent toxic shock syndrome. They may also be used with pads as backup in case they leak. Women can use tampons even if they haven't ever had sexual intercourse, and using tampons does not affect virginity.

Alice

Lost Tampon

Dear Alice,
I had in a tampon, and now I can't find it. It was there. I tried to find it, but I can't. Is that possible? I am really worried about it. It was in for about one day. Please help.

Dear Reader,
A tampon cannot get lost in your body. The vagina is a potential space that can expand, and the tampon can get lodged near the back. It will remain there until you find it. It seems as though the string may have become twisted behind the tampon, or pushed way back in the vagina, making it difficult to reach.

When this happens, it takes some time for the vagina to relax and change position so that the tampon will return to its usual place, or at least to a more accessible location. Try "fishing around" for the tampon or string with your clean index finger. If you're not able to find it, try asking a partner.

Otherwise, see your health care provider. Explain the situation, and tell her/him that you are concerned about the loss, the odor, and toxic shock syndrome (TSS). As a last resort, you can go to the emergency room. It is important to do this not only to regain peace of mind, but because the tampon will begin to smell bad, and ultimately because there may be a small risk of infection, including TSS.

Alice

TOXIC SHOCK SYNDROME (TSS)

Toxic Shock Syndrome is a rare, but life-threatening, bacterial infection that affects between one and seventeen menstruating women per 100,000. Studies have shown that using the super plus tampons, and leaving tampons in the vagina for long amounts of time, increase the risk of developing TSS. Symptoms include a sudden high fever, vomiting, diarrhea, fainting, dizziness, or a sunburnlike rash. To minimize the risk of TSS, wash your hands before inserting a tampon, change your tampon every four to six hours (especially on heavy flow days), and use the lowest absorbency tampon that is reasonable given the amount of your menstrual flow.

Go to Alice at www.goaskalice.columbia.edu for more Sexual Health Q & A's, including these:

- Allergic to Sperm?
- Are Two Condoms Better Than One?
- Burning after Sex without a Condom
- Cold Sores vs. Canker Sores—Oral Sex Risks?
- Contracting HIV from Receiving Oral Sex
- Is Pulling Out Safe?
- Lost (Condon) Condom
- Male Contraceptives?
- Male Yeast Infection?
- Monogamous Couple—Time to Stop Using Condoms?
- Routes of HIV Transmission?
- Sex During Period . . . on the Pill . . . Safe?
- Testing for Herpes and Genital Warts
- Do Two Virgins Need to Use Condoms?
- Yogurt for Yeast Infections?

EMOTIONAL HEALTH

During high school and college, your body brews a constantly changing menu of "hormonal cocktails," serving them up at the exact moment you're facing final exams; falling in love or lust, or both; setting up your very own living space; or, tackling a weight-control problem, a weight-lifting problem, or a wait-too-long-to-start-the-term-paper problem. Meanwhile, you're experiencing separation from parents who may or may not have eased the path to adulthood. If they were great, you may feel devastated and lonely, missing them terribly; if they were inattentive, you may be furious, wishing they'd prepared you better and sent you off with the care packages everyone else seems to have; you may be relieved to be away from them; or you may feel a combination of all of the above. Any change is stressful.

And that's not all: your friends, lovers, classmates, and roommates are just as volatilely juiced as you are. It's a hectic time, but it's also the perfect time to learn coping skills you can draw on for a lifetime.

Typical responses to stress can include depression, panic, anger, and anxiety, in varying levels. These emotions can, in turn, make us feel helpless, hopeless, and devastated, but they are also important signals to let us know when we're "maxed out," need to set limits, or need to ask for help. It's also helpful to know how to respond when one of these alarms is triggered in someone we care about. In this chapter, Alice will shed some light on these situations, in both their major and minor manifestations. She'll discuss shyness, stage fright, performance anxiety, and grief, as well as illnesses such as bipolar disorder.

During our teens and twenties, we learn a lot about our potential limits. We often pack these years with social plans, extracurricular activities, athletics, and dates, not to mention classes, studying, and jobs to help pay for this busy agenda. It's common to feel exhausted, unmotivated, and generally glum when we weigh ourselves down with too many high-pressure obligations. And realizing our limitations can, in itself, be frustrating and immobilizing. It's especially impossible to experience much pleasure if your eyes are constantly on the prize of perfection. It's okay, and necessary, to have at least a few things you do for pure fun.

Sometimes negative emotions cause a severe, self-punishing response. The "outer world" reflects the "inner world," manifested in behaviors such as face-picking, hair pulling, and bloodletting. Thoughts of suicide are especially serious and signal an immediate call to a hotline or counselor.

Alice doesn't just advocate counseling for the deeply depressed. She hopes you'll use all of the mental health resources available to you for emotional maintenance as well. It can be a great relief to have an established relationship with a campus or community counselor, ready and waiting for you during your most stressful turning points.

Learning to maintain your emotional well-being is just as vital as learning to manage your own finances, meals, time, schoolwork, and overall physical health. In fact, emotional well-being is the foundation for all the other aspects of your life. The payoffs include improved physical health, stronger relationships, better productivity, and being content with life in general. But more than just striving to "smile, not worry, and be happy," it's also about developing a strong sense of self—by listening to your emotions, often through that queasy stomach or sleepless night, and by making a commitment to acknowledge and care for that self for the rest of your life.

Stress and Anxiety

Panic Attacks

Dear Alice,
I need some information about panic attacks. My partner moved with me to NY and, at the time of moving, experienced several attacks of extreme fear. This has paralyzed her to the extent that she no longer goes to work, her career is on hold, and she requires help traveling, if she travels at all. As well as being incredibly distressing for her, it's not helping our relationship either. My question relates to my role in helping her recover from this. At present, I frequently "overlook" the problem by going everywhere with her and being as supportive as possible. Am I an "enabler"? Should I make her "tough it out," or will she just get better?

Dear Reader,
Panic attacks are periods of heightened anxiety often coupled with an extreme fear of being in crowded or closed places. At first, these attacks are sudden and unexpected, but, if they continue, are often triggered by environment, like going through tunnels, traveling across bridges, or being in crowded elevators. Accompanying symptoms include a sense of chest pain, shallow breathing, lightheadedness, dizziness, sweating, a pounding heart, chills or flushes, nausea, and even tingling or numbness in the hands. A sense of impending doom is usually part of the experience.

Panic attacks are common, frequently linked to feelings of loss. Panic attacks vary in intensity and tend to be exacerbated by stressful periods. Psychotherapy, with and without medication, is effective for as many as 90 percent of people affected with panic attacks. Cutting back on caffeine may make a difference, too.

While your support may be comforting to your partner, it would be wise for her to get professional counseling, especially since her panic is affecting your relationship. With counseling for yourself as well, you may be better able to help your partner.

Alice

Procrastination

Alice,
I'm a horrible procrastinator and time manager—in school, at work, cleaning my apartment, you name it, I'm somehow always putting it off till tomorrow, or taking forever to finish. Do you have any practical suggestions on time organization and overcoming procrastination habits?

ALWAYS LATE

Dear Always Late,
An inordinate amount of stress in students' lives revolves around time. And procrastination is probably the number one time management problem of all! Procrastination can be a mask for our own unrealistic perfectionist tendencies, self-doubt, or fear of change. It can also simply be a result of poor time management and ineffective study skills.

With patience and determination, you can change some of your procrastinating ways and learn to live with what you can't change. The goal is to learn to fit our daily activities into time's schedule. We cannot manage time; we can only manage ourselves given the time we have. Alice's favorite self-management strategies are:

(1) Be realistic about what you can accomplish in a day— PRIORITIZE two or three major goals or to-do's each day, leaving other activities "lower down" on your list.

(2) Schedule your activities for peak efficiency. Do the things that require more brain power during the times of the day when your energy level is highest.

(3) Divide your projects into small pieces. The job at hand can then become more manageable, and your steady progress might encourage you to move ahead.

(4) Create a schedule that allows flexibility for unanticipated events (e.g., distractions, computer crashes). Remember to leave a 15 percent tip—add extra time into your schedule for each activity because things always seem to take longer than you think.

(5) Forgive yourself if you don't complete all of the things on your to-do list—you're only human.

Remember, this is something you can change.

Alice

Fear of Public Speaking

Dear Alice,
I have an extreme problem with speaking in front of groups of people (especially speeches). I can't do them! My voice either doesn't say anything, or it shakes like I am going to cry or something. I know public speaking is the most common fear, but mine is one I must confront. What kind of options do I have besides books? Any ideas?

FEARFUL PUBLIC SPEAKER

Dear Fearful Public Speaker,
Alice knows about the importance of public speaking. Research shows that a significant factor in people being promoted at work is the ability to effectively and concisely express one's self in public or at a meeting, no matter how large the gathering.

You're not alone. For example, actors with stage fright are coached to transform their feelings of fear into excitement and anticipation. They learn to use their fear to galvanize themselves into doing their absolute best.

Do not berate yourself for what you cannot do, or for what strikes terror in your soul. Think instead about the times you have spoken in public, or when you have told a joke or a meaningful story to a group of friends. These are positive experiences you can build on.

Take a course in speech communication to increase confidence and skills. Also, throughout the country, Toastmasters International holds meetings where ordinary people gather to strengthen their public speaking and communication skills. **RES**

Alice

Athletic Performance Anxiety

Dear Alice,
I compete in an individual sport. The problem is that on the day of a major competition, I have really bad indigestion. Sometimes, I have to run to the bathroom every half hour for a bowel movement! Besides being annoying, disgusting, and a little embarrassing, this interrupts my competition and adds unneeded stress. Why is this happening and what can I do to prevent it?

SIGNED, DASHIN' TO THE BATHROOM

Dear Dashin' to the Bathroom,
It sounds like your angst about competing in athletics is being played out in your gastrointestinal system—not an uncommon arena for nervousness and stress linked to performances of all kinds: athletic,

PRESENTATION POWER POINTS

1. Come up with three or four important messages or headlines that you would like your audience to understand, use, and/or be inspired by.
2. Keep your talk simple; remember, you know much more about your subject than they do—and being overloaded with information can be a burden.
3. Weave stories—personal or made-up ones—through your talk to illustrate points and heighten interest.
4. Try out some of your "material": stories, jokes, ideas, etc., on friends.
5. Practice your presentation formally in front of a mirror or to a group of friends.
6. As teachers have been saying for years about framing your talk:
   • Tell 'em what you're gonna tell 'em.
   • Tell 'em.
   • Tell 'em what you told 'em.
7. Ask your audience members for their names, and find out their goals and experiences as they relate to your presentation.
8. Focus on even eye contact with your attendees—looking just over the tops of their heads or at their noses will work, too.
9. Speak a little more loudly than you think is necessary—talking to the person farthest away from you can help you maintain proper volume.
10. Slow down, smile, and breathe.
11. Allow time for questions and answers.

theatrical, academic, or professional. The short-term stress response, "fight or flight," causes muscle tension and acid production. For some, this leads to stomach discomfort, diarrhea, or constipation.

Rehearsal imagery is a technique widely used by athletes and performance artists. It can also be used successfully by the rest of us who get jittery thinking about the thrill of victory . . . or the agony of defeat. Here's how: a few weeks prior to your competition, make a written list of the who, what, when, where, and how of the upcoming event. Who will be there? What will they be doing, wearing, and saying? What time of day will the event take place? Where will you be: a school, a gym, a stadium? How will you look, stand, run, and perform in comparison to others around you?

When your long list is finished, close your eyes and visualize each of these factors in your mind's eye. Imagine in great detail your actual movements, and how your body will feel as you proceed in your glorious performance. Think of yourself sprinting around the track, following the ball from your hand into the hoop, delivering a slice serve to a specific spot on your opponent's court, passing other bikers, and pacing yourself up and down hills.

Why does rehearsal imagery help reduce performance-related tension and improve the quality of the task at hand? Stress is generated by fear of the unknown, and by new demands and challenges. By imagining that you are really there, even if the actual details are unknown to you, you are familiarizing yourself with what might be, as well as how you see yourself in that situation. This strategy also reduces the element of surprise, which goes a long way when you want to reduce stress. Practice rehearsal imagery once or twice a day right up until your event. You can even tape record your description of the event and play it back, if that's easier. (Leave out the bathroom part.) If possible, make a site visit to where you will be competing. This can make the imagery that much more real. But while you are waiting for the visualization to work, there are over-the-counter antidiarrheal medications you can try. A physician can prescribe an antianxiety medicine that can help, too.

Alice

Stressed-Out Teen with Suicidal Thoughts

Dear Alice,
I will not tell you my age, but I have not yet reached my junior year in high school. Whenever I feel down and very tired, I think about how horrible my life is. I say "Life sucks and then you die," and "What's the point of life since you're going to die anyway." Well, whenever these things come up, I think about suicide. When at home, I open up my window and look all the way down. I think about my body splatting down on the ground, and then I forget about it out of disgust. Well, I hope that you can help me and please hurry up. This is urgent.

DAZED

Dear Dazed,
Please don't commit suicide. Your ability to express your thoughts is impressive. Maybe you could use this talent to talk with someone who is physically closer to you, or more readily accessible than Alice. Talk with a counselor at your school, call a local suicide prevention hotline. Do this now without any delay. With help, the good judgment and caring

of a counselor, and perhaps even medication, your feelings of hopelessness can turn around.   RES

Alice

Stressed Out and Anxious from Schoolwork and Everything

Alice,
I think I just had my breaking point. I don't know how much more stress I can take. I tried to check out stress-reduction workshops, but the next one is next semester. I don't really want to see a psychiatrist. I don't know what to do. Basically, I think a lot of my stress is because it is just so difficult for me to focus or concentrate on anything. My thoughts are running everywhere. I try, I really do. I even moved into a single for it. I feel so incompetent. I don't give a damn about making friends. I'm always feeling lonely. And worst of all, there is always something that makes me so worried, panicked, to the point of just wanting to die to relieve me of it. I have chest pains when I sleep sometimes. When I stand up to do something, I always forget what to do . . . always. This letter that I'm writing has taken me an hour to write because I have to pause so many times to think about my classes. Whenever I do anything away from my desk during my designated "study time," I feel so guilty. Last weekend, I couldn't eat because I didn't want to leave my room to go to the kitchen to eat anything. Yet I am always behind in my schoolwork. Since transferring here this semester, I have never felt confident, relaxed, or satisfied about anything. Everything annoys me. I annoy me. This letter probably sounds really unorganized, but I can't organize my thoughts. I went to see a Broadway play and loved it, but just really hated myself for seeing it when there was so much work I had to do. When I would read my texts, I would try to read faster so I could get all of it done, and a lot of times, just out of nowhere I would get so upset and start crying over my book and myself and my life. I've decided I don't want to live like this anymore. I'm tired of not being able to breathe and get chest pains when I get stressed. Please help me.

FEELINGSUFFOCATEDANDCONFUSED

Dear Feelingsuffocatedandconfused,
You DON'T have to feel the way you do! Think back to your mode before you transferred and know that there is definitely a way to live without the anxiety that you have now. Think about what you can change: Drop a course? Switch to pass/fail grade? Take an incomplete? Right now, do whatever you can to relieve this seemingly unbearable anxiety. No matter what you do, you need to prioritize reducing your

anxiety. Take some action: talk with your resident advisor (RA), dean, and/or someone at the health service. From your letter, it sounds like seeing a counselor (psychologist or psychiatrist) would be a smart next step to addressing your concerns. **RES**

Alice

Blues and Depression

Found College, Lost Goals

Dear Alice,
I have a problem. I used to be a very academic person. I was always careful about my grades and I made A's. I used to be active in a lot of activities, such as basketball and skiing. I used to like hanging out with my friends a lot. I used to have fun. Ever since I have been at college (which has been quite a while), I have changed. Now I don't care about my grades nearly as much as I used to. I don't have any more goals in life. I don't enjoy doing anything. I don't enjoy doing things with my friends. Most people find me boring. And what's worse, I find myself boring. I kind of hate myself. What does that mean?

Dear Reader,
You are at a crossroads in your life and are reaching out because you want to change things. From what you say, there is a relationship between college and your loss of enjoyment, personal goals, and self-esteem. In our imperfect world, there are things over which we have control and things over which we have no control. With some help, people can learn to distinguish between the two, and then begin to make some changes.

Spend some time and energy exploring some of these issues, as well as your feelings, with a professional. Call your school's health service or counseling service for an appointment. Your family doctor also could make a referral. In addition, counseling services may be available at your local mental health department, or in certain community-based organizations.

You are in a kind of crisis. The Chinese symbol for "crisis" has two characters: one represents "danger" and the other represents "opportunity." Your "danger" is that the things that are familiar to you, includ-

ing your sense of purpose, the activities that previously gave you pleasure, and your friends or support network, are no longer satisfying to
you. It's possible that you're depressed. Of course, there are degrees of
depression, and although there are similarities, everyone's depression is
unique. The most vivid description of depression that Alice has seen
is in William Styron's book *Darkness Visible: A Memoir of Madness,*
where he describes powerful, immobilizing hopelessness. Yet as repre-
sented by the two Chinese characters, people who are depressed, or in a
crisis, can also have the "opportunity" to learn, challenge themselves,
and grow.

Depending upon the amount of time and energy you have, you
might think about volunteering your time. Often when students volunteer, they develop a sense of purpose and value since they are contributing to someone else's health or well-being. Tutoring adults in English as
a second language, reading to schoolkids, visiting the homebound
elderly, or working in a kitchen that provides food for the homeless are
some areas where volunteers are needed. It is amazing how much we
can get by giving.

Perhaps, as you work with your therapist, you will decide that school
is not for you, or that this school is not for you. Maybe you will discover
that your passion lies elsewhere. As you get the help you deserve, your
desires will become clearer to you. They may give you the impetus to
approach school with new vigor, since you will need the skills, or ticket
(your diploma), to go on to accomplish these new goals you have identified for yourself.

Your current assignment, should you choose to accept it, is to go
make that call, even if you feel that you can't. Act "as if" you are ready.
Alice is eager for you to find your niche, to strengthen your sense of
self-esteem, and to have your joy return to you. You have an ally in the
universe pulling for you, if that is any comfort, but the steps you take
need to be yours. **RES**

Alice

Friend Is Depressed

Dear Alice,
I am actually asking for a friend of mine since this situation is getting
worse, and I don't know how to help. The problem is that my friend is
very depressed, and has very, very low self-esteem. While sometimes
able to be cheerful and "happy," he claims to rarely feel that way and
mostly just hates himself. He has mentioned suicide, although I think
this is more an expression of the extreme self-hatred he feels than anything. I comfort him and often tell him how wonderful he is—what a
good person, good qualities, etc., but I suspect he does not believe me at

SOME SYMPTOMS OF DEPRESSION

- Feelings of sadness, hopelessness, and irritability that seem to have no cause
- Loss of interest or pleasure in usual activities, including sex
- Poor appetite and weight loss, or increased appetite and weight gain
- Sleep problems (i.e., insomnia, oversleeping)
- Feelings of worthlessness, guilt, and helplessness
- Restlessness
- Decreased energy, fatigue, and feeling slowed down (lethargy)
- Difficulty concentrating or making decisions
- Excessive crying
- Chronic physical aches and pains that don't respond to treatment
- Thoughts of death and suicide
- Alcohol or other drug abuse

all. This has been going on for a long time now, and I think it stems from a somewhat unhappy childhood and adolescence. I don't know how to help him and I don't know what to do. I feel like being strong for him is just not enough, and I can't quite convince him that counseling may do some good. It seems to me that recently, he has been feeling even worse about himself, to the point where nothing will comfort him. He cannot afford counseling, and he has no health insurance. Is there anything you can suggest for me to tell him or suggest to him? Any help will be greatly appreciated, because I just don't know how to help him. Thank you so much.

A Friend on the Line

Dear A Friend on the Line,

Everyone feels "blue" at certain times during his or her life. In fact, transitory feelings of sadness or discouragement are perfectly normal, especially during particularly difficult times. But, a person who can't "snap out of it," or get over these feelings within two weeks, may be suffering from the illness called depression. Depression comes in many kinds and degrees. Demoralization is usually part of depression, but it's not the whole story.

Gently and directly talk with your friend about your concerns while setting limits for yourself because you are not a professional therapist. Let him know that you think he needs and deserves someone's full attention to his feelings and concerns, and that there are many people out there trained and willing to give him just that. You or your friend can call the Samaritans hotline, or log on to their Web site. Both are twenty-four-hour support services.

It is normal for you, yourself, to become frustrated with your friend. You have already offered advice, help, and comfort; and it sounds like your efforts have mostly been to no avail. Remember that persistence can pay off. **RES**

Alice

FINDING AN AFFORDABLE COUNSELOR

1. Check with nearby universities to see if they have graduate programs in psychology or social work. Find out if they have a clinic affiliated with their school, or if they know of community clinics that may be appropriate for you to call. Some major teaching hospitals may also have mental health clinics where they see people at low cost.

2. Many major cities have training institutes for postgraduates in psychology and social work. These therapists-in-training see individuals and couples, usually at low cost. Students are supervised, which helps assure quality care. In addition, call the American Psychological Association or the National Association for Social Workers to see what or whom they may recommend.

3. Not-for-profit organizations can help you find a therapist who sees people on a sliding scale. Check the phone book, or ask someone at the above agencies.

4. Your health care provider can make a referral for you.

Once you select a counselor, call her/him to meet for "an initial assessment"—a one-session meeting where you can determine how you might feel about working with her/him. As a rule, it is useful to learn the background, education, training, and philosophy of the counselor you may choose to see. Plus, you need to feel trust, respect, and a sense that this is someone from whom you can learn. If you feel otherwise, Alice encourages you to find a more suitable professional.

Depressed—No Internship

Dear Alice:

I am a junior. Lately, I have been depressed because of my failure to find an internship for the summer. I feel that I will be at a disadvantage next year when I apply for jobs. I really want a good job when I graduate. I do not know if I am being paranoid over this internship thing that I keep hearing is so invaluable when you go look for jobs.

I feel that I must explain some of my life story to you so that you will better understand my situation. I come from a traditional Chinese family that values education very much. I am depressed because I fear that I will not find a good job when I graduate, and that everyone I know will ridicule me for spending so much money for my education and not being able to get a job. I am also depressed because my father will look down on me for spending all his money. My failure will bring shame to my father and delusion to myself. I am afraid I will not be able to face the humiliation that is forthcoming. Right now, I am spending a lot of time contemplating my future, and I see a bleak road. I have thought of ending everything right here and right now. I say to myself there has got to be a better life after this. So why go through more misery?

DEEPLY DEPRESSED

Dear Deeply Depressed,

It sounds like you're under enormous pressure. Many people get jobs without having an internship during college. Make an appointment with your school's career service to find a position that meets your needs as well as to talk with them about the pressure you feel.

You haven't even finished your university studies yet and you've decided that you're going to be unemployed forever. After speaking with someone at your school's career service, why not also talk with someone at your school's counseling service? This may be uncomfortable given your traditional background, but it may very well help you sort out some of the conflicts you're feeling between your family and cultural values. You may benefit from the experience and perspective of others to help bring honor to your family and to you.

Alice

Roommate Seriously Depressed—Is it Contagious?

Dear Alice,

This is more of a coping question. I am a first-year who applied for a single room over the summer and was denied. I figured that everything would be okay nevertheless. I tried to look at the situation as a character-builder. Well, that is not the case. My roommate is very depressed. I talked to the RA on my floor, but she didn't take any action, except to talk with her. Unfortunately, my roommate is so ashamed of what's happening that she denied the facts, and the RA believed her. No one except me has realized yet that she is sleeping most of the day and all of the night, and that it is indeed a real problem. I have expressed my concern to her and encouraged her to go to counseling services. She went a couple of times and then started canceling appointments left and right. I have worried about her, but I have no backup whatsoever, so there is really nothing I can do to help at this point. We get along relatively well otherwise.

Right now, the concern I have is that her depression is pulling me down, too. I literally have not been alone anywhere for more than two to three minutes in weeks. I wanted a single because it's a requirement that I spend some time by myself, and I'm going crazy these days. The lights are always out in the room, and I've noticed that I'm sleeping more than usual myself as the situation has progressed. Also, I am having to deal with some personal issues of my own this semester, and I simply don't have the energy to take care of someone else who desperately wishes that I would do so. Any ideas would be greatly appreciated.

WISH I WERE A LONER

Dear Wish I Were a Loner,
There are two levels to your problem: (1) getting help for your roommate, and (2) getting relief and support for yourself. As for your roommate, Alice has to wonder how she can maintain her grades in school if she's sleeping all the time. Have her professors and/or dean not noticed? You said that you spoke with the resident adviser (RA)—how about the residence hall director (RD)? Or one of the deans? This seems to call for more intervention than a brief talk. Is there anyone on campus who your roommate respects aside from you? If so, walk with her to that person's office. If not, go the RD or dean route and take some action that may not be to your roommate's liking, but certainly is in her best interest.

Now, on to you. It is above and beyond the call of duty to baby-sit your depressed roommate. You need to draw your own boundaries so that you don't get so emotionally involved that you become incapacitated, too. Remember—and, if necessary, reorder your priorities—you came here to be a student; your schoolwork comes first. If this is becoming too much for you, call your campus's peer support and referral service/hotline, call a depression hotline, or go to your school's health and counseling service. Find an outlet for your emotions in dealing with your roommate and a structure that will work so that you don't get so involved. Alice hopes that you get some alone time soon. **RES**

Alice

Seasonal Affective Disorder (SAD)?

Alice,

Every winter, especially when the days are short, I feel tired, depressed, and unproductive. Then the spring comes and I start feeling myself again. Is this just a normal seasonal cycle? I've heard about SAD, Seasonal Affective Disorder, but don't know much about it.

MELANCHOLY BABY

Dear Melancholy Baby,

Nobody knows how common Seasonal Affective Disorder (SAD) is, but researchers estimate that it may affect as many as 5 percent of all Americans, or about 14 million people. And many more experience some of these same symptoms, though more or less mildly or consistently—sometimes merely because they work in dark or windowless offices. It's amazing, but it's long been known that the short dark days of winter can cause people to experience a distinctive type of depression and malaise. SAD, in particular, has been defined as follows: fall and winter depressions for at least two years, alternating with non-depressed periods during spring and summer; at least one disabling depressive episode; no other major psychiatric disorder; and no other possible explanation for the mood change.

People with SAD tend to sleep more, be less productive at work, have less energy for recreational activities, including sex, and feel down in the dumps for no particular reason. They tend to eat more (especially sweets and starches) which, together with a low activity level, generally leads to winter weight gain. Generally, the SAD months are November through March, January and February being the worst. Of course, this reflects the population average. At the extremes, annual SAD relapses can begin as early as August and end in January, or they can begin as late as January and last through June. Do not rule SAD out as a possible explanation for the above symptoms if you experience them beginning in, say, October.

If you think you might have SAD, or a milder form of seasonal depression, here are some initial steps you can take, according to the National Institute of Mental Health (NIMH):

- Make your house, apartment, or room bright. Keep the curtains open. Use bright colors on walls, upholstery, and bedding.
- If you are in an office, ask if you can work near a window.
- Try to go away on vacation in the winter—somewhere sunny and warm!
- Exercise outdoors. If you exercise indoors, try to do so near a window.

Light therapy is another method of SAD treatment. It requires regulated exposure to intense light: a light box consisting of fluorescent bulbs and a diffusion screen. The box is placed on a desk or tabletop where users face the light for about fifteen minutes or more, usually while reading, writing, eating, etc. It is not necessary, or even recommended, to look directly into the light, but the eyes must be open for light therapy to be effective. The degree of light intensity, length of therapy sessions, and the time of day that this treatment is used have a major impact on the success of this treatment, according to preliminary research findings.

If you find that you are unable to remedy your winter depression on your own, you might consider consulting a psychologist or psychiatrist. S/he can coordinate your anti-SAD efforts, from stress management techniques to antidepressants to light therapy.

The Center for Environmental Therapeutics (CET) and the Society for Light Treatment and Biological Rhythms (SLTBR) can provide additional information about light therapy and SAD.   RES

Alice

Manic-Depression?

Dear Alice,
I'm worried that I might be manic-depressive, or bipolar-depressive, though I'm not quite sure what the exact medical definitions of those terms are. From time to time—sometimes over a couple of hours, sometimes over a couple of weeks, I can get very depressed, and everything in my life seems like it's going wrong—school, work, relationships, etc. These happen at night and during the winter more often than usual, but they happen fairly regularly all year round, for at least the last three or four years. Other times, even for weeks at a time, I'll feel fine; get really happy with certain things; not ecstatic, but happy. I also find that these depressive states can be brought on by certain things, like an argument with someone or just something that pissed me off. But then they get better, usually before I have a chance to see a counselor, and I feel silly for having felt that way at all; things seem much rosier at those times. I've seen counselors before, but never wanted to bring it up—I was hoping they'd guess at it on their own; I did describe all my feelings, just not that I thought I might be manic-depressive. I always thought that I was just being a hypochondriac. What do you think?

SIGNED, BIPOLAR?

Dear Bipolar?,
Affective bipolar disorder has two extremes: on the depressive end, you don't feel pleasure in anything, have no energy, are lethargic, cry for no reason, don't feel good about yourself, feel lonely, irritable, have difficulty concentrating, feel unloved, etc.; on the manic end, a mild form is expressed in increased motor activity, little sleep, rapid thoughts, confi-

dence, and noninhibition. Those who experience this disorder usually like the euphoria, happy feelings, and fast pace. However, the manic behavior usually evolves into a dangerous state—exhaustion from extreme hyperactivity, flight of ideas, poor judgment, and distraction are common symptoms of manic periods. While bipolar difficulties are one very specific form of difficulty, it's important for you to know that there are many other variations on that theme that are related to "mood swings" as well.

It seems as though you *are* having difficulties that need attention. A psychologist or psychiatrist can distinguish between mood swings and/or a condition that could be helped by medication. When you do find a professional you think will work for you, do yourself justice and tell her/him everything. Therapy will likely be more effective for you if your therapist doesn't have to guess what's on your mind. So, be as open and honest as you possibly can.

Alice

Falling from Faith?

Alice,
I come from a small town in Nevada. I came on the suggestion of one of the elders in the church, partly as a means of becoming a stronger voice of the church and partly to become more familiar with my own faith. Over the past couple of months, I have begun to question many things the church says and does, and many of the things I believe. I find myself doing things that I never would have dreamt of doing only six months ago. I'm not sure that this process is reversible or where it is headed. I am really confused and not sure what I want. I am afraid that relations with my family will become difficult if they find out how much I have been questioning my faith. I am really confused and don't know what I want. Are there any organizations on campus that I can talk to about this? Do you have any advice?

SIGNED FALLING FROM FAITH

Dear Falling from Faith,
As you move away from home and enter college, you are gaining independence and discovering how you want to live your life. Now that you are not as immersed in your family and church, you have the opportunity to take a step back and look at your faith from a unique, more objective view. With this new view, you may see things you never saw before. You may also find yourself in new situations, dealing with issues that you've not yet faced. It's okay to examine, explore, and question your faith and the teachings of your church. The seemingly "simple" teachings of your faith may not fit into your new, more complex world.

Most likely, the confusion you feel will be with you for a while. The answers you want may not come easily or quickly. Accept that you are going through a period of questioning, and that this does not have to mean you have "fallen" from your faith. You could speak with your pastor or your parents about some of the things you've thought about. You don't have to tell them about what you've been doing at school. Tell them about the questions and doubts you have—they may have gone through something similar when they were younger. Or if you are sure this won't go over well, you could speak with a pastor on your campus.

Think about the pros and cons of your religion. What works for you and what doesn't? Why? Do you think it will have relevance in your life in the future? Can you come to terms with the aspects of your church with which you do not agree? Sometimes, it is better to recognize and reconcile with what you do not believe in, agree with, or support, than to discard your religion lock, stock, and barrel. For example, some Catholics support the use of artificial birth control—they are vocal in their disagreement with the Church's teaching on birth control and are working toward change in this area, but they haven't completely left their religion.

Faith is an extremely personal matter. It can add to, and complement, your life; and it can help guide you through difficult times. You may decide to keep your faith, but not your religion. With time and patience, you'll decide what is best for you.

Alice

"Getting Over" an Abortion

Dear Alice,
I had an abortion almost a year ago and I have pretty much recovered emotionally from it, but every so often, I have "relapses." In these relapses, I become very upset for an hour or so and withdraw from the world. I in no way regret my decision—I did what I had to do—but it still upsets me. What advice do you have for me that will help me to get entirely over the abortion?

DOWNHEARTED BUT HOPEFUL

Dear Downhearted but Hopeful,
The psychological side effects of abortion are not clearly defined. Each woman's responses vary depending upon the unique factors in her life. These emotions may change in the context of your life, disappearing rapidly after the abortion or lingering for a while, becoming stronger at moments and dissipating at others. They may change with your hormonal cycle. Particular times of the year may provoke feelings, such as the abortion anniversary, the conception anniversary, or the expected

birth date of the fetus. Any feelings you might have are natural, and, sometimes, just getting them off your chest may help you better understand how you feel. Talking with a close friend or relative, writing in a journal, or going back and speaking with the counselor in the clinic where you had your abortion are some things you can do. Some clinics offer counseling and/or support groups for women who have had abortions. If the feelings are still unresolved, and the periods of withdrawing continue to linger, you may want to talk with a therapist. You can go for just one appointment to talk things through, or you can go for a while. The feelings may never go away completely, but with time, they can naturally lessen in intensity and frequency.

Alice

Leaving the Call Girl Business

Dear Alice,

Three years ago, in my freshman year, I ran out of tuition money in the middle of the spring semester. There was no one to help. Financial aid told me I was maxed out on my loans, and I had no place to go. I did not want to drop out. I had traveled two thousand miles to go to school here. I could not go home. As a last resort, I started working as a call girl and I have been working on the weekends doing that ever since. I really want to get out of the business—but if I do, I will have no way of paying for school. I have no family to speak of to look to for either financial or emotional support. Even with loans and aid, I still have to pay $15,000 to $17,000 a year. I know it sounds like it's easy to get out, but it's not. I'm afraid of so many things. I'm out here all by myself. I have no friends here at school. The pressure from school is enough; if I had to worry about money too, I'd never make it.

I am double majoring, so I will be here next year as well, and then law school comes next. I'm beginning to think that I will never get out of the business. I can't see the end of the tunnel. I'm depressed. I can't have a relationship. I can't date. Help me—just give me direction.

JEZEBEL

P.S.: I don't want to be perceived as some two-bit street hooker. I work for a respectable agency, and it is strictly in-call (not escort), and I am very safe and do not do any drugs or alcohol. I really am a nice person—I just got caught up in this work. I guess it came easy for me because of a very sexually and physically abusive childhood.

Dear Jezebel,

You have your direction. You want to get out of the call girl business, you want to pay for school, and you want to feel more in control.

Your first step is to see your dean. Your dean can act as a problem-solver. S/he can open doors for you at financial aid, career services, or academic advisement by generating ideas, and by suggesting the names of people who can work with you in your best interests. Discuss your willingness to work to pay for school, as well as your need for financial and academic strategy. Once you've developed a plan for paying for school, your next step is to tell your boss you quit. Quitting may seem less daunting once you have your plan in place.

In addition, make an appointment with your school's counseling service to talk about your feelings of hopelessness, helplessness, loss of control, current situation and goals, and childhood abuse. Support groups are available for many of these issues. The transition will be challenging, but with your strength, new direction, and desire to change, Alice is confident you'll be able to achieve your goals.

Alice

Bisexual to Straight = Black Hole

Dear Alice,

I have read all your advice to others and have learned a lot. However, I have a problem that I do not know how to handle. It started when I decided to turn myself around from being bisexual to straight (nobody knew what I was, except my best friend, who is also bisexual). I now have a big hole inside me that is being filled by the dark things of life (such as hatred). I had good qualities, such as a great personality, being open-minded, and I would rather go through life without it than turn back to the "bad" habits (please do not get me wrong, I will never judge gays for I have been close to being one). Please help me to fill the hole with life, to get back or improve on my qualities, and to gain the knowledge to approach and attract someone of the opposite sex. And one last thing, do you think it is wise to let my future girlfriend know what I used to be?

THANK YOU, BLACK HOLE

Dear Black Hole,

Having feelings toward men or having sex with men are not "bad habits." They are feelings, your feelings, which deserve to be felt, and, if you choose, expressed and enjoyed in either fantasy, reality, or both. Human sexuality is more complex than many of us realize, and Alice has a lot of respect for this fact.

Alice is also aching with compassion concerning your decision to turn away from your bisexual self to be exclusively heterosexual. If this decision were making you happy, Alice would support you fully. However, since you appear to be so unhappy, it seems that there is a negative impact from denying yourself your feelings.

Before you think about how to handle disclosing your feelings with a future girlfriend, make peace with yourself. There are counselors who help people manage their feelings concerning their sexual orientation, as well as any feelings of depression they may be experiencing. Seeing one, even for a short while, can help.   **RES**

Alice

Prozac Side Effects

Dear Alice,
What are the long-term effects of taking Prozac? I've been taking 20 mg/day for almost a year.

HAPPY BUT AT WHAT COST?

Dear Happy but at What Cost?,
In the last several years, Prozac has become the most widely prescribed antidepressant in the United States. Besides treating depression, Prozac is used to treat obsessive-compulsive and panic disorders. Prozac is the oldest drug of this kind, with twenty years of research behind it showing no known long-term side effects. Prozac has few side effects when compared to other antidepressant drugs. These side effects may include dry mouth, constipation, urinary retention, sedation, and weight gain.

Prozac is however associated with insomnia, restlessness, nausea, and tension headaches, which normally go away within one to two weeks from the time it was first taken. One possible side effect, which remains for the time Prozac is taken, is its effect on your sex life. It often reduces desire and can delay or interfere with orgasm, in both women and men. Fatigue and memory loss are other possible problems. These side effects subside when you stop taking the drug. In some people, the effectiveness of Prozac seems to diminish with time, and an increase in dosage is necessary. In these cases, talk with your prescribing doctor, who may alter your medication.

Stopping Prozac's use needs to be supervised by a physician. It is not advised to take this drug if you are pregnant or breast-feeding. So, talk with your doctor for an alternative.   **RES**

Alice

Communication Concerns

Shyness?

Dear Alice,

I'm a graduate student who is still trying to cope with shyness. I have extreme difficulty talking to people—even people I see and work with every day. I know making friends takes time and patience, but I seem to be at a loss as to how to develop acquaintances too. I've always been antisocial, but I never wanted to be. Who does, right? But I just don't know how not to be.

I'm studying a profession that requires a lot of personal communication; so, it's making me nervous and depressed whenever I can't overcome my introvertedness. But it's not my career that worries me the most. I sense my emotional well-being deteriorating every time I feel myself lost around others. Is there anything I can do to overcome shyness? I've been reading articles about the antidepressant drug Prozac and its success on passive people—should I consider it? Or are there places I can go for therapy? Thanks.

WANT TO BREAK OUT OF THE SHELL!

Dear Want to Break Out of the Shell!,

You are not alone in feeling shy—although it probably feels that way. Millions suffer from shyness, even though as a concept, it is difficult to define. It seems to be a form of social anxiety, where a person may experience a range of feelings from mild anxiety in the presence of others to a pronounced anxiety disorder. For shy people, it is anxiety-producing to have to interact with others at all, and, at the same time, the loneliness of limited relationships is profoundly painful.

Shyness relates to one's exaggerated sense of self. Shy individuals are often absorbed in themselves, and constantly focused on how they affect others and how others feel about them. They worry about themselves and become so absorbed in their own discomfort and inadequacies that they cannot focus on or feel toward others. This cycle further isolates shy people from the mainstream of warm, giving relationships.

Since shyness is now recognized as a real social problem, there is considerable research being conducted toward identifying ways to help shy people. Look around for a shyness clinic—incorporating methods of treatment ranging from building social and cognitive skills, to assertiveness training, techniques to reduce anxiety, and systematic desensitization. You may always be shy, but with professional help, you can learn concrete behaviors that will benefit your professional and personal life. Rather than using Prozac as a first step, another alternative is to use your school or neighborhood's counseling service.

Alice

Difficulty Maintaining Eye Contact

Dear Alice,
I've been experiencing in the past few months something that I understand, but am unable to deal with effectively. It is the difficulty to maintain eye contact while conversing with others. Usually my thinking drifts from paying attention to the conversation into concentrating on where should I look. It's really annoying and sometimes it makes me avoid people just because I'll be unable to have eye contact with them. What is also annoying is that I feel that the person I'm talking to is getting unnecessary tension because of my "looks" that I'm sure do not carry any bad feelings or insinuations. I've read an article suggesting that this could be part of a "shyness syndrome," however, I do not consider myself to be shy. Finally, this phenomenon fluctuates, but I haven't been able to relate this fluctuation to any specific factor (i.e., it does not change whether talking to men or women). Thanks for your valuable answer.

Yours, The Appreciative Inquirer

Dear Appreciative Inquirer,
Alice understands that you do not consider yourself to be shy, but one thing you might have in common with shy people is that you attach more meaning to your own words and actions (in this case, eye contact) than do those around you. It sounds like you get so overly concerned with your behavior and how it is interpreted that it distracts you from the conversation or issue at hand. As you explained, this then shifts your focus to the "unnecessary tension" that you feel is created by your eye contact, or lack of it. Perhaps your belief system (usually irrational beliefs) is causing your tension, annoyance, and/or other emotional issues. Some of your irrational beliefs might be that people won't

respond to you unless you have direct eye contact, or that you're not good at socializing, and never will be because you can't maintain eye contact.

Alice suggests that rather than focus on the other person, think of what you'd like to know about her/him, and ask. Smile. Compliment her/him. Pay attention to what s/he tells you. This changes your focus from you to her/him, and will help alleviate some of your stress and anxiety. A course in conversation or social skills, which might be offered at the YM/YWCA or at a local community college, might also help you. Two books come to mind that may be useful to you as well: Dale Carnegie's *The Leader in You: How to Stop Worrying and Start Living* and *How to Win Friends and Influence People*. Accept your inability to initiate or maintain eye contact, keep it from becoming worse, and actively try to change it for the better.

If none of these suggestions help, you may want to talk with a counselor, because this may be a symptom of something else. **RES**

Alice

Obsessive and Compulsive Behavior

Obsessive Face Picking

Dear Alice,

My girlfriend has a terrible obsession with picking her face. It is not that she has bad skin or acne, but, when she is in a certain state, she will stand in front of the mirror for hours and pick her face to shreds. It leaves her with horrible sores and open cuts covering her face. One day, she will be fine, and the next day, she will look like a war casualty. After she does this, she feels that she has to hide for days. Aside from these concentrated sessions in front of the mirror, she is constantly picking her face while she is studying or reading or talking on the phone. Often, the state of her picked face affects our plans—for example, she may not come with me to see my family even though we had planned to go together. When she is particularly self-conscious about it, she forbids me to look at her. She will cover her face with her hand or hair if I am even gazing anywhere near her. It is hard to communicate when I cannot see her face, and it affects our kissing and other intimacy.

We are very close and have been together for two years. We have talked about this many times and it does not seem like there has been any change. Mostly, I have been supportive by listening to her and comforting her. But, at times, I have been upset and have let her know. Some of her family members do not hesitate to be cruel to her when she "looks like shit." But she is well aware of her problem, but cannot seem to stop. She has had this obsession for over three years, and it is really making her miserable and is making me wonder if it will ever go away on its own.

We have talked about the possibility of some kind of therapy, but she does not feel that it could help. She seems to be terrified of having to see any kind of therapist. I feel that somewhere inside, she needs to stay feeling miserable even though she is clearly genuine when she is cursing the terrible life this habit makes for her.

I have every intention of staying with her, but I feel that her obsession and the self-consciousness and misery that come with it are keeping us from getting closer. How can I have more of a role in affecting some kind of change in this? I feel that there are things that I have no control over, but they affect me and the one I love deeply.

No Pock Marks

Dear No Pock Marks,
What you are describing is a basic compulsive disorder. Compulsions fall under the rubric of anxiety disorders. Remember that fear is a basic and useful human emotion—it provides motivation for self-protection and learning to cope with new or dangerous situations. Only when fear is out of proportion to real danger can it be considered a problem, and this seems to be what's happening to your girlfriend. Anxiety is another word for fear, referring especially to a feeling of fear that is not directed toward any definite threat. When anxiety is experienced almost daily, or is related to life situations that recur and cannot be avoided, it becomes an anxiety disorder. Compulsions, such as excessive face picking and hair pulling, are repetitive actions, difficult to resist actions, and often associated with obsessions (recurrent, unwanted thoughts or impulses).

Treatment for compulsions ranges from medications to psychological interventions that concentrate on a person's conscious or unconscious thoughts or overt behavior. Fill your girlfriend in on this when she says she doesn't think therapy will help—there are so many therapeutic models that she is sure to find one that will help her overcome her face picking. Strongly encourage your girlfriend to see a therapist. Finding a good therapist—someone you can trust and believe you can learn from—is important. You can offer to go with her to keep her company at her appointment, and/or to meet her afterward. Make her feel safe in the knowledge that you support her. It's commendable that you are willing to stick with her through this; it's also important that she get some help so that she can regain control over her own life.

Alice

Self-Mutilation

Dear Alice,
I am very concerned about a friend of mine who recently has taken to self-mutilation. She makes multiple scratches on her arm on a daily basis with a knife or scissors. I asked her why she does this, and she is not sure; she just feels like it. PLEASE, PLEASE tell me if my concern is warranted and what I should do.

What's Normal?

Dear What's Normal?,

Your concern is definitely warranted. Some psychological disturbance is causing your friend to do this.

Self-mutilation occurs mostly in young people, and it is three times more common in women than in men. Although your friend self-injures by scratching her skin with a sharp object, others intentionally cut or burn themselves, jab themselves with needles, rub glass into their skin, or pull out their head and body hairs (trichotillomania). People who self-mutilate can be drug and alcohol abusers, and often have a history of violence and/or sexual abuse in their past that they haven't told anyone about. They could also be suffering from an eating disorder.

Some teens say that they feel numb, unable to feel or experience anything. Self-mutilation is an attempt to feel something in their lives—a check-in that they're still alive. For others, self-mutilation is a way of temporarily coping with pain that seems to dissipate as they see blood flow from their self-inflicted wounds.

Your friend's self-mutilation is her way of asking for help. She needs to speak with someone not only to help heal her visible wounds, but her invisible wounds as well. Tell her of your concern, and see if she'd like you to accompany her to a counseling service. Your willingness to go with her may be the support she needs. **RES**

Alice

Child Abuse

Full of Hate about Childhood Sexual Abuse

Dear Alice,
I have a problem with hate. I hate my older brother. He molested me when I was young, and now I'm nineteen and I still have to live in the same house as him. My parents know what happened, but they just don't talk about it. I understand that it's hard to deal with. However, I never talk to my brother, and when I move out of my house, I don't plan on ever talking to him again. I don't think this is healthy, but there is nothing that I can do about my hate.

FULL OF HATE

Dear Full of Hate,
You owe it to yourself to find someone you can talk with and work with to help you understand and resolve your feelings, as well as protect yourself. Perhaps you need a plan to help you move out of the house. Clearly, you are angry, hurt, and, perhaps, fearful, and these powerful feelings are translating into hate. It is understandable, since your feelings are most likely the direct result of your molestation; however, these feelings can be destructive *to you*. That is why it is so important to get the help you need and deserve. Of course, you need to set your own goals; however, Alice's goal for you is to learn to minimize the hate you feel so that it doesn't interfere with living your life in a rich and satisfying way. Many women and men have been molested by family members, and more people than we realize have been able to find the assistance they need. This assistance has made a huge difference in their ability to live loving, productive, and satisfying lives. Reading Ellen Bass and Laura Davis's *The Courage to Heal: A Guide to Women Survivors of Child Sexual Abuse*, may also be helpful to you. RES

Alice

Possible Childhood Sexual Abuse

Dear Alice,

This may seem like a stupid question, but I'm eighteen years old, and I recently read a book in which there was a girl who had been molested by her father. One of the things that she did was poke holes in the female genitals of her dolls. Now I distinctly remember doing that with my dolls when I was a lot younger. Is this normal, or could there be "something" in my past? I don't remember anything, and don't want to try and make up something that was never there, but how can I be sure?

Dear Reader,

This is not a stupid question. Truthfully, there is no way of knowing for sure. The fact that you had the same doll play as a woman in a story who was molested by her father may be coincidence, or it may have meaning. There are questions that you can ask yourself to help you see if this situation, or a related one, may have occurred and had some impact. For example, if you had an unwanted childhood sexual experience, what might it mean to you? How is your current level of functioning? How is your life unfolding? For example, are you in school? Do you have a job? Do you have friends? How is your relationship with your mother? Father? Family? Have you had meaningful relationships or friendships with both girls and boys (when you were younger), or men and women (currently)? How happy are you in life? Do you have goals for yourself? Self-worth? A sense of humor?

Positive answers to these questions are some indicators of a well-balanced and productive life. If you have these, or elements of these, then it really may not matter whether or not you were molested. Alice is not minimizing the important issue of molestation. Alice is letting you know that being molested is an issue when it interferes with the quality of your life.

To learn more about childhood molestation and its impact, you can look at many books on the subject. As you read them, see if anything seems somehow familiar. If it does, or if your quality of life is somehow compromised, then it would be important—in fact, an investment in yourself—to get help.   RES

Alice

Grief and Loss

Friend's Mother Has Cancer

Dear Alice,

The mother of one of my best friends from high school was diagnosed with liver cancer a few months ago. She is quite ill and in a lot of pain. She's been in and out of the hospital lately and things don't look so good. My own father was diagnosed with prostate cancer a year and a half ago, but he is really doing quite well (with medication, treatment, etc.). My friend's mother will probably be dead within six months to a year, so I'm not going through an immediate crisis.

My question is: What things should (and shouldn't) I be saying to, and doing for, my friend? I try so hard to be there for her but I really don't know what she's going through. She is very matter of fact about the fact that her mom is going to die. But I'm sure there's something I could be doing, isn't there? I hate feeling like I'm actually making her feel worse! Could you give me some idea of what she might be going through right now and how I could help? Even if it's methods of taking her mind off it occasionally (if that's a good idea).

THANKS, JUST TRYING TO HELP

Dear Just Trying to Help,

You sound like you are a good friend. What you really need to do right now is take your cues from your friend. If she's at the point of it all being "matter of fact," you can't push her into feeling her emotions. What you can do is let her know that you're willing to talk with her about anything, at any time, so that when she's ready, or if she'd like to, she knows she can rely on you. In terms of taking her mind off her mother's illness—ask her. Would she like to go to the movies one night? Or visit a museum? Maybe go shopping? Or meet for coffee, etc.? It will all depend on how she's feeling at that moment, whether or not life seems frivolous and she'd rather not take her mind off her mother's illness, or whether she's at the point where she really would appreciate a break.

The other thing to think about is expressing your *own* feelings with your friend—telling her how you feel, with respect to your father's illness, her mother's illness, and your day-to-day life. Being real with *your* feelings will help nurture your friendship, the way it was in the past.

There is no one right or wrong thing to do when someone's going through a crisis like this. Continue being her friend—don't abandon her no matter how distant she seems to be getting. You don't have to force your companionship down her throat, either; just let her know you're around for whatever she needs—for talking, listening, or laughing; or for a good night out to forget. Knowing that she has a good friend can make all the difference.

Alice

Grieving a Parent's Death

Dear Alice,
My mother just died and I just started my freshman year of high school. If this was on paper, you would see my teardrops covering it. I feel like I have no one to talk to. I see the school grief counselor once every three or four weeks, but I was wondering if there is anything else that I might be able to do to lessen my feelings of depression and the feeling that I've been abandoned.

SIGNED, LONELY AND DEPRESSED

Dear Lonely and Depressed,
You are experiencing normal feelings of grief. Grieving for a loved one, especially a mother, takes time, energy, and caring. Life has changed irrevocably. Your family structure has changed. You may feel that you are growing up faster than you had ever anticipated. You may feel as if there is no one to take care of you, and it is difficult and painful to feel abandoned.

During this time, it is especially important that you seek out and talk with people you feel close to. Often, people are happy to help; however, they may not know how. They also may be waiting for you to seek them out. You could choose someone, and ask her/him to do something very specific: to listen to you, sit with you quietly, hug you, see a movie, or take a walk with you. Just sitting quietly or reading different books together can be comforting. Sometimes, exercise can make a difference. It is important to get your feelings out and take care of yourself more frequently than every three or four weeks. By the way, maybe you could talk with your school's grief counselor more often—at least for now.

Think about your family, friends, and neighbors. Who is already close to you? Who can you talk with? Who do you feel might understand? Your father? A sister or brother? An aunt or uncle? Cousins? A close family friend? A good friend's mother? A neighbor, or someone you feel close to or admire who lives nearby? Someone from synagogue, temple, or church could be understanding and helpful. Perhaps you can open up to a teacher.

There are also books you can read. Your school librarian or local bookstore will be able to steer you in the direction of books that are written for young adults about death. After all, death is a normal part of the life cycle, and something we all face sooner or later. There are also fiction books that deal with similar issues. Reading these kinds of books can help people experience, understand, and manage their feelings in a full and complete way.

You can also keep a grief and healing journal to compose your thoughts when you are happy, unhappy, or when you want to tell your mother something—just like you've done here. You can write her letters that express your feelings—this outlet will help you heal more quickly.

Finally, make an appointment with your pediatrician or family doctor, who can talk with you about your grieving process, assess your coping skills, and make a referral for counseling. You can also read Hope Edelman's *Motherless Daughters: The Legacy of Loss*. In addition, grief and loss groups are held at local community centers and churches. Alice will be thinking of you.　　**RES**

Alice

COPING WITH YOUR GRIEF

- Realize and recognize your loss.
- Take time for nature's slow, sure, stuttering process of healing.
- Give yourself doses of relaxation and routine busyness.
- Know that the powerful, overwhelming feelings will lessen with time.
- Be vulnerable, share your pain, and be humble enough to accept support.
- Surround yourself with life—plants, animals, and friends.
- Avoid rebound relationships, big decisions, and anything addictive.
- Recognize that forgiveness (of ourselves and others) is a vital part of the healing process.
- Know that holidays and anniversaries—sometimes for decades after a loss—can bring up the painful feelings that you thought you had successfully worked through.

(Adapted from The Centre for Living with Dying)

How Long Does Mourning Last?

Dear Alice,

I'm sorta new at this but I'll give it a shot anyway. My dad died of a massive heart attack just over a year ago. I went through a pretty rough mourning period but it didn't seem to last very long. My mom is still very much in mourning to this day. I guess my question is: How can you tell if you've mourned enough? And how can you tell if you're avoiding it?

They say the worst is over when the pain stops and the good memories start. But how do I know I didn't just skip to the good memories?

A DISTRESSED NITTANY LION

Dear Distressed Nittany Lion,

There is no formula for grief and mourning. Each person does it at his/her own pace. It's not like there's a designated period of mourning with an abrupt end. Good memories and sad moments will be with you throughout your life as you think of your dad. Sometimes, the anniversary of your dad's death, birthdays, holidays, a favorite song or food, and/or someone's smell will be reminders of your loss; and, at other times, these events will evoke warm, loving, tender, and even joyous feelings.

Obviously, your mourning is different from your mother's—your relationship with your dad was different and you're a different person from your mother. Your mom lost her partner, and her entire daily life has changed.

After a year, however, it may be your *mother* who needs some help with her mourning, not you. Perhaps the two of you could read some books about grief and loss—for you, it's to see how well you've coped to better understand your mother; and, for your mother, it's to help her move on with her life—a challenging step. Lynn Caine's *Being a Widow* is a good book, as is Harold S. Kushner's *When Bad Things Happen to Good People*. Perhaps your mother has a close friend you could talk with. Or a clergy person could visit her, assess where she is, and make a recommendation for her to see a grief counselor or participate in a loss group. Sometimes, these are even available at a neighborhood YM/YWCA.

Alice has great respect for your grief and ability to move on. Hopefully, your mother will get strength from you as well. **RES**

Alice

Go to Alice at www.goaskalice.columbia.edu for more Emotional Health Q & A's, including these:

- Always Late
- Attention Deficit Disorder
- Disappointed with Therapist?
- Divorce Pain
- Life Management
- Molested as a Child—Promiscuous as an Adult?
- Nightmares
- Number One Cause of Stress
- Prozac and Libido?
- Stress at the Start of School
- Stress Management
- Struggling with Low Self-Esteem
- Talking to Yourself
- Wedding Bell Butterflies
- What is Mental Illness?

FITNESS AND NUTRITION

No matter what your fitness level is, exercise can be a challenge. If you're a gung-ho athlete, your body probably sends you constant feedback on your workout, but how do you know if you're reading the messages correctly? Or maybe you suffer from exercise phobia: not everyone was a team captain in elementary school. There are plenty of P.E. survivors who still get queasy at the mention of "dodgeball." Athletic ability and overall body type can be highly individual traits. Not everyone has the stamina required to win Olympic gold, and not everyone is born with the proportions needed to look like a supermodel.

Even if you're a dietitian in training, selecting the best fuel for your body has never been more complicated than it is today. Newsstands shout out the latest cancer-causing or cancer-preventing foods; weight-loss books, some with conflicting strategies, duke it out on the bestseller lists; health food stores and vitamin shops boast the next new quick-fix diet pill, muscle-builder, or nutritional supplement trend; the corner grocery store now offers enough choices to make Betty Crocker's head spin. What do you want to eat today? What do you have time to eat? What *should* you eat?

In this chapter, Alice will offer realistic ways to enhance your physical fitness, which is key to emotional well-being, too. Fitness and nutrition also play a vital role in making your brain fire away with optimum precision, so if you think you need to cut out exercise so you'll have more time to study, think again. The same time-management concept applies to so-called "fast food." Alice will discuss reasonable weight-loss strategies, along with signposts to help you recognize when a weight-loss plan becomes an eating disorder.

Alice will also take the mystery (or misery) out of gym workouts, beginning with locker-room etiquette. She'll explore a range of exercise options—what the benefits are, how you can expect them to affect your body, and ways to prevent injury while you're in action.

Alice will also consider the source of all this energy: your diet. Recent food-labeling regulations have made it easier than ever to see how much fat, carbohydrate, sugar, protein, vitamins, and minerals are in that can of Coke or bag of green peas. But how do you apply all this data to the numbers you see when you hop on the scale, or to your menu and food choices? Alice will help you cope with the smorgasbord of completely unlabeled edibles available. How can you prevent gaining those "first-year fifteen" pounds as you forage through the school cafeteria or dining hall?

Even if you prefer home cooking to fast food, it helps to know a few basic ground rules about nutritious eating. Whether you crave tofu or tamales, applying the U.S. Department of Agriculture/U.S. Department of Health and Human Services Food Pyramid to your entire food philosophy will insure that you give your body the fuel it needs to think fast during exams, gyrate on the dance floor, and feel better about life in general.

Do you tend to choose sleep over breakfast, then gorge at noon because your stomach's empty—or is midnight your main mealtime? By becoming aware of your actual eating routines and hunger pangs you can find ways to custom-build not only a nutritious plan, but also a healthy, appealing, energizing, easy-to-follow, and tasty one suitable for you—one that you can work into your schedule and that will also see you through the most hectic, demanding weeks.

As Alice recommends, listen to your body's signals. Which foods seem to get you overly charged up or sleepy? Which workouts leave you achy and pooped, rather than rejuvenated? With Alice's help, and the advice of your health care provider, a nutritionist, and/or an exercise physiologist/trainer, you can start creating your personal "owner's manual" for your body. So why not begin today?

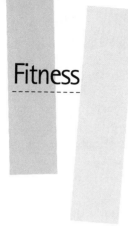

Fitness

Exercise Motivation ... for Stress Reduction

Dear Alice,

Does exercise really reduce stress? I recently took a new job that is very high stress, and I need a release. My friend says I should take up mountain biking, that it will reduce my stress (and keep me from gaining weight at this desk job).

Dear Reader,

A high-impact *yes* to your question! In fact, Alice can't think of many better pursuits for stress reduction than exercise, for several reasons. First, let's make sure we're on the same treadmill about our definition of "exercise." The National Heart, Lung, and Blood Institute (NHLBI) recommends increased and sustained cardiovascular elevation for fifteen to thirty minutes, three to four times a week. The American College of Sports Medicine recommends twenty to sixty minutes of aerobic exercise (same thing), three to five times a week, for optimal fitness, with two or three strength workouts per week.

Now, before you run in the other direction, let Alice dazzle you with some of the health-promoting and stress-controlling benefits of aerobic activity. Most notably, this type of exercise strengthens your heart and lungs. These two vital organs—especially the heart—bear the brunt of the body's physiological stress response, constantly being called upon to "fight or flee" from job, school, family, financial, relationship, and every other kind of stressor we confront daily.

You brought up another exercise plus: weight loss and maintenance— a healthy goal. For many of us, looking good also means feeling good. Exercise improves physical appearance, enhances self-esteem and self-confidence, and offers other mental health goodies. Regular exercisers report more energy and better ability to concentrate. Oh, and we can't forget about improved quality of sleep, reduced stress reactivity (not getting as stressed out about things as you usually do), and, yes, maybe even slowing the aging process!

Now, Alice knows that this exercise-as-stress-management thing is easier said than done, so here are some strategies that have helped many would-be health-seekers to start and stick with their exercise programs:

- Begin slowly. If you are not used to exercising, start out with ten to fifteen minutes twice a week and build up from there.
- Snag a workout partner—there's nothing like the motivation of another sweaty, panting humanoid to keep you going.
- If the gym will be "workout central" for you, take a quick lesson from a trainer on proper equipment use. Simple direction from experienced health club personnel can reduce gymphobia (and possibly injuries) while improving the quality of your workout. Your gym should offer this one-time service free of charge to newcomers. But this doesn't mean that you can't ask for guidance down the line, too.
- Let friends and family know that you are exercising for your health—let them cheer you on.
- Last, but not least, make your workout sessions regular and real. Schedule them in your calendar, just as you would record business appointments, classes, and social engagements. Exercise is just as important.

And, before Alice forgets, if you are thirty-five or older (some college students are), or have any heart trouble, blood pressure problems, or other medical conditions, you will want to get a medical clearance from your physician before you choose your exercise plan.

By the way, your exercise options are wide open, and you don't have to join a gym to partake. Walking briskly, running, biking (mountain if it sustains your heart rate), swimming, calisthenics, playing tennis or basketball, and cross-country skiing are just a few possibilities.

In addition to exercise, try to take breaks from your high-stress job. Walk around outside, take lunch, or sit in the bathroom for a few minutes if that's the only way to get away. Just a few breathers during a hectic day can go a long way toward stress relief.

Okay? Get moving!   RES

Alice

Gym Manners

Alice,

I'm looking for some helpful pointers you might have on the subject of health club etiquette (i.e., don't wear perfume because others will leave workout equipment wearing your perfume). I would appreciate anything you have to offer on the subject. Thank you!

Dear Reader,
Glad you asked this question. Given how much Alice goes on about the benefits of exercise, it's also important to make working out more enjoyable for everyone.

So, let's start in the locker room:

(1) Exercise control when loading and unloading your gym bag and locker. Remember, you are in a locker room, not at a picnic, so refrain from spreading your towels, clothes, shoes, and toiletries all over the benches and floor around you.

(2) In the name of prevention, pop on some extra deodorant before your workout begins. Even the freshest-smelling folks can have others reaching for their gas masks during a vigorous workout.

(3) Before hitting the gym floor, wash your hands, and, yes, wipe off some of that cologne/perfume.

Now, we're ready for our workout:

(4) Do you have an extra towel with you? Wipe off aerobic equipment, free weights, weight machines, and mats after you use them—even if you don't sweat.

(5) If you're a multi-set kinda gal or guy, glance around to see if someone else is waiting to use the machine or area you currently occupy. Offer to let them work in (alternate) with you, and if you're feeling particularly generous, ask if they'd like you to "spot" them.

(6) If you are waiting for equipment currently in use, DON'T HOVER! Give the dude or dudess some space to move and breathe—you'd probably appreciate that same courtesy.

(7) Put free weights back in their proper place after you use them. Who wants to clean up after others or search high and low for equipment scattered far and wide?

(8) Distracting other gymrats with loud grunts, sing-alongs with one's Walkman, and social hours with friends and neighbors should be avoided.

(9) Gyms and health clubs can be great places to meet that special someone. But if an object of your desire doesn't return your winks and smiles, take a hint: they are probably there to work out, not to hook up.

(10) Finally, timeliness to classes, racquetball games, and training sessions not only gives you more exercise time, but also reduces back-

ups and waiting time—helping the whole darn place run like a well-oiled stairclimber.

Here's to a good workout . . . and many more!

Alice

Body Fat and Exercise Intensity

Dear Alice,

I am a little confused as to which way is best to burn off the most fat. Will you burn more fat cells by keeping your heart rate at 125 for thirty minutes or at 160 for thirty minutes? I was under the impression the more calories you burn, the more fat you will lose. Is that true?

CONFUSED FAT BURNER

Dear Confused Fat Burner,

Whenever we exercise, we are burning *both* fat and carbohydrate. We also burn more energy (calories) at higher levels of intensity. So, when our heart rate is higher, we are using a higher percentage of carbohydrate; and, since we are using more energy overall, we will use more fat, too. Regarding your question, what this means is that we will be burning a larger number of fat calories at a higher intensity, given an equal amount of time. In others words, in thirty minutes, we will burn more fat calories at 160 beats per minute than at 125 (assuming you are able to keep your heart rate at 160 for 30 minutes).

Also consider energy balance. To burn fat and lower body fat, the calories we eat *cannot* exceed the calories we expend, because if they do, they will be stored as *fat*. If this is the case, you will be adding, not losing, fat.

To burn as much fat as possible in a set amount of time, work at a challenging intensity you can comfortably manage for the entire duration. An easy measure is being able to talk, but not sing, while exercising. For most people who exercise regularly, this is about 70 to 75 percent of maximum heart rate (MHR). As your fitness level improves, you may be able to increase exercise intensity and/or duration *and* your fat burning abilities.

Alice

CALCULATE YOUR APPROPRIATE EXERCISING HEART RATE

USE THE FOLLOWING FORMULA:

Maximum Heart Rate (MHR), calculated by subtracting your age from 220, is an accepted indicator of exercise intensity. For example, MHR for a twenty-year-old is: 220–20 = 200. His/her range should be 65 to 85 percent of MHR. For a twenty-year-old person, this is 130 (65 percent of 200) to 170 (85 percent) beats per minute.

Muscle Soreness and Weightlifting

Dear Alice,

I am an avid weightlifter. I want to know how to prevent muscle soreness, or flush out the lactic acid from my system. Thank you.

Dear Reader,

Muscle soreness can happen to any of us at any time. It usually always happens to people who are just beginning an exercise program, but can also happen to trained exercise enthusiasts who overload excessively, or who change from one activity to another, or work the same set of muscles in a new and different way. Are you providing ample time for your muscles to recover from lifting—generally forty-eight hours? This means that your strength workouts should be every second or third day. If you lift every day, don't work the same muscle groups, or work opposing groups and secondary muscles. For example, work chest and triceps one day, back and biceps the next.

Although at one time lactic acid was believed to be involved in muscle soreness, exercise physiologists no longer believe this is so. Lactic acid is long gone from the muscles before soreness occurs. Soreness may be caused by several factors, including small tears in the muscle fibers or connective tissue, muscle spasms, and perhaps overstretching.

To prevent soreness, don't overload and gradually increase the amount of weight or number of repetitions you do. Give yourself time between sets . . . one to three minutes, and include warm-up and cool-down stretching exercises in addition to your lifting.

Alice

CHOOSING THE RIGHT ATHLETIC SHOES FOR YOUR FEET

What you wear on your feet is important not only for your feet, but for the health of your back, legs, and hips.

It's a good idea to get properly fitted for athletic shoes. The shape of the shoe needs to correspond with the shape of your foot, without pressure or pain, or a feeling of binding. Improperly fitted or worn-out shoes can contribute to injury.

Each type of athletic shoe has a specialization. When purchasing shoes, take into consideration your prior experience with athletic shoes, your foot type (i.e., normal, rigid, or flat), your intended use (for instance, mostly for running or divided among a few sports activities), and the surface on which you will play or practice (for example, concrete or asphalt running needs shoes that provide maximum cushioning). Also solicit advice from friends and from a few specialty stores about what brands and styles are best. Spend what you need to in order to get the proper fit and help prevent or alleviate injuries.

All Torn Up over Stretching

Dear Alice,

In the past I have injured myself by overextending myself either when lifting weights, or playing sports. I feel this is due to not understanding how to stretch properly. Could you tell me the most effective ways to stretch before any physical activity?

THANKS!
ALL TORN UP

Dear All Torn Up,

Sports injuries occur for a variety of reasons. Contrary to popular belief, *inadequate* stretching is *not* the cause of all injuries. A true relationship between stretching and injury has never been conclusively proven because there are so many variables involved in causes of injury. Scientific proof involves controlling for all other factors that may contribute to, or cause, injuries—a difficult (if not impossible) task.

We have proof that stretching improves flexibility. A stretching program over a period of time—months, for example—can lead to an increase in range of motion. For those wishing to stretch *before* exercise, the conventional wisdom is that stretching should follow a mild warm-up, such as calisthenics, walking, very light jogging, or any activity that slowly raises heart rate. A warm-up will increase body temperature, which also warms the body's muscles and tendons. Warm muscles and tendons may extend more easily than cold ones, making them less likely to tear or pull easily. Stretching *after* exercise relaxes muscles and may prevent tightness. Conclusive evidence does not exist to prove that post-exercise stretching reduces soreness; however, some people feel better after stretching.

Three types of stretching exist: ballistic stretching, which involves bouncing motions and is generally less safe and effective than the other types; static stretching, which involves stretching a muscle to the point of resistance (when you feel the stretch, not the pain); and, proprioceptive neuromuscular facilitation, which uses alternate contractions and stretches of the muscle.

It's difficult for Alice to recommend specific stretches because she does not know what sports you play and what your weightlifting routine involves. Stretches should be specific to a person's sport or physical activity so that flexibility and range of motion are improved in the muscles and joints used in an exercise routine.

Key points on stretching:

- Stretching may or may not prevent injury.
- Over a period of time, regular stretching will improve flexibility.
- *Improper* stretching can cause injuries.
- Stretch after a warm-up. A higher core body temperature will increase muscle and tendon extensibility.
- Stretches should not cause pain, but should be felt (i.e., as some tension).

For more information on this subject, check out Bob Anderson's book *Stretching*. RES

Alice

Swimming: Good for Weight Loss?

Dear Alice,
I've read that swimming may be a great exercise, but not for weight loss. Is it true?

FAT SWIMMER

Dear Fat Swimmer,
Swimming is a wonderful form of exercise. It uses almost all the major muscle groups, and places a vigorous demand on your heart and lungs. It develops muscle strength and endurance, and improves posture and flexibility. The buoyancy factor makes it especially useful for people

who are overweight, pregnant, or have leg or lower back problems. It is a great sport for people of all ages and all proficiency levels. In order to lose weight, you might want to keep your swimming regime (speeding up your pace a little bit and increasing the length of your swimming sessions, if necessary), and supplement it with some good-paced, arm-swinging walks.

Research on swimming and weight loss, however, have produced inconsistent and contradictory results. Studies have found that swim-mers lost weight (and body fat), gained a few pounds, and had no weight changes at all. In most of the cases where swimmers gained weight, it was lean body mass (muscle) and not fat. If your primary rea-son for swimming is to lose weight, cut down on your calorie intake. In addition, speed up your strokes and increase your duration—sometimes, people don't swim fast enough or long enough. At a slow pace, twenty laps may burn only fifty calories—little more than simply staying afloat. On the other hand, a swimmer doing a brisk forward crawl will often burn as much as eleven calories per minute.

Alice

KUDOS FOR THE CRAWL STROKE

Best stroke . . . the forward crawl! You'll get all the benefits of swim-ming from the crawl. It fully uses your upper and lower body; it's nonimpact; it's aerobic (improving circulation and the health of your heart, lungs, and vascular system); and it's relaxing—swimming is a perfect stress reduction activity.

Optimal Nutrition

Food Pyramid—How Much Is a Serving?

Alice,

Is there a chart that lists how much of various foods constitute a "serving" under the new Food Pyramid guidelines?

Trying to Eat Healthy

Dear Trying to Eat Healthy,

The Food Pyramid, created by the U.S. Department of Agriculture/ U.S. Department of Health and Human Services, is a recommendation of types of foods to eat to maintain a healthy diet. The food pyramid shows that no one food is absolutely essential to good nutrition, and that no one food group provides all the essential nutrients adequately. *Variety*, *balance*, and *moderation* are the keys to the plan.

Alice has listed the Food Pyramid's suggested number of daily servings and serving size by group below:

- **Breads, Cereals, Rice, and Pasta**—6 to 11 servings a day. One serving equals 1 slice bread; 1/2 cup cooked rice, pasta, or cereal; 1 ounce cold cereal.
- **Vegetables**—3 to 5 servings a day. One serving equals 1/2 cup raw or cooked vegetables; 1 cup leafy raw vegetables.
- **Fruits**—2 to 4 servings a day. One serving equals 1 piece of fruit or a melon wedge; 3/4 cup juice; 1/2 cup canned fruit; 1/4 cup dried fruit.
- **Milk, Yogurt, and Cheese**—2 to 3 servings a day. One serving equals 1 cup milk or yogurt; 1.5 to 2 ounces cheese. Choose low-fat options from this group.
- **Meat, Poultry, Fish, Dry Beans, Eggs, and Nuts**—2 to 3 servings a

day. One serving equals 1.5 to 3 ounces cooked lean meat, poultry, or fish; 1 to 1.5 cup cooked beans; 2 eggs; 4 tablespoons peanut butter.
* **Fats, Oils, and Sugar**—use sparingly.
  This includes alcoholic beverages and high fat and/or sugar in foods, such as cheese, ice cream, and french fries.

Make an appointment with a registered dietitian or nutritionist for more info.

Alice

WHAT'S A SERVING?

* $^1/_2$ cup vegetables = 1 tennis ball
* 3 ounces cooked meat = 1 deck of cards, 1 quart jar lid, or palm of your hand
* 1 ounce piece of cheese = 1 ping-pong ball

Interested In Becoming a Vegetarian

Dear Alice,
I am a first-year graduate student planning to become a vegetarian for ethical reasons. Since I've eaten and cooked meat for many years, I'm not exactly sure what a good vegetarian diet includes. I don't want to do anything unhealthy, of course. Is there someone with whom I can arrange to talk about and plan a vegetarian diet? Thanks!

FUTURE VEGGIE

Dear Future Veggie,
Choose generously from different whole grains, fruits, and vegetables; moderately from the legume, nut, seed, and meat alternative group; and sparingly from the vegetable fats, oils, and sweets group. Since no one food contains every nutrient our body needs, it is important to include a wide variety of foods in our diets. Other important nutrients found in more abundant, and bioavailable (meaning in a form that is more readily absorbed by the body), amounts in animal (vs. plant) foods are Vitamin B_{12} and D, calcium, iron, and zinc, just to name a few. Make sure you get enough calories to meet your energy needs.

Vegetarians need to eat enough complete protein to repair and replace worn-out body cells and supply sufficient nutrients. Complete proteins are those that contain all of the amino acids our bodies require from food in order to synthesize human proteins. Animal foods have all of these; plant foods, however, do not. For example, to get complete protein on a vegetarian diet, eat several servings of grains each day along with one or two servings of legumes, nuts, or seeds. You can eat them during the same meal, or during different meals, within a day.

Many of these foods are high in fiber. To avoid possible gas and bloating, increase fiber intake gradually. Also make sure you drink lots of water to move it on through.

In planning a vegetarian diet, specific recommendations depend upon a number of variables. These include your body size, activity level, health status, food preferences, and lifestyle. Meet with a registered dietitian, through your student health service, who can help create a healthy (vegetarian) eating plan that meets your particular nutritional and physiological needs and wants.

Alice

NOT ALL VEGETARIANS ARE THE SAME

Lacto-vegetarians do not eat any animal flesh, but do eat dairy products.

Ovo-vegetarians do not eat flesh or milk products, but do eat eggs.

Lacto-ovo-vegetarians do not eat flesh meats, but do eat eggs and dairy.

Semi-vegetarians do not eat beef, veal, pork, or similar meats, but do eat eggs, dairy, fish, and maybe chicken.

Vegans do not eat animal products at all, but rely on plant-based foods.

Why Are Whole Grains Healthier?

Dear Alice,

Can you explain the difference in healthiness of breads and grains? Are all darker grains better for you than lighter counterparts? Why? If all bread is low in fat, how can it be bad for dieters, etc.? Thanks!

Dear Reader,

Whole grains are healthier because they contain higher amounts of vitamins, minerals, and fiber than refined grains, primarily because the bran of the kernel has not been removed. When the bran becomes part of the product, such as a 100 percent whole wheat bread or brown rice, it is healthier.

Even though most breads are low in fat, someone could still overeat, taking in more calories than s/he needs. So for the most part, you're right: it isn't the bread that is fattening, but the quantities you eat. And, of course, those in the know would never go on a diet that suggests cutting out bread and potatoes—two healthy, low-fat food choices. With all the "fat watching" going on, people have forgotten that overall caloric intake still counts. The extra calories, if not used up through activity, can, and probably will, be converted and stored as fat.

Alice

BUYERS BEWARE

A dark color is no guarantee that a product is made from whole grains. Some food companies have been known to add burnt sugar or molasses to their products to make them look darker and seem healthier. Check the label. For it to be labeled whole grain and for you to make sure you are eating nutrient-dense food (more nutrients and fewer calories), the first ingredient must be 100 percent whole wheat or other whole grain.

Which Are Better: Desserts High in Fat or in Sugar?

Alice,
I realize dessert products labeled fat free are high in sugar (which can be converted into fat). But which is the lesser of the two evils: high fat or high sugar content?

Sweet Tooth

Dear Sweet Tooth,
If you're making a choice between two desserts, both containing 300 calories, where one has most of its calories from fat, and the other from sugar, you would be better off going for the sugary one. Your body's first choice for fuel is sugar, making it more likely that the calories from that dessert would be usable. Excess calories from the sugar also have a slightly lower chance of winding up as stored fat. However, one thing to take into consideration is that rarely are two desserts equal in caloric content and ingredients used.

Your body needs some fat to work properly. Fat also helps us feel satisfied. So it will probably take many more desserts of the fat-free variety for you to feel satisfied and full than it would of a traditional rich dessert. It's not hard to go through a whole box of fat-free treats in one sitting and still feel like your sweet tooth isn't satisfied (particularly when you're thinking, "There's no fat here, so why not?"). You may even end up eating more empty calories than if you ate one or two of the regular chocolate chip variety.

If you're going to eat fat-free foods, go for those that are naturally fat-free—such as fruits or fruit salads, or products that are made without fat at all, rather than with a fat substitute. It's fine to eat regular desserts (medium- to high-fat) once in a while or in smaller portions, especially if the rest of your diet is healthy and balanced.

Alice

Five or Six Meals a Day vs. Three?

Alice,
What are the advantages of eating five or six smaller meals per day, as opposed to three meals per day? I've heard it helps to lose body fat. Also, are there advantages to eating more of your calories early in the day?

Grazer

Dear Grazer,
Most of the articles on "nutrition" in fashion magazines suggest the "right" times to eat and the number of meals to eat to prevent weight gain. It is common to hear that eating late at night causes excess fat to be produced. This is not true—it is OVEReating at any time, not simply eating at night, that causes someone to gain weight, particularly if they're not exercising or expending enough energy during the day. These articles also suggest that manipulating the number of meals per day could increase your metabolism and help you lose weight. Realistically, there is no magic number of times you should eat, nor are there specific types of foods you should eat or a particular time to eat to lose weight.

The bottom line is: eat when you're hungry and avoid overeating. The number of meals you have per day and when should depend upon your schedule and the total number of calories you want to take in. If you lead a typical student lifestyle, three meals a day may not work best for you. A classic example: let's say you grab a bagel at about 7 A.M. You may not have lunch until 2 P.M. and dinner until 8 P.M. This is a long time between meals. Chances are that you would be very hungry before both lunch and dinner. Being overly hungry, or "starving!" as some might say, could easily lead you to overeat at both meals. Many of us not only overeat when we are too hungry, but we also end up eating too fast, which is bad for our digestion.

Carrying healthy snacks during the day is the best way to avoid overeating at meals. Take a bag of carrot sticks, pieces of fruit, nuts and raisins, half a sandwich, or a granola bar with you during your next long day on campus. You'll find that when you don't deny yourself food when you're hungry, you'll be much more in control of eating the amounts that are right for you. Stay in touch with your body and your hunger signals. And remember, a healthy diet includes moderation, variety, and some tasty foods, too.

Alice

Eating Poorly, No Exercise

Dear Alice,

I feel I am getting fat, am eating poorly, and not getting enough exercise. I feel generally unhealthy. I have no time for exercise. Though I'm in physical education, the only class that fit into my schedule was yoga. This is a great form of meditation, but I'm unhappy with my body shape. I have to eat in the cafeterias, and I try to eat healthy, but I'm always hungry, especially late at night, and tend to go to inexpensive diners, where the food is not exactly first rate, and I order too much (such as tonight), and consequently feel ill, full, greasy, and like I'm going to sleep with it all in my system—yuck!

I'm a vegetarian. I don't eat very poorly, but I'm still getting flabby. I want to exercise but either have too much to do, forget about it, have no time, am too worried about stuff, etc., and I don't really know what or how to exercise to tone up and feel good. I know that if I exercise, I'll feel better about myself, eat healthier, etc. I refuse to diet. It's such a waste of time and I know it's worse for me than anything else. What can I do?

FLABBY

Dear Flabby,

Although the way you feel about your body is valid, sometimes it is helpful to remember that we are harder on ourselves than we need to be. You are smart for not wanting to "diet." Restricting food intake usually backfires because you end up eating more in the long run. This is especially true for college students with late-night study schedules. Take a more holistic approach to your health, eating habits, and lifestyle, and make realistic changes considering your current situation at school.

Even if it's true that you feel better when you're exercising and now you're not, you can still benefit from eating healthfully. Many school dining services now offer more healthy and low-fat choices and can alter portion sizes to meet your needs.

For a healthy vegetarian diet, choose a variety of grains—brown rice, breads (whole grain when possible), pasta, cereals, and bulgur. Beans and peas—kidney, pinto, lentils, chick peas—are a great way to balance grains and get a complete protein source. This category also includes tofu and tempeh, available at health food stores, and probably in some meal choices at your school's dining service. Fruits and veggies are also an important source of vitamins and minerals. If you eat dairy products, another good nutritious food source, eat them in moderation or try low-fat or nonfat varieties.

With whatever food choices you make, eat enough throughout the day so you are hungry, not starving, at night. Do you eat breakfast? If not, a bowl of cereal with fruit can help jump-start your day. If you are living in a residence hall, keep some food in your room, such as fresh fruit, yogurt, cereal, and milk. You can also bring food with you to classes. Throw a piece of fruit in your bag for later, or carry some trail mix and dried fruit, graham crackers, rice cakes, or breadsticks, which won't spoil in your backpack. And you may want to eat several smaller meals throughout the day rather than three larger ones, if that's the case.

Additionally, plan for and allow yourself a late-night study snack, roughly two hours before going to bed. With this plan, you'll know you are supposed to have a snack, so you'll be more likely to make a wise choice no matter where you are. Try a piece of fresh fruit, air-popped popcorn, nuts and raisins, or cut-up veggies. Avoid a highly sugared item, like a candy bar, because it can leave you feeling more hungry, and even tired. And watch how much you eat because calories can add up quickly.

As you know, eating healthy at a cafeteria is only part of the challenge. Making time for physical activity is important, too. If you feel you don't have time to formally integrate exercise into your schedule, walking and climbing stairs are a great way to get some exercise without taking up extra time. Walk an extra few blocks to mass transit or that special store, and climb the stairs instead of taking the elevator all the time. You can also check out the exercise classes offered at your school's fitness center. They are usually free for students, and can complement your yoga class. Maybe you and a friend can sign up together and motivate each other to go; or the two of you can agree to work out together twice a week. It sounds like you know what to do. The next step is to make a plan and follow through with it. Take it slowly, and don't get down on yourself if you miss a workout.

Alice

First-Year Fifteen—Can It Be Avoided?

Alice,
HELP! I'm terrified of the Freshman Fifteen! How do I not put on the weight during my first semester? I have to go now, the school dining service is about to close and I need a donut!

HOPELESSLY HUNGRY

Dear Hopelessly Hungry,

Often, students put on weight when they first come to college. For many, it's their first time away from home, making choices about what to eat, how much, and how often. And first-year students eat for more than hunger—they're coping with stress and loneliness.

You can, however, make good food choices. Watch out for fried foods, including donuts, or anything with a high fat content. Fit some exercise into your schedule, more than just walking for a sweet treat. Call your school's health service and make an appointment with, or get a referral for, a nutritionist to create an appropriate food plan for your individual needs.

During the first year at college, students often consume much more alcohol than in the past. Although there is no fat in alcohol (fat being the source of much weight gain), calories from alcohol are unusual in that they can't be stored or converted to energy for later use. Calories from alcohol are used first, and other calories that might be burned up are not, contributing to weight gain.

Gaining a few pounds may feel like the worst thing that can happen to you; however, it's important to learn how to take care of yourself, stay healthy, listen to your body, and *eat because you're hungry*—not because you don't want to study, you just got in a fight with your roommate, or you think you may have flunked a test! Think about what you can do to maintain control over your eating routine and have a great first year.

Alice

Eat varied and well-balanced meals at your school's eateries. Besides what you choose to eat, watch how much you eat as well, because calories count and can add up quickly.

Breakfast
- Low- or nonfat yogurt with fresh fruit or cold cereal
- Cold cereal (especially whole grain varieties) with skim milk
- Hot cereal (such as oatmeal)
- Waffles with fruit
- Whole grain toast

Lunch
- Sandwich—choose lean meats (such as fresh roasted turkey, roast beef, or ham), grilled or fresh veggies, and low- or nonfat cheeses; top with whole wheat, rye, or whole grain breads; spread on some mustard rather than mayo or other dressing (unless low- or nonfat is available)
- Salad—include beans, peas, grains, and sweet potatoes (if offered), as well as a variety of fresh veggies (including different types of lettuce, if available) and fruits; choose low-fat dressings and get them on the side
- Soup—choose broth-based rather than cream-based
- Pasta—stick with tomato-based rather than cream-based sauces, and try to get them on the side
- A meat entree—choose baked, broiled, steamed, stewed, or roasted skinless and de-fatted meats

Dinner
- Vary your entree selection—meat once a week, fish once or twice a week, pasta once or twice a week, chicken once or twice a week, and vegetarian once a week
- Steamed veggies
- Salad or soup (see above for hints)

Food Choices and Health

Calcium—How Much Is Enough?

Hi Alice,
I drink about three cups of coffee and one cup of milk a day. I was wondering if one cup of milk contains enough calcium to keep my bones strong. I am twenty-three years old.

Dear Reader,
One cup of milk a day is not enough to keep your bones strong and healthy. A cup of milk contains about 300 mg of calcium. Teenagers and twentysomethings need about 1200 mg of calcium each day. So, four cups of milk a day, or the equivalent, is more like it.

Why do we need so much calcium? The short and sweet answer is: to maintain strong, healthy bones and good general nutrition, as well as to prevent osteoporosis. Calcium is an essential component in the lifelong process of laying down new bone. Later in life, calcium helps our bodies maintain bone mass. Before you reach thirty, more bone is made than lost; after thirty, this trend reverses.

Women need to be especially vigilant about calcium. On average, women make less bone and lose it at a greater rate than men. A woman's calcium stores are drawn on during pregnancy and lactation. Adding to this, women generally live longer than men, giving their bones more time to become brittle, less dense, and prone to fracture (i.e., to develop osteoporosis).

The two best things you can do now to prevent future osteoporosis are: (1) include enough calcium in your diet; and (2) exercise often, and include weight-bearing activities in your exercise routine. A family history of osteoporosis and your body's ability to absorb calcium are other risk factors for osteoporosis. You have no control over these risk factors, but you can control how much calcium is in your diet and how much you exercise.

If drinking three to four cups of milk a day does not appeal to you, you can get calcium from a range of other dairy and nondairy sources. An eight-ounce cup of milk or yogurt, or half an ounce of cheese, each contain roughly 300 mg of calcium. Some nondairy sources of calcium include:

- 1 orange; 1 cup sweet potatoes, green beans, lentils, chick peas, navy beans, or pinto beans; 3 oz. shrimp, crab meat, or clams **(less than 100 mg)**
- 1 cup cottage cheese, cooked dandelion greens, or kale; 3 oz. canned salmon with bones; 1 (2.5″) cube tofu **(100–199 mg)**
- 1 cup cooked broccoli, turnip greens, or oysters **(200–299 mg)**
- 1 cup cooked collard greens; 3 oz. canned sardines with bones **(300+ mg)**

Calcium in foods, versus supplements, is a better way to get calcium into your body. Lactose-intolerant folks, however, may need to take calcium supplements. A few other pointers on how to maximize the calcium in your diet: calcium is absorbed better in the presence of vitamins C and D and lactose (a sugar found in milk and dairy products); excess dietary fat, and certain acids found in whole grains and leafy veggies, actually hinder calcium absorption. For instance, only a small percentage of the calcium in foods like spinach, kale, lentils and other beans, and whole grains will be absorbed by your body because the calcium is locked into the food in a way that makes it hard to absorb. Alice doesn't recommend cutting them out of your diet—they are excellent sources of other vitamins, minerals, and fiber—just don't eat them along with other calcium-rich foods, because they can prevent calcium absorption from calcium-rich foods as well.

Two final thoughts on osteoporosis and calcium: salt and phosphorous. Regardless of how much calcium you get from your diet, researchers have found that adding a lot of salt to your food or eating foods high in sodium can lead to a loss of calcium. And most sodas are high in phosphorous, which has the potential to replace calcium in bones. If you drink lots of soda (and not enough milk), or if your diet has too much salt in it, consider ways you can cut back on sodas and salty foods. Your bones will thank you.

Alice

Low Blood Sugar

Dear Alice,

Is there any chance that because I get low blood sugar occasionally, I may become a diabetic someday? And what can you keep with you to take when your levels do drop, and you can't get to any food or juice?

THANKS, SHAKY SHARON

Dear Shaky Sharon,

Hypoglycemia, or low blood sugar, often happens because we go too long without eating. Some symptoms of hypoglycemia may include dizziness, mental confusion, anxiety, shakiness, and weakness. To determine the cause of your hypoglycemia, see your health care provider. S/he may better discuss your individual risk factors for diabetes. S/he may also refer you to a nutritionist.

In a Hypoglycemic Diet Plan, you would eat every two to three hours. Mixed meals and snacks, including carbohydrate, protein, and a little fat, are recommended. An easy snack to keep with you that fits this bill is peanut butter crackers, prepackaged or ones you make yourself. Other appropriate snacks include low-fat yogurt and low-fat trail mix. Avoid eating a concentrated sweet, such as a candy bar or a sugary drink like soda, because this causes our blood sugar to drop even further. Drink plenty of water because many symptoms of between meal "lows" are caused by dehydration.

As for your question on diabetes, sometimes hypoglycemia is a precursor for people who eventually will develop diabetes; however, many people who are hypoglycemic never develop diabetes.

Alice

Sources of Iron

Dear Alice,

What are the major sources of iron (especially vegetables, if any)? Thank you.

POPEYE

Dear Popeye,

Iron is an essential mineral our body needs to function well. If you don't take in enough iron, you can become iron-deficient. Women are at particular risk for this because of blood loss during their periods. Iron deficiency is most common when iron needs are greatest in your life cycle—during infancy, preschool years, and puberty, and during childbearing years for women. Pregnancy and disease also increase iron needs.

Our ability to absorb iron from foods varies, depending on its form in the food, the body's need for it, and a variety of other factors. Iron from animal proteins is better absorbed by the body than iron from plant foods.

Animal sources of iron include liver, kidneys, red meat, poultry, fish (especially oysters and clams), and eggs. Plant sources of iron include peas, beans, nuts, dried fruits, leafy green vegetables (especially spinach), enriched pastas and breads, and fortified cereals.

To optimize the amount of iron you get from plant foods, eat them with vitamin C at the same meal. Keep your dietary fiber intake to under 35 mg a day, and reduce tea consumption, especially at mealtime, to increase iron absorption.

For people who may be anemic, get a physical examination from a health care provider to determine the cause. Iron supplements are often all that's needed for a cure.

Alice

FOLIC ACID RESOURCES

Besides iron, pregnant women are also at particular risk for folic acid deficiency. Folic acid, also known as folate, is an important B vitamin that significantly lowers the risk of serious birth defects of the brain and spinal cord. **Women of childbearing age (approximately fifteen to forty-five years) are recommended to include 400 micrograms of folic acid in their diets, particularly important before and during pregnancy to prevent these birth defects.** Rich dietary sources of folate, such as dark green, leafy vegetables; whole wheat bread; lightly cooked beans and peas; nuts and seeds; sprouts; oranges and grapefruits; liver and other organ meats; poultry; and, fortified breakfast cereals, are recommended. Pregnant women can supplement with a prenatal vitamin to be sure to get a sufficient amount. Check with your obstetrician or midwife to be sure.

Folic acid and vitamins B_6 and B_{12} could also help lower and control homocysteine (an amino acid) levels in the blood, recently gaining recognition as a risk factor for heart disease.

Cancer and Diet

Dear Alice,

I guess I am kind of obsessed about cancer because my grandfather died of stomach cancer two years ago and I was with him for several months before he died. What are the major causes of cancer? How can we avoid them? If we eat some cancer-causing substance, are we more likely to get stomach or intestinal cancer because that's where the food passes through, or are we equally likely to get other cancers? I mean, do a person's digestive organs have a particularly high susceptibility to cancer compared to other parts of the body because they are exposed to the food, which is where almost all the carcinogens come from?

WORRIES ABOUT CANCER AND DIET

Dear Worries about Cancer and Diet,

Cancer is not one disease, but is actually a group of diseases caused by the unrestrained growth of cells in one of the body's organs or tissues. Who gets cancer, when they get it, and which organs it affects are questions still difficult to answer. One factor that increases a person's risk of contracting cancer is genetic makeup. Environmental triggers (i.e., food choices, sunlight, alcohol, viruses, tar in tobacco smoke, pollutants in the air) also play a part in cancerous formations.

Two out of every five Americans will be diagnosed with cancer at some point in their lives. Cancer risk increases with age, with half of all cancer diagnoses being made in people over sixty-seven. Four cancer sites—lung, colon, breast, and prostate—account for more than half of cancer deaths in the United States, with lung cancer alone accounting for 25 percent.

Worldwide, stomach cancer is second only to lung cancer in number of deaths. People at increased risk for stomach cancer include smokers, men, African Americans, people with a family history of stomach cancer, those who eat few fruits and vegetables, and those whose stomachs are infected with *Helicobacter pylori* bacteria, which usually causes peptic ulcer disease. High intakes of pickled, cured, or smoked foods may also increase risk, but it has not been proven in humans to date.

One third of colon/rectal cancers are found when the cancer is still localized, which means the patient's chances of five-year survival are 90 percent. Those who are at highest risk are people whose diets are high in fat, heavy in red meats, and low in fruits and vegetables. Also, anyone with a family history of colon or rectal cancer, polyps, or inflammatory bowel disease is at risk. Research on vitamin supplements, including beta carotene, vitamin E, and vitamin C, did not demonstrate a decrease in risk of potentially precancerous polyps. **To reduce your risk, you simply need to eat a variety of whole grains, fruits, and vegetables regularly.**

Alice

CANCER PREVENTION STRATEGIES

RECOMMENDATIONS THAT MAY HELP PREVENT CANCER:

- Don't smoke or use smokeless tobacco.
- Limit alcoholic beverages to less than one a day for women, or two a day for men.
- Eat five or more servings of fruits and vegetables every day.
- Cut back on fats, especially saturated fats and red meats.
- Eat whole grains and legumes (beans and peas) whenever possible.
- Include at least thirty minutes of moderate activity in your daily routine.
- Limit cured or smoked foods, like bacon, ham, smoked salmon, and hot dogs. If you choose to eat these foods, have them with a glass of orange juice or another rich source of vitamin C.
- Limit sodium to 2400 mg a day or less.
- Maintain a healthy weight.
- Manage your stress.

(Adapted from the American Cancer Society's Guidelines on Diet, Nutrition, and Cancer Prevention)

Eating Disorders

Friend Has a Weight Complex

Dear Alice,

My best friend has a weight complex. She constantly asks me if I think she's fat and even asks my boyfriend what he thinks of her weight. She isn't overweight and I just wish she would stop worrying about it all the time. Is there anything I can do to convince her she isn't fat?

SINCERELY, WANT TO HELP

Dear Want to Help,

Your best friend's behavior is not normal. Her obsession with her weight is her attempt to cope with life and its problems. It is possible that this is her way of letting others know that she feels unaccepted and unacceptable for who she is, and that she needs some sense of control in her life. She may even have an eating disorder. When we care about someone who only seems to care about her/his weight, our natural tendency is to see the behavior (saying s/he's fat) as the problem and try to help her/him solve that problem.

It is important for you not to take responsibility for her behavior and whether or not she will change. You can express your concern to her as a friend. You can let her know *not only* that she's not fat, but that you're concerned because she seems so preoccupied with her weight and body image. Tell her that she has a right to a life without worrying so much about how she looks and how much she weighs, that the amount of time she spends worrying about her weight could be used in many constructive ways. If she needs to talk with a counselor or therapist, that may be another option for you to mention.

Alice

No Period and Underweight—Anorexia?

Alice,

What should my normal body weight be? I am 4 feet 11 inches tall and I weigh 75 pounds presently. I think that I am underweight because I haven't had my period in almost a year. If I were of normal weight, what percentage of my calories should come from fat?

WEIGHT CONSCIOUS

Dear Weight Conscious,

The fact that your menstrual cycle has stopped is a telltale sign that your weight has gone too low. Alice wonders if you've experienced any of the signs of anorexia over the last year? Few people experience all of them, but if you have a cluster of anorexia's warning signs, it's important to see a health care provider.

Anorexia is a disease with no simple causes or solutions. It may begin as an attempt to lose weight, and, over time, may become a life-threatening disease.

SIGNS OF ANOREXIA

- Your sense of taste is different from before, changing your appetite.
- You've been constipated.
- You feel bloated, which makes you get full earlier in a meal.
- You're expending less energy than you used to.
- Your hair is falling out.
- You have mood swings and difficulty concentrating.
- You are preoccupied with food.
- You're growing new downy (soft) hairs on parts of your body.
- You've lost muscle mass.
- You fear becoming fat.
- You constantly think about food.
- Your skin is rough, dry, scaly, and cold.
- You get dizzy, and may have blacked out.
- You have become preoccupied with cooking and preparing food, often fixing meals for others without actually eating.
- You and/or other people have become concerned that you are too thin.

Talk with a nurse practitioner or physician who specializes in eating issues about your loss of menstrual cycle and concern about weight; or with a nutritionist about your weight issues and percentage of calories from fat; or with a counselor about your feelings associated with your weight loss and cessation of period. Please talk with someone and take care of your health before serious long-term effects (i.e., fatigue, electrolyte imbalance, low pulse rate, kidney failure, heart arrhythmias, and heart failure) on your body set in.

Alice

Dangers of Bulimia

Dear Alice,
I am bulimic and I would like to know exactly what harmful things this does to your body. Can you die from it? Can you actually be cured?

Dear Reader,
Bulimics eat enormous amounts of food rapidly and in secret, without much appreciation for its taste, texture, or quality. Following these binges, they feel guilty, ashamed, and out of control, and try to get rid of the food through vomiting; overexercising; abusing laxatives, diuretics, or enemas; or not eating for several days. These practices may take place daily or weekly and go on for years.

Is it harmful? YES. Even though people may be bulimic for years, there are dangers associated with bulimia. The most notable is cardiac arrest or heart attack, which is caused by an electrolyte imbalance of the mineral potassium, a consequence of vomiting or the use of certain diuretics. People who vomit frequently will also lose the enamel from their teeth, which subsequently become sensitive to heat, cold, and acids. Their teeth may eventually decay and fall out. Those who abuse laxatives will find that their own natural body processes cannot function properly when they stop using laxatives, and constipation will result. Stomach ulcers and irritation of the esophagus result from vomiting. More scary, an esophageal rupture could happen the first time, or the two hundredth time, you vomit, and this could kill you. Psychologically, there is depression.

People *can* be cured of bulimia, although the road to recovery is gradual and difficult. The sooner you talk with a mental health professional who specializes in eating disorders, the better. Treatment methods vary, including learning to like and accept yourself, establishing regular eating patterns (so you don't get so hungry that it triggers a binge), alternative coping strategies for stressful or lonely times, and, in some instances, taking antidepressant medication. The good news is that you can change this self-destructive pattern, with commitment and help.

Alice

Laxative Abuse—Any Side Effects?

Dear Alice,

A friend of mine takes laxatives to keep her weight under control. The directions on the box say that you should only take two a day for no more than a week. She has been taking two to six a day for two months now. I was wondering what possible physical side effects might result from this kind of activity.

THANK YOU, A CONCERNED FRIEND

Dear Concerned Friend,

When laxatives are taken regularly for a prolonged period of time, one or more adverse effects, some of which are serious and/or dangerous, can occur. The person may experience abdominal cramping and pain, or diarrhea and vomiting (which can cause dehydration, potassium deficiency, and, in some of the worst cases, heart failure, among other things). Excessive laxative use can impair absorption of vitamin D and calcium, which can cause osteomalacia (bone disease characterized by softening of the bones), and can also impair absorption of fat, which can cause greasy diarrhea and weight loss. Laxative abuse can also lead to gastrointestinal (GI) tract damage, including weakening of intestinal musculature, loss of GI protein, and cathartic colon, which is a poorly functioning colon that develops after years of laxative abuse. This can lead to an inability to have a bowel movement when not taking laxatives. Permanent bowel damage usually results if not treated in time. Liver disease is also possible.

Some of these side effects may indicate other serious health problems as well, such as an eating disorder, which would require a visit to a health care provider. When, and if, the time is right, you may want to share this information with your friend.

Alice

ABOUT LAXATIVES

Two types of over-the-counter laxatives that are commonly used include stimulant laxatives, which irritate the colon to induce bowel movements using bisacodyl or senna, among other things; and, bulk-forming laxatives, such as those containing psyllium or wheat bran, which add bulk to the bowel. Use of stimulant laxatives, in particular, is not recommended for more than one week, or at a dosage greater than recommended on the package.

Men with Eating Disorders?

Dear Alice:

Is it possible for a male to have an eating disorder? I mean, I know it's possible, but I've never heard of any documented cases. All I've seen are connected to females.

WONDERING

Dear Wondering,

Unfortunately, yes, men do have eating disorders. However, eating disorders in men are masked, less common, and not talked about.

Both men and women can fit the diagnostic criteria for anorexia and bulimia. In addition to the general factors thought to contribute to the development of eating disorders, men appear to diet for different reasons than women: the presence of actual pre-illness obesity; weight loss related to greater sports attainment or the fear of gaining weight because of a sports injury; and weight loss in order to avoid weight-related medical illnesses found in other family members.

Other reasons men with eating disorders diet: a desire to improve athletic performance; a history of being teased, criticized, or picked on for being overweight; wanting to change a specific body part (to reduce "flab" and promote muscle definition); to make required weight for a specific sport (i.e., wrestling or crew); to be more attractive to a potential partner; to look less like one's father; vegetarianism; and, to develop the appearance of a model in magazines.

For further reading, try Arnold E. Andersen's *Males with Eating Disorders*. **RES**

Alice

How to Help a Roommate with an Eating Disorder

Dear Alice,

I am writing in hopes that your answer to this question will help other readers. A few years ago, when I was in college, I discovered that my college roommate was bulimic. My boyfriend and I found evidence in the mornings that she had been vomiting on a daily basis; she also developed weird eating habits (at 6 A.M., she would wake up and buy two pints of ice cream and eat it all, and then not eat for the rest of the day). We didn't know how to address the problem, and were afraid of hurting her. When we called the Health Service, they took the "my best friend is bulimic" line to suggest that I was bulimic instead! I didn't want to become the food "hall monitor"—are you eating? What did you eat today? etc.—but we tried to include her in healthy meals. Eventually, some other stress factors in her life calmed down and her binge/purge behavior seemed to subside. However, I've always regretted that I couldn't attack this situation head-on. Do you have any advice for people that might be in a similar situation?

SIGNED, FOR FUTURE REFERENCE

Dear For Future Reference,
Alice is certain there are many people who've noticed strange eating patterns among certain friends or roommates that they later learned were signs of an eating disorder.

If this were an emergency situation, for example, if the person is blacking out, has lost significant amounts of weight, is sleeping all day, or has suicidal thoughts or attempts, do not try to deal with the situation politely or gently. Tell your resident adviser (RA) or residence hall director (RD) to get the assistance and support you need.

If this were not an emergency situation, a good friend or roommate is the best person to make the first approach, rather than an authority figure. You can leave pamphlets on eating disorders around the room, attend a seminar on eating disorders, body image, or healthy eating and invite your roommate to come with you, or talk with her yourself. What action you take is a judgment call depending on the particulars of the situation, and your personal style.

To talk directly with your roommate, pick a time to talk when you are feeling calm and both of you have plenty of time.

Cover the following three things in your conversation:

- *Why you suspect a problem:* Be specific about what you see regarding her eating, purging, exercising, or starving behaviors. Your observations, rather than evidence of wrongdoing, can be discussed gently as a basis for your concern.
- *How you feel:* Use "I" statements to express your feelings about what's happening to your roommate. "I'm upset because I've noticed that you don't eat meals with us anymore"; or, "I'm tired of hearing you complain about how fat you are all the time. I think there's something wrong."
- *What your goals are:* Make sure that your goals for the conversation are attainable. Your goal is NOT to stop your roommate from bingeing, purging, or starving. You would probably end up in an ineffective control battle. A realistic goal is simply opening the door to talk, and, either now or in the future, helping her get the help she needs.

You can stop the conversation before it gets out of control. This may be a difficult conversation, and you can keep it from becoming a fight. If you get upset, ask if you can continue the conversation at another time. Try to anticipate her potential reactions. Common responses include relief; admission of a problem; or defense and denial, including "how dare you!," "mind your own business," "you're not so great yourself," and "you're wrong." No matter what the reaction, know that you have tried to get your roommate to talk, and let her know that you care. Keep your cool. For your own backup, call a nutritionist, counselor, or therapist.

Alice

Go to Alice at www.goaskalice.columbia.edu for more Fitness and Nutrition Q & A's, including these:

- Abdominal Fat
- Antioxidants
- Best Thing to Drink Before a Workout? After?
- Breast Cancer Prevention and Nutrition
- Build Muscle Mass?
- Chocolate—Good or Bad?
- Cholesterol-lowering Methods
- Do I Have an Eating Disorder?
- Fast All Day and Feast at Night—Healthy?
- Gas, Bloating, Fiber?
- Greasy Foods and Acne? Gall Bladder?
- How to Gain Weight
- I Want a Flat Stomach!
- Ideal Caloric Intake?
- Jogging Injury
- Milk—Bad or Good?
- No Time to Cook?
- Nonmeat Proteins
- Serotonin and Foods?
- Vitamins for Health?

ALCOHOL, NICOTINE, AND OTHER DRUGS

No matter which side of America's drug war you're on, mind-altering substances probably make up a part of your world. Alcohol and other drugs have been a part of the human experience throughout the ages. From the sacred wine of antiquity to opium dens in vogue during the nineteenth century, the urge to expand consciousness has never been permanently snuffed out (so to speak) by any group of legislators.

The average American consumes about three gallons of alcohol a year, while the average college student downs a whopping thirty gallons a year—the main reason that this chapter focuses on what seems to be a social fact of life.

Statistics don't seem to deter drug use either. Every year, approximately 100,000 Americans die from alcohol-related causes, and about 400,000 die from tobacco-related causes. Despite the threats—lung cancer, emphysema, stroke, heart attack, central nervous system and liver damage, not to mention the possibility of personal harm while your alertness and judgment are impaired—you can see alcohol and tobacco users everywhere you turn.

With other drugs, even more contradictory scenes abound. Public health campaigns portray the horrors of heroin addiction, but at parties, you may encounter plenty of trustworthy-looking peers lighting up to "cook" a hit. Dance clubs are perhaps the "best" places to find carefree, sexy crowds doing drugs, defying every stereotyped image of unattractive side effects.

Decisions about alcohol and drugs are deeply personal; in this section, Alice and her readers recognize the variety of reasons (and many of the benefits) for use of these products. There are unquestionable payoffs for entering a more relaxed, optimistic state. Some people say they achieve their creative peak only through some "chemical massaging" of their brains. Couples on a first date feel less anxious about opening up if they have a drink or two or three. For those pulling an all-nighter, a stimulant can help them survive the shift—and Alice doesn't just mean speed: coffee and cigarettes count, too.

There are just as many reasons to opt against, or at least to think seriously about curtailing, illicit drug, nicotine, and alcohol use. Children of alcoholics, who are genetically predisposed to alcoholism, may choose to avoid alcohol in all situations. Others may want to stay in complete control, especially at parties. Can the people around you be trusted to take care of you if something goes wrong? Do you know anyone who turns solely to a beer or a bong to deal with a bad grade or a bad day?

Not everyone does drugs. The numbers of people around us who we *think* are drinking, smoking, snorting, and injecting are much higher than the actual numbers of those who do. But the perception that everyone's on something, and the pressure sometimes applied by friends and acquaintances to use, overuse, or incorrectly use drugs, can be just as, if not more, destructive than the substances themselves. Your own body chemistry, psychological makeup, life experiences, and expectations will profoundly affect your reaction to the drugs discussed in this chapter. It's also important to realize that what one of your friends appears to swallow with ease, you may not be able to handle at all, and vice versa.

And no matter how well you know your body, there's no way to tell exactly what's in any illegal substance you buy. Alice can tell you what the chemical compounds are expected to be, but it's impossible to predict whether you'll walk away with a $200 bag of baking soda or a tainted powder that will keep you from ever breathing again.

Legal substances may be easier to get, but they're not necessarily much friendlier. For instance, some say the addiction to nicotine rivals the addiction to far more potent substances, and many people don't want to quit smoking until the harmful side effects begin setting in. But by then, it can be a frustrating experience to cope with nicotine withdrawal. Smokeless tobacco poses the same dilemma. Alice will give quitting strategies to those of you out there who really do want to stop smoking (or chewing) tobacco.

In this chapter, Alice will also discuss some burning issues, such as hangover prevention, which can also prevent your dorm room from turning into a vomiteria. More serious health concerns will be addressed as well, including memory loss, binge drinking, and identifying problems and helping friends. Alice will also cover marijuana myths and facts, plus inquiries about other currently chic street drugs: coke, speed, 'shrooms, GHB, and even cover-up fluid, to name a few.

In many cases, this chapter's most stimulating moments come from the real-life stories of Alice's readers, who provide plenty of thought-provoking perspectives.

Alcohol

Hangover Helper

Dear Alice,

Do you have any tips for hangovers?

HUNGOVER

Dear Hungover,

Hangovers are a set of symptoms that are thought to be brought on by withdrawal from a temporary drug addiction, or they may result from alcohol's chemical contents.

One of the best ways to minimize the headaches, nausea, diarrhea, fatigue, and other all-around gross hangover products is to practice some prevention before, and during, your drinking episodes. Here are some popular tips on how to do just that:

Chow down. Eat a substantial meal before you go out to a party or bar. Bread and fatty foods, like milk and cheese, provide temporary storage space for alcohol and slow hangover-producing intoxication.

Hold that line. You're probably familiar with your tolerance of alcoholic beverages (the point when the alcohol you've consumed begins to cause noticeable physical and psychological changes). Crossing your line can easily send you into hangover land the next morning. Challenge yourself to hold that line—set and state a drink max before you go out—your body and friends will thank you tomorrow.

Pace yourself. Hangover helpers and healthy drinkers recommend one or two drinks per hour as a guide. This rate gives your body a chance to process the alcohol without sending it special delivery to your head.

Alternate. Start your partying with some food, then have a beer, then down some water or juice, then have another beer (remember to pace yourself along the way). Don't switch off with carbonated drinks—they can speed up intoxication and heighten hangovers.

Mix, not! Avoid alternating the types of alcohol you consume. If you begin with beer, stick with beer to the end. Starting with Scotch? Stay with Scotch, and so on. For many, downing different kinds of drinks leads to hellatious headaches and sick stomachs. It's challenging enough for your body to react to one type of foreign substance, so why give it a harder time with two, three, or four?

Sip or sink. Drink each alcoholic beverage slowly. Remember, your liver can handle only ¾ ounce of alcohol an hour. Rapid consumption of alcohol via shots, funnels, and drinking games are sure to win you a big hangover.

CHEERS,
Alice

Alcohol Use and Memory Loss

Dear Alice,
What exactly does "blacking out" from alcohol mean? Can people get so drunk that it is physiologically impossible for them to remember what happened the next day? Also, is it possible for someone to walk around, talk to people, etc., and then have no way of remembering those actions?

Dear Reader,
Yes, indeed. Blackouts, defined as periods of amnesia (memory loss), are caused when alcohol consumption levels prevent the formation of memories in the brain. These levels vary from person to person, and the time frame of these memory lapses is not always marked by visible altered states of consciousness. For example, you and your friends could go to a bar tonight, have some drinks, and talk about politics. But tomorrow, when your friends recall in detail the previous evening's discourse, you may not recall the actual conversation even though you were a full and competent participant. This point is important because blackouts are often confused with passing out, which does constitute a change in consciousness.

Blackouts are common among alcohol abusers and can be a warning sign to drinkers and their friends that alcohol-related problems exist. Blackouts are also considered an early high-risk indicator of alcoholism. For problem and healthy drinkers alike, blackouts are often

What percentage of the total American college student population do you think drinks alcohol (in any quantity—legally and illegally)? If you're like most people to whom Alice has asked this question, you guessed between 95 and 100 percent. WRONG. A still-reliable early '90s national college survey put the answer to that question at about 84 percent—with higher numbers at rural schools and lower ones at urban institutions, generally speaking. This means that if you decide not to drink, or choose to drink responsibly, you're neither alone nor a geek.

Now, for those of you who can't come up with one good reason for why anybody in her/his right mind would choose to drink healthily, or abstain from alcohol altogether, here are some creative ideas Alice has heard over the years:

- *"My father was an alcoholic, and it's too risky for me to drink right now."*
- *"I'm on medication that can't be mixed with alcohol."*
- *"I'm trying to fight off a cold."*
- *"It's against my religion."*
- *"It makes me sick."*
- *"I'm in rehab."*
- *"I have a game tomorrow."*
- *"I'm broke."*
- *"I don't want to."*
- *"None of your business."*

Because perception and peer pressure drive drinking and other drug use—sometimes to tragic and irreversible ends—a reality check about numbers and norms, and total respect for someone's right to limit or eliminate drug use for whatever reason, should be our own rule of law.

troubling or traumatic when serious and typically unforgettable occurrences are impossible to remember, such as . . . I don't recall slapping her! You're kidding, I took my pants off and danced on the bar? Did I have sex with that guy last night? . . . Or even, was he wearing a condom? It can be pretty sobering to realize that, in the end, we are responsible for our actions, whether we remember them or not. It's too bad when we forget, for life, really pleasurable things like a party, meeting new people, or intimate moments of sexual pleasure.

If you are concerned about your own blackouts, or the memory-challenging episodes of others, cutting back or setting limits on your alcohol intake would be wise and responsible. If the problem is chronic, and a symptom of more serious drinking or other drug use, professional support or assistance is the next step.

Alice

Trouble Controlling My Drinking

Dear Alice,

I have just realized that I am not able to handle alcohol. Whenever I go to a bar or a club, I drink to excess. I do not have any urge to drink. However, when I am in a club or a bar, the same thing happens: I drink too much! This is making me think that I am an alcoholic. My question is: Where can I go for help? Thanx.

BINGER

Dear Binger,

It's really great that you've taken time to think about your drinking, but before you diagnose yourself as an alcoholic, take a look at these three definitions:

- An *abuser* uses alcohol and/or other drugs in ways that threaten her/his health and well-being, and compromises her/his ability to function in social, family, and work situations.
- Someone *addicted* to alcohol and/or other drugs *needs* to take these drugs and *needs* to increase her/his dosage over time to maintain the effects of the drugs. An addict's pattern of use is compulsive, and withdrawal symptoms occur when drug use has stopped—and disappear when drug use has resumed.
- *Alcoholics* have the disease of alcoholism, which can be defined by the interaction of biological, psychological, and social factors. Here are examples of these factors:
  - *Biological*: Genetic differences that predispose someone to alcohol abuse. Sons, daughters, brothers, and sisters of alcoholics are more likely to become alcohol abusers themselves.
  - *Psychological*: Personality and psychological traits that predispose someone to alcohol abuse, including self-medicating unpleasant feelings and depression.
  - *Social*: Environmental factors supporting alcohol abuse—things like job stress, insufficient employment and/or financial resources, relationship problems, and peer pressure to drink.

- Getting in trouble with family, roommates, significant others, friends, a resident adviser (RA), or the law as a result of drinking.
- Drinking to escape worries or troubles.
- Becoming unreasonably angry or aggressive—fighting, vandalizing, forcing sex, etc.
- Having to drink more and more to get the "desired effect," or drinking more than you planned to.
- Not remembering parts of what happened the night before (having blackouts), or wanting to forget parts of what happened.
- Trying to cut down, but not being able to.
- Missing class or work due to drinking.
- Frequently drinking until you're drunk, or drinking solely to get drunk.
- Beginning to experience unexplained anxiety, sleeping trouble, lethargy, depression, or feelings of alienation or isolation.
- Rapidly drinking the first two or three drinks in an effort to get drunk quickly.
- Joking about your drinking, or avoiding discussion of your usage.
- Having unsafe sex, which could result in an STD or unintended pregnancy.
- Driving while intoxicated.

No one person would exhibit all of these signs, but if you feel that a cluster of them applies to you, speak with a counselor, or call a hotline. These resources would also help you if you're concerned about the alcohol or other drug use of a friend, family member, teammate, or partner. RES

Alice

Friend of an Alcohol Abuser

Dear Alice,
Last year, I became very good friends with a guy on my floor. He was a little out of the ordinary in the way he dressed, as well as in some of his opinions and habits. I had the feeling that he did drink more than he should, and he also did pot. I did not worry too much about it, because it appeared to be more of a lifestyle choice than an addiction, and did not cause him major troubles.

Unfortunately, he started to have academic problems. He did not do his work, missed classes, and eventually exams as well. I still did not relate these things to his alcohol and drug habits, and hoped that once he got over the adjustment everyone needed to make in freshman year, he would be fine. Well, he wasn't. He did not come back to school this

PROFILE OF A "HEALTHY DRINKER"

- Know your family history of alcohol use, because children of parents who abused alcohol may be predisposed to alcohol dependency.
- Be aware that alcohol is a powerful, potent, and potentially harmful drug. Excessive, long-term alcohol consumption is a factor in cirrhosis, ulcers, strokes, heart disease, certain types of cancer, and birth defects. It is also a major factor in homicides, assaults, rapes, suicides, family violence, and traffic accidents.
- Limit your intake to two drinks or less at one sitting (a drink being one twelve-ounce beer, a five-ounce glass of wine, or a normal cocktail, which is one and a half ounces of 80 proof); drink slowly, about one or two drinks per hour; alternate alcoholic with nonalcoholic beverages; sip rather than chug; and eat a substantial meal before drinking, all of which help to limit hangover symptoms associated with heavy short-term drinking.
- Know that there are times when the body and spirit are more vulnerable to the negative effects of alcohol and abstain during those times. The difficulties of coping with life crises are exacerbated by alcohol.
- Drink for positive reasons, such as celebrations and cultural and religious events, rather than for escape from problems or proving your worth.
- Believe alcohol is a complement to an activity, not the primary focus.

fall, and when I called him, I learned that he had gone through a lot that summer. He was diagnosed for depression and a cocaine addiction, and put on Prozac as well as sent to therapy. At that point, I thought that he was on the right track, because he was also going to get a job, and planning to take classes at a nearby college. However, when he came to visit me a month later, he had already had two beers before he even came here, and got more and more drunk as the evening progressed. I would not let him drive home, but he ignored my warnings and left anyway. I was very disturbed, because a friend of his had just been in a drunk driving accident. I was very mad at him, told him clearly that I will always be his friend, but prefer not to talk to him or see him if he showed up drunk again. He did not call for a while and neither did I. When he called me yesterday and I told him that I thought he should do something about his alcohol problem, he kept repeating his excuses, that he drinks because he is Irish, that he doesn't care if he dies early as long as he had fun in life, etc. On the other hand, he can't find a job and seems to be very depressed. I want to help him, but I don't know how. Any ideas?

CONCERNED

Dear Concerned,

You are in a difficult, yet common, situation. You are a friend of an addict. The best thing you can do is be supportive, let him know you care, but don't take on his problem. It sounds as if you have already started doing that by telling him you don't want to see him when he's drunk. Talk with him when you both are sober, and be clear and specific about what's going on for you and what you see is going on with him. If your friend doesn't want help, or continues to deny that he has a problem, *it is not* your responsibility to change his mind or behavior. He is the only one who can make the decision to change.

When you speak with him, follow these steps:

- Tell him that you care about him, and that you are concerned about how he's been acting.
- Tell him exactly what he's been doing that concerns you. "You came to visit me after drinking, and proceeded to get more drunk and then drove home."
- Listen to his response, no matter what.
- Tell him what you would like to see him do. "Only come and visit me if you're going to be sober." Or, "I'd like to see you go into rehab, or get some kind of professional help that will work for you."
- Tell him what you are willing and able to do to help him. This can range from simply being a good listener, to helping to arrange a meeting with a professional who can help. Alice knows he's already seeing a therapist, but he may need to be working with someone different—someone with whom he can relate and not manipulate.

Talk with him again if it doesn't work the first time. It often takes time and repetition for a person with a drug and alcohol problem to accept what you have to say.

You may need help yourself, if being supportive of your friend becomes too exhausting or time-consuming. If you don't take care of yourself, you can't help your friend. **RES**

Alice

Child of an Alcoholic

Dear Alice,

My father is an alcoholic and I've been told that I should stay away from drinking altogether. I'm a freshman this year and it seems like most of my friends always want to go to keg parties or hang out and drink. Sometimes I drink with them, but then I feel guilty and worried afterward thinking about my dad. It's hard to avoid alcohol here, but I don't want to follow in my father's footsteps either. Any advice or support you can give would help. Thanks.

SOUTHERN COMFORT

Dear Southern Comfort,

You've already gotten beyond one of the hardest steps to healing that children of alcoholics have to take: admitting that a parent has the disease of alcoholism. Often, sons, daughters, wives, and husbands of alcoholic households learn early on to deny that any problem exists and to cover things up.

It's good that you've thought about your drinking in terms of your family history. In fact, this is one facet of the "Profile of a Healthy Drinker" (see page 215). Because of genetic and environmental influences, children of alcoholics are about three to four times more likely to become alcoholic than the rest of the population. That's why it may help you and others in your shoes to evaluate your alcohol use: how much, how frequently, and whether or not you should drink at all.

Children of alcoholics tend to take on roles that help them adapt to the chaos at home. In an alcoholic household, there is a severe lack of role models for positively expressing emotions. So, some children become "placaters," doing anything to keep peace and to comfort others at their own expense. Some assume an adult role, taking care of younger siblings and even their parents. Others will always adjust to whatever's going on, while there are some who act out at home and/or school as a way to get attention and deflect attention from their parents' drinking. It is common among children of alcoholics to continue in these roles as adults. Many marry or make lifelong commitments to other alcoholics (about 50 percent), and many more develop compulsive behavior patterns, such as alcohol or other drug abuse and/or overeating (about 70 percent).

Young and adult children of alcoholics may also face a range of emotional problems. These include a strong sense of guilt, particularly for the parent's drinking; constant anxiety and/or fear of what will happen at home; embarrassment and confusion; an inability to trust others and self; anger; and depression.

It is important for you to develop a healthy sense of self-esteem. Your father's problem is his problem—you are in no way at fault. Recognize his illness and know how it can influence certain aspects of your life, like right now with drinking at school. In the United States, there are an estimated 30 million people who grow up in alcoholic households. Yes, about 10 percent of our total population can relate to your concerns. Many of them have gotten help and worked through the difficult issues they face. There are many organizations nationwide that you can contact to find support, help, and other resources. Among them: Al-Anon, Alateen, the National Association for Children of Alcoholics, and the Children of Alcoholics Foundation, Inc. Your school's counseling service is another place for short- and long-term assistance.

RES

Alice

Nicotine

Quitting Smokeless Tobacco?

Alice,

How can a person get help quitting the use of smokeless tobacco? All of the resources in this general area are geared toward helping smokers stop smoking, but a smokeless tobacco nicotine addict does not have a similar usage ritual as a smoker, but does have a similar, or worse, addiction than a smoker because the nicotine absorption levels are many times greater. Any suggestions as to how a smokeless tobacco user can get help stopping this addiction would be greatly appreciated.

SNUFF HEAD

Dear Snuff Head,

Smokeless tobacco appears in two common forms, chewing tobacco and snuff, and contains nicotine that is absorbed through the gums and lining of the mouth. The nicotine dose in smokeless tobacco is comparable to the amount found in cigarettes, making smokeless tobacco highly addictive. Common side effects of smokeless tobacco use include tooth decay, gingivitis, and recession of the gums. Oral cancers occur more frequently in users of smokeless tobacco, and long-term use can increase the risk of cancer of the cheek and gums.

You're right—most smoking cessation programs focus on cigarette smokers. Some of these programs may be transferable to smokeless tobacco. There are self-help booklets, videotapes, and quit kits available which offer privacy, low cost, and flexibility in quitting. You can also try talking with your doctor and working out a plan for quitting with him/her. The nicotine patch is another possibility. It is applied to the user's body and releases a continuous flow of nicotine through the user's skin to help reduce the craving for nicotine and other withdrawal symptoms. Use is tapered to make sure that you also don't get addicted to using the patch. There are behavior modification programs, which provide built-in support for quitting. Although the majority of group participants are cigarette smokers, the skills taught in this course can be applied to all tobacco users. Getting comfortable with a tobacco-free life is a process that takes time.

Other cessation techniques include conditioning methods that employ using more tobacco than you could possibly stand in order to try to develop an aversion to it. Hypnosis is an alternative possibility, as is acupuncture. Over-the-counter products can be useful, but in actuality, few have been shown to be effective in helping smokers quit.

A good "quit tobacco" program would include at least a few of the following tips:

- Be patient with yourself.
- Reward yourself for each week and month you stay off tobacco.
- Be positive.
- Get support from others.
- Avoid "triggers"—those certain times, places, and situations that make you want to use tobacco.
- Plan alternatives to tobacco use for coping with stress.
- Don't be defeated.

Alice

SMOKELESS TOBACCO FACTS FROM THE AMERICAN CANCER SOCIETY

- All tobacco can cause cancer.
- People who use smokeless tobacco are several times more likely to be at risk for oral cancer than people who don't use tobacco.
- Increased heart rate, blood pressure, and blood levels of nicotine of smokeless tobacco users are similar to those of cigarette smokers.
- After only a few years of smokeless tobacco use, a permanent sore can develop in the mouth.
- The nicotine in smokeless tobacco has addictive properties, and can cause chemical dependence.

Weight Gain and Quitting Smoking

Dear Alice,

I've been a smoker for eight years and now I want to quit smoking. But there's one thing that annoys me—I've heard that if one quits smoking, s/he will gain weight. Is it really true? Thanks in advance.

Dear Reader,

To begin with, a note of congratulations on the first step toward becoming a nonsmoker. A strong personal resolve to kick the habit is a primary factor in quitting smoking successfully. Many people gain weight when they stop smoking, and, for that reason, they may light up again. However, a normal, healthy person would have to gain close to a hundred pounds in order to equal the health risks s/he takes with smoking. Also, it is not a given that everyone who quits smoking gains weight. Regardless, you can strategize to fend off unwanted pounds.

Use common sense to maintain your weight while quitting smoking. Obviously, if you substitute a candy bar each time you crave a cigarette, you will gain weight. Eating a well-balanced, low-calorie diet with three meals a day, and increasing your activity level, will probably prove effective in maintaining your weight.

If you think this won't be enough, figure out your current average daily caloric intake and use this as a guideline for weight maintenance after you quit. Plan meals and shop ahead at first. Stock your kitchen and office with healthy, low-calorie snack foods, such as carrot and celery sticks, air-popped popcorn, dry cereals, or crackers. Don't give yourself carte blanche with snack foods, however. View them as aids to getting beyond the craving to smoke. Other things that you can use to put in your mouth include toothpicks, plastic straws, gum, and hard candy.

Think about when you normally smoke and decide what you'll do instead. For instance, if you always have a cigarette with your coffee, plan to have something else on hand. If you find that the nonsmoking causes you to want to eat more at meals, drink a glass of water before and during the meal. Chew your food well, eat slowly, and concentrate on how much better food tastes now. After a meal is a great time for a cigarette, right? Well, then get up and moving right away—wash the dishes, go for a walk, brush your teeth . . .

Nicotine addiction can be monumentally difficult to overcome. Whatever your reasons for wanting to quit, know that there are many sources of assistance. To start, your school or office may have smoking cessation groups and/or integrated practices, such as hypnosis. **RES**

Alice

WHY DO SOME PEOPLE GAIN WEIGHT WHEN THEY QUIT SMOKING?

Nicotine suppresses the appetite and causes the liver to release glycogen, which raises the blood sugar level slightly. With nicotine out of your system, you may feel hungry more often. Smoking artificially elevates heart rate and increases your metabolism. When you stop smoking, your body has to readjust to a lower metabolic rate. If you eat the same as you did when you were smoking, your body will end up using less and storing more (as fat) of the food. Smoking dulls the taste buds. Food begins to taste better to new nonsmokers; this can increase food intake. And then there's oral fixation—some ex-smokers may want something to fill the void of cigarettes.

Marijuana

Marijuana and Health

Dear Alice,
Just how dangerous is light to moderate use of marijuana (one joint per week)? I have heard that it is less dangerous than alcohol or tobacco use. Also, its metabolites are stored in fatty tissues, but do they cause any harm?

THANKS.

Dear Reader,
The long-term physiological and psychological effects of smoking pot are complicated. Further clouding this issue is the absence of a clear definition of "light," "moderate," and "heavy" use. Based on a range of research, however, a few joints a year can be considered light use, lighting up a few times a month constitutes moderate use, and daily hits or multiple uses per week spell heavy use. The duration of marijuana use over time may be the major player when it comes to unhealthy effects: long-term, heavy use of the drug may result in the illnesses and diseases associated with long-term cigarette smoking. Cigarettes have been linked to an increased incidence of heart disease and lung cancer (marijuana smoke contains the same cancer-causing chemicals as tobacco smoke—actually four times as much tar); emphysema; gum disease; and cancers of the mouth, jaw, and tongue.

Additionally, short-term memory loss, reduced fertility in men and women, and personality changes may occur in some long-term pot smokers. The more immediate effects of moderate and heavy marijuana use are better known: congestion, sore throat, dry mouth, impaired thinking and motor skill ability (including reaction time essential for driving), fatigue, anxiety, dilated pupils, and more. Some research links a rare childhood leukemia with mothers who lit up while they were pregnant.

Storage-wise, about half of the marijuana metabolites—the substances that result from pot's breakdown by the liver and kidneys—pass through the body hours after the first hit. The rest of the metabolites are stored away, sometimes for weeks, in fatty tissue, where their effect is unknown. We do know that pot, by itself and not when it is combined with other unknown substances, is not physically addictive, nor does it appear to impair intelligence.

Is pot more dangerous than alcohol? On an individual level, it depends on many factors, including reasons for use (as part of a healthy celebration, or as an unhealthy coping crutch), family history of alcohol and other drug use (drugs are often more dangerous if one or both parents are/were abusers), and your comfort level in the environment and situation in which drug use occurs.

Let's go somewhere else with your pot query. Like cigarettes, pipes, and cigars, joints and bongs deliver secondhand smoke to nonusers around them—through the air, under doors, and via air vents. And a nonsmoker in a very smoky room theoretically can get high, too. Likewise, urine can test positive via a drug test for innocent bystanders within a day or two of breathing secondhand pot smoke. Weed and other drug use can also impact relationships with friends, roommates, parents, etc., in ways that you might not have predicted before you lit up.

Alice

Marijuana: How Long Does It Hang Out in the Body?

Dear Alice,

How long does marijuana stay in the body?

Dear Reader,

The longevity of THC (tetrahydrocannabinol, the active chemical in marijuana) in the body depends mostly on the user and the mode of use. Generally, half of the THC that comes from smoking weed passes out of the body within a day. The other 50 percent either stays connected to blood proteins, enters cells, or moves into fat before it says good-bye for good. Many marijuana users who are concerned about passing drug tests allow a full month between their last toke and "D-day." Of course, random drug testing makes this period impossible to plan.

Speaking of drug testing, mandatory exams primarily test urine (THC can remain in urine for one month). Some private companies test hair samples for marijuana remains (THC supposedly remains in hair indefinitely, until the affected/exposed hair is removed). However, the utility of these tests is controversial because other factors, such as being in the presence of secondhand pot smoke, can leave pot residue on the hair of a non–pot user.

Alice

Club Drugs

Ecstasy Effects

Dear Alice,
I heard that the first reaction you have to taking Ecstasy is to become violently ill, after which the party can continue. This sounds like an urban legend to me. Could you clarify please?

Dear Reader,
Ecstasy (N-methyl-3,4-methylenedioxyamphetamine or MDMA), a hallucinogenic amphetamine, is a recreational drug that's widely used in many countries. Limited research exists about the nature of effects, with nothing about "violent illness" for first-time use. First-time heroin use, however, often produces acute sickness, and perhaps your "urban legend" evolved from there. This does not mean that sickness cannot result from initial use of Ecstasy or any other drug. Dosage, preexisting health conditions, and drug combinations (including alcohol and prescription drugs) can all adversely impact one's drug experiences. FYI, the effects of one dose of "X" (usually taken in pill form) last for four to six hours.

Ecstasy is popular as a companion at parties and nightclubs because it produces a combination of heightened arousal, mellowing effects, and enhanced self- and group-consciousness. The drug, illegal and considered to have no legitimate use by the government since 1985, when some users' problems with X made headlines, has been most associated with a rise in body temperature—usually resulting in acute dehydration. This is important since dancing for hours without enough breaks and water is pretty common while on X.

Studies have shown that ecstasy uses serotonin, a chemical in your brain that affects your moods, so that after the initial high, you may feel tired, depressed, or moody. Your body will eventually produce more serotonin, but it may take some time to get it back to normal levels. So, after a weekend of heavy partying, you may have trouble getting up and going to class or work, and, once there, you may be irritable. (True for many non-Xers, too.)

Heavy use has been linked to speedlike symptoms of paranoia, and in some cases, liver damage and heart attacks. Although research has not yielded evidence of Ecstasy-induced brain damage in humans, heavy administration of the drug has produced neurological damage in rats and monkeys.

Alice

Rohypnol "Roofie" and Rape

Dear Alice,
I have heard about pills one can take to increase the effects of alcohol while lowering the actual consumption level (in essence, getting drunk off of one beer). I think the pill might be called roche (I don't know how it is spelled—pronounced *row-shay*). Could you describe more about this pill and its dangers?

Curious and Concerned

Dear Curious and Concerned,
You may be referring to a drug called Rohypnol (flunitrazepam), street-named "roofies," "roachies," "rophies," "ruffies," "roofenol," "roche," "La Rocha," "rope," and "the forget pill." But as we know, drug street names change all the time. This hypnotic sedative enhances the effects of alcohol: decreased inhibition, sleepiness, and memory loss. However, the drug's medical purpose is quite different; Rohypnol is primarily used as a surgical anesthetic or sleeping pill in about eighty countries, although the United States is not one of them. Drug enforcement officials say that Rohypnol is illegally coming into the United States from Mexico, Colombia, and Europe.

Unfortunately, the use of drugs, mostly alcohol, by sex abusers to sedate their "prey" has been practiced for centuries. Rohypnol is potentially a more dangerous addition to their arsenal. Many other drugs, primarily from the same family of drugs as Rohypnol (benzodiazepines), can also be used as "rape drugs." Beware. Rohypnol is a cheap and powerful drug—a white, dime-sized pill that dissolves quickly in alcoholic and other beverages, such as soft drinks. Known as a "date rape drug" in high schools, on college campuses, and in other communities across the country, it's being used (mostly by men, according to recent criminal cases) to secretly sedate and sexually assault women and men. Roofie is dropped into drinks at bars and parties, leaving roofie recipients open to suggestion, physically weak, and perhaps most troubling of all, without memory of events that transpire after the drug takes effect. This has made prosecution of "roofie-rape" cases challenging, as people report waking up naked and alone in strange hotel rooms, for example, without any idea of how they got there and who was involved. And it doesn't stop there. One of the newer club drugs, GHB (gamma hydroxybutyrate), is also being slipped into drinks and has become known as "Easy Lay." GHB, which produces psychedelic effects for the recreational user, has a sedating effect at higher doses.

Rohypnol creates a bitter taste when dissolved in alcohol. By now, lots of red warning lights should be flashing in your head. For starters, be aware of the color, texture, and taste of your drinks; accepting pre-purchased, open drinks of any kind from strangers and casual acquaintances should be avoided (unfortunately, this may harken back to mom and dad saying, "Don't accept candy from strangers"). Rohypnol's misuse also makes it advisable not to leave drinks unattended, even in familiar surroundings.

It's possible for people who were sexually assaulted and suspect that they were drugged to be tested for the presence of Rohypnol and other drugs. These drugs can usually be detected in urine for about three days after ingestion, sometimes even a little longer. However, the sooner someone is tested, the better. Most rape crisis centers and hospitals will be able to run these tests.

Alice recognizes that this may be a *big* drag, but until roofie is run out of town, or loses its status as a drug of the day, prevention and education is the best way to protect yourself and others. So, spread the word.

Alice

NEWS FLASH ABOUT ROHYPNOL

There is good news about Rohypnol: its manufacturer recently reformulated the drug to make it more detectable. When put in a light-colored drink, new Rohypnol will now turn the beverage bright blue. Consumers of darker-colored beverages should be tipped off by a cloudy appearance. The drug will also dissolve more slowly and form small chunky pieces (how pleasant).

GHB / "Liquid Ecstasy"

Dear Alice,
A lot of my friends have made the switch from Ecstasy to GHB. I do X sometimes when I go to clubs, and this is fine for me. I'm just wonder-

ing what GHB is, and if I'm missing a good time by sticking with tradition.

X Is Enough

Dear X Is Enough,
In the constantly changing, and sometimes oh-so-trendy, club and party drug scene, GHB (Gamma hydroxybutyrate), street-named "Grievous Bodily Harm," appears to have blown Ecstasy (N-methyl-3,4-methyl-enedioxyamphetamine, or MDMA, and X for short) right off the dance floor over the past year or so. GHB, like many other drugs du jour, has been around for a long time; it was developed in the 1980s as a surgical anesthetic, but then it became popular as a muscle-building and weight-loss potion. The sometimes unpredictable effects of GHB vary from one person to the next, which, along with its potential to cause memory loss, vertigo, reduced heart rate, seizures, respiratory failure, and even coma, prompted the government to ban its use and sale, except for licensed research. GHB is commonly used with other drugs, including X, and this fact of drug life today clouds both certainty about its effects, and whether serious incidents associated with GHB were caused by that drug, or its combination with other substances. GHB seems to be particularly dangerous when mixed with alcohol.

GHB is often called "Liquid Ecstasy" because it comes in small bottles, with a capful of GHB providing users with X-like desires to be "touchy-feely"; however, its overall impact is likened more to that of acid than Ecstasy. This makes sense because GHB is a psychedelic sleep-inducer, whereas X is a speedy amphetamine. GHB is a powerful sedative that can leave the body limp and tired. X is frequently taken along with GHB to counteract this sedation.

GHB may or may not be addictive, but our society's addiction to the "better time," the "bigger TV," the "fancier car," etc., drives most of us, sometimes, to forget our present satisfaction in the pursuit of an even peachier life. Yes, different, stronger drugs can produce higher highs, but they can also bring on new risks, responsibilities, expectations, and relationships—including how your drug use affects people close to you.

Alice

Special K

Dear Alice,
Lately, I have been doing a relatively new drug called Special K. I know it is a sedative/tranquilizer (what's the difference?), but very little about side effects, etc. Can you go over this information?

Thanks
Crankin'

Dear Crankin',
Sedatives are depressant drugs. They cause restfulness in low doses, sleep in higher doses, and death in high to very high doses. High dose sedatives are called hypnotics. Sedatives include alcohol, barbiturates, and minor tranquilizers. A tranquilizer is a drug used to calm or pacify.

Special K is the street name for the drug Ketamine. Other names by which it is known are Ketalar, Ketaject, and Super-K. Ketamine is closely related to PCP, and it produces similar effects. Like PCP, Ketamine use produces a reaction called a dissociative state, and also like PCP, Ketamine is known to cause bad reactions in some of its users. However, unlike PCP, Special K is a legal prescription drug intended for use as an anesthetic for people and large animals. In recent years, Ketamine has begun to be used recreationally. Similar to PCP, Ketamine can have a significant impact on coordination, thought, and judgment, and it can produce agitation, violence, confusion, and communication difficulties.

Alice

"Hard" Drugs

Cocaine

Alice,

My friend recently smoked some pot laced with cocaine. First of all, is this possible? Whatever the case may be, he seems to be infatuated with the idea of trying straight coke. I've heard that trying coke for the first time is quite dangerous, true? Also, what are the effects of the high? And how detrimental is coke in general?

SINCERELY, CONCERNED FRIEND

Dear Concerned Friend,

Cocaine is a stimulant drug, and also a naturally occurring anesthetic. Most of the effects of coke, however, occur when the drug interrupts the neurotransmitter balance in the central nervous system. The initial effects of this interruption are pleasant—increased confidence, a willingness to work, greater motivation, increased libido, and a euphoric rush or high. At the same time, coke raises blood pressure, increases heart rate, causes rapid breathing, tenses muscles, and causes the jitters (although many don't notice it because they're feeling so alert and euphoric). Over time, and with regular use, people may get paranoid, anxious, and confused, and sometimes they hallucinate. Insomnia, agitation, and depression can also result from frequent cocaine use.

Cocaine is extracted from the coca plant, which grows on the mountain slopes of the Andes in South America, in certain parts of the Amazon jungle, and on the island of Java in Indonesia. Native cultures have used coca leaves, in chewed and brewed forms, for thousands of years for social and religious occasions. In 1860, cocaine was isolated from all the other chemicals in the coca leaf, and a pure form of cocaine was extracted. Cocaine is much more potent when injected than when chewing the leaf. The drug readily dissolves in water, allowing users to inject it and dissolve it directly into drinks. Injecting cocaine results in an intense rush in fifteen to thirty seconds, while drinking it results in a milder, yet longer lasting, stimulation thirty to forty-five minutes after ingestion. Both these methods of using cocaine popularized the drug in the United States at the turn of the century.

The physical effects of coke are the same as any other stimulant drug—except that the first rush is possibly much more intense. The problems with cocaine come from doing too much, its mixture with other drugs, and the crash after binge use. The latter arrives when the initial feelings of well-being and confidence, the sense of omnipotence, and the satisfied feelings disappear as suddenly as the rush appeared, leaving the user with the desire to have *more*. Usually, after a night, or a few nights, of snorting coke, the user crashes—sleeping all day long, trying to put energy back into the body—and decides never to do the drug again. Anywhere from a few hours to a few weeks later, the person wants to do it again, searching for that good feeling from the last time.

Cocaine use can easily slide into abuse—and yes, this can occur shortly after one's first cocaine experience. The brain's pleasure centers that cocaine short-circuits makes its use a mighty hard habit to kick—despite the side effects of chronic nasal irritation, nosebleeds, paranoia, and bank account depletion.

Alice

Where's the Freaking Info about Speed?

Okay Alice,
I am a recovering speed freak. I was all whacked out of my skull for too long. Literally too long, like seven or eight days at a time, and I don't see one freaking bit of info on what I see to be a major problem in the youth of today, and I would like it if you could put something in here about speed.

THANK YOU, SPUN CHICKEN!

Dear SPUN CHICKEN!,
Glad to hear you're less whacked.

Amphetamines are used legally (with a doctor's prescription) as appetite suppressants for weight control, and for treatment of attention deficit and hyperactivity disorders, narcolepsy, and depression. In low doses, amphetamines temporarily increase alertness and reduce fatigue. Illegally, speed, also called crank, meth, crystal, and ice, is mostly snorted, smoked, injected, or swallowed to produce feelings of exhilaration, excitement, and euphoria. Speed literally speeds you up: it increases heart and respiratory rates, and can produce an irregular heartbeat, increase perspiration, and raise body temperature. Paranoia, anxiety, and panic are the most common negative psychological effects of speed. By the way, all of these effects add up to a chemically induced stress response. Long-term use can lead to hallucinations, delusions, and violent and self-destructive behavior. OD'ing on speed can send you into convulsions, high fevers, coma, and possibly death, from heart failure, ruptured blood vessels in the brain, or hyperthermia.

Alice usually considers specific questions about drugs, sex, stress, nutrition, and other health topics, rather than waxing philosophical about social issues, politics, and legal policy. Alice put your letter up because your testimonial is educational in and of itself. Thanks.

Alice

Interested in Trying LSD

Dear Alice,
I have become interested in trying LSD. But I am worried about what the side effects are and the consequences later in life. I only want to try and have no real need to continue, or desire to, for that matter. I am just really curious. What could happen to me?

Signed, Mr. LSD

Dear Mr. LSD,
LSD (*d*-lysergic acid diethylamide) stimulates the nervous system. Physically, this results in a rise in pulse rate and blood pressure. It may produce sweating and palpitations, or trigger nausea. Mentally, LSD overloads the brainstem—the sensory switchboard for the mind—causing sensory distortions, better known as hallucinations. There is a loss of judgment and impairment of one's self-preservation mechanisms. This, coupled with slowed reaction time and visual distortions, can make everyday tasks a chancy proposition. There is also the possibility that you may experience a "bad trip." The amount of acid, the surroundings, and the user's mental state and physical condition all determine one's reaction to a drug. Because of its effects on the emotional center of the brain, someone on LSD may experience the extremes of euphoria and panic. People who take too high a dose, or a tainted dose, can feel acute anxiety, fear over loss of control, paranoia, and delusions of persecution or grandeur.

The popular picture of someone using LSD just one time and becoming permanently psychotic or schizophrenic is incorrect. Why do some people have extreme reactions the first time they use the drug? These users have a predisposition to mental illness and the drug may precipitate an episode of that illness at an earlier age. Also, some otherwise normal users can be thrown into a temporary, but prolonged, psychotic reaction, or severe depression, that requires psychological treatment.

Alice

Bad Trips with LSD, 'Shrooms, and Hash

Dear Alice,

I am writing to you regarding drugs. I have always enjoyed dropping hits of LSD, liquid or tabs (never the junky stuff with plenty of strich in it that's here in New York. I always get it sent to me from northern California—Berkeley or Santa Cruz). I've never been a big 'shroomer though. A couple of months ago I did some 'shrooms with my boyfriend at our apartment and had a really bad trip—my first ever—and it was *très* scary: I lost completely my sense of reality and felt at once like I was just a part of someone's dream and that when they woke up, I would die into nothingness, then I reverted back into a childlike state, and even though I was a happy child, I still had no grasp on reality. I didn't trip for a couple of months and then a few weeks ago, I was with two of my girlfriends and we made some hash brownies—I had another awful trip, and even though it was more physically sickening, I still had terrible thoughts while I was tripping . . . For many months, I have been having a rough time with my boyfriend, whom I live with. Could this be affecting my trips? We also used about half an ounce of hash in three small brownies, and I had more 'shrooms than my boyfriend did. Could the quantity be affecting me adversely? I am trying to figure out why I'm having bad trips. What am I overlooking, and will I be able to have happy trails again? (And, please don't say I should go into rehab . . .) Thanx.

DAZED AND CONFUSED

Dear Dazed and Confused,

Alice can't say for sure why your trips have suddenly gone bad. The dope and purity (or lack of purity) could certainly be a factor, but unless you run your stuff through lab tests before you use it, their effects may be hard to pin down. In any case, whenever you're on psychedelics, there's always a moment of panic—a moment of, "Will I ever see the world the same way again?" or "Will the world ever see me the same way again?" etc., etc. These panic thoughts can last for moments, or for what seems to be a lifetime. For people who like to trip and do it often, these feelings usually last for moments. When it starts to feel like the anxiety and fear are lasting a lifetime, it's usually time to stop tripping. Why trip if it's no fun anymore?

Your stress level, your relationship with your boyfriend, your school pressures—all of these cloud one's mind and may affect your state when tripping. Try taking a break, cleaning up your daily life, and then see-ing how you feel. Do you still need the drugs? Have you experienced enough tripping to alter your perceptions in a positive, lasting way? Do you want to try one more time, in a safe, supportive environment? Or are you entering a new phase of life, with increased awareness and sensitivity because of your previous drug use? These are questions to think about.

Alice will honor your request to refrain from recommending rehab, but she will take the opportunity to plug professional assistance or twelve-step groups—whether it's short-term counseling or long-term rehabilitation—as an option for anyone who wants to cut back, or cut out, drug use. Such an endeavor is often very difficult to go alone, for reasons that sometimes have little to do with the drugs themselves. Having some help—a coach, if you will, or taking a break from "regu-lar" life for a while—may be the only way to get back on the track you want to be on.

Alice

Heroin Hell

Hey Alice,
What do you know about heroin? Is it really as addictive as they say? My friend keeps buggin' me to try it, but I'm not sure I want to move from weed to smack. Any guidance would be groovy.

Dear Reader,
Addiction is a real danger when it comes to using heroin. Depending on how much you use and for how long, mild to severe addiction is almost inevitable. This is because a heroin addiction has both a physio-logical (primarily involving the central nervous system) and a psycho-logical component. If you use somewhat weak heroin for a few weeks, you could develop a mild dependence; use something a little purer (which is quite common these days), for a little while longer, and you may find you've got a pretty tough habit to kick.

Heroin is a narcotic derivative of morphine, a common painkilling sedative. Heroin is potent and fast-acting, producing a pleasant sick feeling (nausea) and indifference to pain. Pleasure seeking and pain re-duction can become an all-consuming way of life, and the reason to live, for many heroin users. Such an addiction is not cheap to overcome and is extremely difficult to break.

Many new heroin users get high by smoking and sniffing the drug's cooked byproducts, but some may soon find that real satisfaction can come only from intravenous injection (usually in the arms and legs). If that stops doing the trick, addicts sometimes resort to injecting heroin into their necks, groins, and penises because the vessels in their arms and legs are no longer useful conduits.

Movies like *Pulp Fiction* and *Trainspotting* don't lie about the dark, ugly side of heroin. Overdosing is a possibility—the heroin you can buy today is generally more pure, and therefore deadlier, than ever before. OD'ing aside, you can count on experiencing some nausea and constipation when you do heroin—the nausea will hit before the high does. To relieve constipation, heroin users often become dependent on laxatives as well. If you inject, HIV/AIDS and infectious hepatitis are obviously big concerns, especially if you share or use unsterilized needles.

To be fair, there are heroin users who remain productive, maintaining their grades, work responsibilities, and social and family affairs. "Managing" heroin use, however, can become impossible as a constant craving for this very powerful drug becomes stronger and more difficult to resist.

Only you can decide if you want to take the risk with heroin. Alice is one for informed decisions—perhaps you'll share what you learn with your friend, too. Compared to pot, heroin is a beast of a completely different nature.

Alice

Inhalants

Sniffing Lighter Fluid

Dear Alice,
What are the effects of sniffing lighter fluid? I recently had a friend sit in a car to listen to music and smell lighter fluid. He tells me he gets a high from this. What are the effects of doing this? I would appreciate this to educate my friend.

Dear Reader,
Lighter fluid, like gasoline, model airplane glue, paint thinner, varnish, nail polish remover, and even some types of cover-up products, are members of the organic solvent, or volatile organic compound (VOC) family. Like the effects of low-dose anesthesia, the pungent fumes of these chemicals produce a lightheaded and hot feeling. Because of their toxicity, organic solvents can also lead to dizziness and nausea. Many heavy solvent sniffers report altered states of consciousness, complete with visual hallucinations and vivid dreamlike experiences while awake.

For many young people—especially eleven- to thirteen-year-olds—inhalation of solvent fumes, also called "huffing," is their first chemically induced high. This makes sense given that these agents are legal, cheap, and readily available around the house. For the most part, light use of solvents for getting high does not directly cause mental or physical harm; since 1970, however, there has been a steady rise in "sudden sniffing death" due to VOC-induced heart attacks and asphyxiation. Other problems arise when disoriented users drive, cross busy streets, and do other things that require sharp judgment and reflexes. Some links have been made between birth defects and mothers who sniffed solvents while pregnant.

Serious consequences are more likely as exposure to these compounds rises—particularly among workers in industrial plants, where ventilation and protective equipment are inadequate. The fumes produced by these substances are taxing to the respiratory system and liver, and can cause loss of consciousness and brain damage in extreme cases. By the way, good ventilation is critical, wherever and however organic solvents in any quantity are being used.

Good luck with your lesson plan, and more power to your educational efforts.

Alice

Nitrous Oxide

Alice,

I am wondering about the direct effects nitrous oxide has on the brain, and if it is a fallacy that it kills brain cells.

SINCERELY, HIPPI CRACK

Dear Hippi Crack,

Nitrous oxide has been around for a couple of hundred years and has a long medical history as a mild anesthetic. More popularly known as "laughing gas," "poppers," or "whippets," nitrous oxide is a colorless, sweet-smelling gas that produces giddiness, a dreamy or floating sensation, and a mild, pain-free state. Because nitrous oxide relieves anxiety and indirectly blocks pain, it's used most often for minor oral surgery and dental work.

When administration of nitrous oxide is monitored in a doctor's office as an anesthetic, it is considered a safe pharmacological agent. But when it is used recreationally, hazards exist. Nitrous oxide rapidly affects motor control, so you are likely to fall down soon after inhaling it. Sitting down while inhaling it, to avoid a major fall, reduces one of the potential negative effects. Nitrous oxide needs to be mixed with oxygen if it is used for more than a few minutes, as breathing straight nitrous oxide can cause asphyxiation. When the gas comes from a pressurized tank, it's freezing and can cause frostbite of the nose, lips, and possibly of the vocal cords, which the anesthetized user might not be able to feel as it is occurring.

Immediate effects following use include nausea, fatigue, lack of coordination, disorientation, and loss of appetite. Long-term use of inhalants can result in organic brain syndrome, which is characterized by loss of muscular coordination, irritability, disorientation, nerve injury, and liver and kidney disease. There is some evidence that excessive or prolonged use of nitrous oxide can also damage the central nervous system (brain and spinal cord) and bone marrow.

Alice

Caffeine and Energy-Boosting Drugs

Long-Term Effects of Caffeine-Based Drugs

Dear Alice,
What are the long-term side effects of substituting Vivarin for sleep? Last semester, I averaged only about three hours of sleep a day, and it doesn't look like this semester will be terribly different. Thanks in advance.

WEARY GRADUATE STUDENT

Dear Weary Graduate Student,
Vivarin is one of many over-the-counter drugs with caffeine as its main ingredient. Each dose (two pills) contains the amount of caffeine found in approximately two cups of dripped coffee. Caffeine is probably the most popular psychoactive drug in use today, and also one of the most ancient. In ordinary doses, caffeine increases alertness and produces a sense of well-being. It cuts down on feelings of fatigue and boredom, and allows you to maintain physically exhausting or repetitive tasks longer.

Caffeine mildly stimulates the heart and respiratory system, increases muscular tremor, and produces more stomach acid. Higher doses may cause nervousness, anxiety, irritability, headache, disturbed sleep, and stomach upset or peptic ulcers. In women, excessive caffeine consumption may aggravate the symptoms of premenstrual syndrome. With high doses over time, people become "wired"—hyperactive and sensitive to stimulation in their environment. In a few cases, the disturbance is so severe that a person may misperceive her/his surroundings—a toxic psychosis. So there *is* a level of caffeine that causes toxicity.

Withdrawal symptoms can occur when people stop taking caffeine-based drugs or drinking caffeinated beverages. Symptoms of irritability, headaches, and even mild depression do occur. You might want to start by slowly decreasing your daily intake of caffeine, and then working toward quitting caffeine. Your study habits will clearly improve with sleep (which we need mentally, physically, and spiritually to replenish our bodies), and you will probably be more able to effectively prioritize your responsibilities. It is absolutely imperative to eat, sleep, and have some "down" time while you're a student. It will greatly increase your acuity when you're studying and conceptualizing, and allow you to formulate good work habits for after you graduate.

Alice

Coffee Withdrawal Symptoms?

Hi Alice,

Been reading your site for a while and wanted to first thank you for an excellent site! So anyway, here's the question: I've been having headaches off and on for the past year and noticed that it seems to coincide with days that I don't drink coffee in the morning. I've heard of becoming "addicted" to caffeine, so I decided I should just go ahead and quit for a while. This past week, I cut out coffee and all caffeine-related products from my diet, and have been suffering from pounding headaches every day. Today (six days from my last cup of coffee) is the first day that I don't seem to have a headache. Is this common? And also, any ideas on what will happen if I do have some coffee? Will my system require coffee every day again (at the sake of a pounding headache)? I'm completely clueless on this, and I *love* coffee, so any advice would be helpful.

DECAFFEINATED AND HATING IT

Dear Decaffeinated and Hating It,

Headaches are a normal response to an abrupt and drastic cut in the supply of caffeine to the system (i.e., your body). If you drink lots of coffee, or somehow provide your body with a steady, high supply of caffeine, with time, your body will develop a tolerance to caffeine. When you deprive your body of the caffeine it has grown accustomed to, your body struggles to cope with this sudden change. In the coping process, you end up with a pounding headache. Headaches, irritability, lethargy, nervousness, and mild depression are all fairly common withdrawal symptoms associated with cessation of caffeine intake.

Withdrawal symptoms from caffeine "detox" are nowhere near as severe as symptoms of withdrawal from other drugs. Although it does produce physical dependence, most of us would not identify caffeine as a dependency-producing drug.

As for your other issue, it's not a question of "if I do have some coffee . . ."—rather it's one of "can I have some coffee without having some more, and then maybe one more cup for the road?" Alice's point is that it's possible to drink a cup of coffee every now and then, or even one a day, without developing such a strong tolerance that your headaches will be back to haunt you on your first coffeeless morning. The key here is moderation. It's also important to be aware of the caffeine content of other beverages you drink, primarily teas and sodas. Make sure you're not substituting one form of caffeine for another.

If you really can't live without coffee, drink one cup of full strength and then switch to decaf for the rest of the day. Or, like Alice, make your pots half decaf and half caf (and use good coffees, like French Roast, Viennese, Yukon Gold . . . get the aroma?).

Bottoms up!

Alice

CAFFEINE, A STIMULANT CONSUMED BY AN ESTIMATED 90 PERCENT OF THE WORLD'S POPULATION, IS FOUND IN THESE PRODUCTS:

PRODUCT	CAFFEINE (IN MILLIGRAMS)
• Coffee [1 cup (8 oz.): brewed, dripped]	115
• Coffee (1 cup: percolated)	80
• Tea (iced, 12 oz. glass)	70
• Coffee (1 cup: instant)	65
• Caffeinated soft drinks (12 oz. glass, range of brands)	45–60
• Tea [1 cup (8 oz.): brewed]	40–60
• Milk chocolate candy bar (average size)	6
• Chocolate milk (8 oz. glass)	5
• Coffee (1 cup: decaffeinated)	3

FUN WITHOUT DRUGS?

Dear Alice,

I think it would be a good idea for me to stop smoking marijuana and cut down on my drinking, at least during the school year. The problem is, I have been doing it for so long it is almost as though I have forgotten how to have fun without it. Contributing to this problem is the fact that many of my friends smoke or drink to have fun. Many of my other friends just do not seem to have fun at all; they stay in Friday and Saturday nights to do work. I've found it difficult to quit, I think because I'm just not sure of what's out there to do that's fun without being stoned or drunk. Can you recommend anything that's fun whether you're intoxicated or sober, so that I don't have to stop hanging out with certain friends if I want to relax and have fun? I know, it's NYC and there are a *bazillion* things to do, so why am I bored? Well, another factor is expense—it costs around $20 to go to a nightclub, for example, and I don't really like "the scene." I want to finally enjoy life without relying on an altered state of consciousness. What's there to do when you're sick of renting movies? Also, any tips for resisting the urge to take people up on their offer to toke up? (I'm never pressured into it, but it's like the dieter who's offered some chocolate cake—it's there, it looks sooo good, and the fact that other people are doing it makes it seem more "okay.") Thanks so much.

Baked or Bored

Dear Baked or Bored,

It is exciting and refreshing to picture you at the beginning of your journey to fun and fulfillment without always tanking and toking up to reach this destination. You acknowledge at the outset that your trip (no pun intended) will be full of obstacles, challenges, temptations, and other potholes that might slow you down, or send you back to the starting line. Reducing any degree of psychological or physical dependence does not occur overnight, and can be realized through measured reductions in use of, in your case, alcohol and marijuana.

With your question to Alice, you have clearly begun to consult a map and ask for directions before your cast off. You don't have to stop here! Talking with a counselor at your school who can help you define specific goals, like how much you want to cut back, and at what pace, might also make for a smoother ride. Sharpening your awareness of your social, academic, professional, and spiritual interests can go a long way toward finding a few of those "bazillion" activities you mentioned. And make pit stops along the way, checking in with your counselor, or a supportive friend or relative, who can help you stay on course.

Tempting detours, like ever-present alcohol or that stray joint, might also be averted by some planning. Think about how you will respond if someone encourages you to have a drink or take a hit: maybe you could say, "Thanks, but I'm cutting back for a while," or "No, I have a big urine test tomorrow." Set limits for yourself (and state them to others, if appropriate) if you choose to place yourself in situations where alcohol and other drugs are present. Learning yoga, meditation, and other relaxation techniques have helped many on the same road to "dry fun" cope with stress resulting from this change in lifestyle, as well as provide motivation for improving mind-body health. Don't forget to consider physical exercise in this category, too.

As you may know, Alice is a big fan of searching for groups whose activities match some of your non-drug interests. Maybe organizations that work toward a cause in which you strongly believe, athletic groups, political campaigns, reading circles, writing and theatrical clubs, or professional organizations will be the ticket. These groups are usually free and full of people who fall somewhere between "drug-reliant" and "bookworm." Staying on this trail, how about activities where drugs just wouldn't quite cut it: working out at the gym (also free at most universities); museum hopping (most are heavily discounted for students with IDs); in-line skating or biking; taking tours of different NYC neighborhoods; or going up to the top of the Empire State Building or World Trade Center (natural highs, if you ask Alice). Peruse the New York City section of bookstores for publications about cheap and free offerings. Last, but not least, keep your eyes open for flyers and posters on bulletin boards for similar samplings.

If you are at a school or university, contact student activities for information about student organizations you can use as resources. If none of this works, you may have a different problem from the one you have described. Thanks for your question . . . and your perspective.   **RES**   Alice

Go to Alice at www.goaskalice.columbia.edu for more Alcohol, Nicotine, & Other Drugs Q & A's, including these:

- Alcohol and Liver Damage
- Difference between Pot and Hash
- Drinking Addiction—Psychological or Physical?
- Effects of Marijuana on Libido and Fertility
- Lightweight Drinker
- Little Sister Doing Coke?
- Low Tar and Nicotine Cigarette?
- LSD: Nirvana or Burnt Out?
- Marijuana and Sex
- More on Alcohol Tolerance
- Nauseated from Smoking
- Secondhand Marijuana Smoke and Drug Tests
- Spontaneous Tripping
- Supporting a Loved One After Drug Rehab
- Tested Positive for Cocaine, but Never Touched the Stuff
- Trying Psychedelics
- What Are Blunts?

GENERAL HEALTH QUESTIONS

From head to toe, Alice readers open the lines of discussion on some of the most typically troubling, but seldom-discussed, aspects of keeping a human body up and running. If you've found the other chapters eye-opening, you'll really hear yourself saying, "Gee, I always wondered about that," as you read this part. Alice will shed some light on a wide range of nitty-gritty issues, including headaches, athlete's foot, and most parts of the anatomy in between. Alice will also touch on the effects of some common over-the-counter offerings, including acne cleansers and creams.

But first, Alice will build on one piece of advice you've read often throughout this book: consult a health care provider. How do you choose a doctor or specialist after graduation? That's one of the most important decisions you'll make when school's behind you. Alice can help you change your view of health care providers, from sometimes seeming more like intimidating authority figures to sensitive, open-minded professionals working *for* you. If you're interested in becoming a more active, involved, and informed patient, then read through the *Patients' Bill of Rights*.

This chapter goes into general hygiene, too. "Gas mask" topics include body aroma (How often to bathe? What can be done to cut the stench of smelly feet? What causes someone to pass gas all day long?). You'll also learn how to control unwanted body hair, sunbathe more safely, and cut back on nail-biting. And for you avid nose-pickers, grab a tissue: Alice will share some advice you're not likely to find in the next issue of *Glamour* or *GQ*.

Alice will dig even deeper (into her medicine cabinet, that is) to find answers for those of you who want information about chronic hemorrhoids or ringing in the ears. She'll also recommend ways to relieve backache and eyestrain (especially useful for anyone who logs lots of hours at a desk studying or tapping away on a computer).

Throughout this chapter, you'll find references to stress-related symptoms as well. Mental health and physical health go hand in hand, so Alice's repertoire includes a menu of stress-reduction techniques, which not only boost your immune system, but could possibly keep you from getting gassy to boot. Getting a good night's sleep is a must for stress management, and Alice has information to help both insomniacs and sleepyheads.

This chapter couldn't possibly cover all of the glitches encountered by the mind-bogglingly complex human body, so Alice hopes you'll keep exploring the infinite range of information sources out there to learn more about any part of your body that's perplexing, painful, or just intriguing to you. In any case, keep in mind that the best specialist in maintaining your overall health is *you*.

Body Maintenance

After Graduation, How Do I Find a Doctor?

Alice,

After I graduate and move away from home, from town, from anyone I've ever known: how do I pick a doctor? How do I even *find* a doctor to pick?

Looking for a Doctor

Dear Looking for a Doctor,

These days, it's likely your health insurance will influence your choice of physician(s). For example, if you are a member of a health maintenance organization (HMO), you'll be given a list of primary health care doctors to choose from. You'll have to pick one as your Primary Care Physician (PCP). Some plans allow women to choose a gynecologist whom they can see once a year without having to see the PCP first. At any rate, ask people at work about the doctors in the plan. Look for one near your home or workplace. You can also find out if there is a college or university in the area. If there is one, call its medical school or teaching hospital for referrals in the community. Then, see if they're on your plan's list of doctors.

Once you have a few referrals that seem good to you, choose one and make an appointment to meet with him/her. If s/he seems competent, confident, and caring, then you've made a good choice.

Many health insurance companies provide the following important information if you ask for it:

- What specialty is the doctor in?
- Does the doctor practice by her/himself or in a group? If s/he practices in a group, can you request to see that doctor?
- Is the doctor involved in teaching medicine?

- What are the doctor's hours? Does s/he have evening or weekend appointments?
- What is the doctor's availability in emergencies?
- Will the doctor give advice over the phone?
- Is the doctor's office wheelchair-accessible?
- With which hospital is the doctor affiliated?
- What are the doctor's fees? Does s/he accept your insurance? Will s/he bill you or the insurance company?

To get the most out of your doctor's visit:

- Tell the receptionist why you are making the appointment.
- Tell the doctor why you're there, list your symptoms, and say what you're worried about. Be specific.
- Learn about your own medical history, such as dates of major or chronic illnesses, operations, hospitalizations, allergies, pregnancies, and physical and/or learning disabilities.
- Know the background of your family's health, including cancer, heart disease, high blood pressure, diabetes, genetic disorders, and alcohol or other drug abuse.
- Inform the doctor of any over-the-counter or prescription drugs, as well as vitamins, minerals, and other nutritional supplements you are taking. Bring the bottles or labels with you.
- Make sure your doctor hears and understands your symptoms and concerns. Make sure you know and understand your diagnosis and treatment.
- Tell your doctor about *any* changes in your life because they may affect your health. *Alice*

HEALTH CARE PROVIDERS INCLUDE:

- doctors
- nurses
- nurse practitioners
- psychiatrists
- psychologists
- mental health counselors
- registered dietitians or nutritionists
- social workers
- complementary, alternative, or integrated medicine specialists
- other clinicians, including gynecologists, obstetricians, midwives, and urologists

Doctor's Wrongs, Patient's Rights

Alice,
On a recent gynecological visit, I requested an HIV test. The doctor, a woman, responded with the question "Why, too many New York nights?" I was shocked by her response, but, because I felt intimidated by her, I disregarded her remark. After I told her that I had never been tested and thought it was time, she looked at me and said, "I think you're okay." Needless to say, I did not get tested by her.

During my exam, a Pap smear, she put on her rubber gloves and then realized that she couldn't find an instrument. So she rummaged through the drawer, went to the door and turned the knob, requested something from the nurse, closed the door, and proceeded with the exam. She never changed her gloves. I was appalled, but never said anything. I don't know why, but she totally intimidated me—one of those women who seem to have it all, brains, beauty, family, wealth, etc.

My question to you is, do I report this woman? If so, to whom? It happened several months ago and it was outside of NY state. I appreciate any reply. Thank you.

INTIMIDATED BY UNIFORMS

Dear Intimidated by Uniforms,
Alice agrees. It is difficult to be assertive with doctors. When you see a doctor, you are paying for a service, and ideally, at the moment, that doctor needs to act responsibly toward you. As difficult as it is, Alice encourages you to speak up. If after you speak up, the doctor is still unresponsive, Alice suggests you take your business and medical records elsewhere.

In terms of your recent experience, as a courtesy, you could inform the doctor of how you perceived her manner and delivery of services. You may write a letter or call the office, whichever is more comfortable for you.

Alice

Bathing—How Often?

Dear Alice,
How many times a week should one bathe?

Dear Reader,
Bathe or shower as regularly as you feel comfortable. How often is a matter of who you are as a person—your culture, gender, ethnicity, and/or where you live. Some people like to shower or bathe every day, and others do it less often.

THE PRECEPTS OF THE PATIENTS' BILL OF RIGHTS HOLD TRUE FOR ANY DOCTOR-PATIENT RELATIONSHIP.

THE PATIENT HAS THE RIGHT TO:

- Be treated fairly and openly in all matters, including sexual identity, race, gender, age, and socioeconomic status.
- Considerate, respectful, and confidential care.
- Obtain all information regarding his/her visit.
- Receive information necessary to give informed consent prior to the start of any office procedure and/or treatment.
- Refuse treatment and be informed of the medical consequences of his/her action.
- Receive a copy of his/her medical records, consistent with the state statutes on this matter.

(Adapted from *Patients' Bill of Rights*, New York State Hospital Code Law, New York State Department of Health—varies by state and province)

The main purposes of bathing or showering are to remove dirt and odors and slough off dead skin cells—basically, to maintain good hygiene. In addition, people bathe or shower to feel clean, smell fresh, and revitalize or relax.

Bathing or showering is a personal choice with social and cultural influences. People from other countries hold different views on personal hygiene and body aroma, none of which are right or wrong, only different. For example, Americans are smell-conscious and cleanliness-oriented ("cleanliness is next to godliness").

There may be times when other people will object, either by verbal or facial expression, to the way you smell and vice versa. If you are affected by this, and are living with someone or are in close quarters with other people on a regular basis, you may want to consider bathing more often (at least every other day), and bathing after any activity that involves perspiration.

If it weren't for the revolutionary changes in hygiene, sanitation, and the environment at the turn of the century in the United States, certain infectious diseases would continue to be a burden on the public health of our society. Alice is certain that good hygiene practices don't hurt one's social life either.

Alice

Body Aroma

Hey Alice,
What can be done about excessive body odor? I shower every day, yet sometimes, I catch a whiff of myself and it isn't pleasant.

SKUNKY

Dear Skunky,
Sweat glands, imbedded in your skin, produce a liquid as our body gets hot. Evaporation of the liquid cools the body, keeping your body's temperature regulated. This perspiration usually has a distinctive aroma, but it is not terribly offensive.

Offensive odor is caused by bacteria on your skin and clothing. The bacteria tends to survive in the warm, moist environment your armpit provides, for example. You said that you shower every day. How about using a deodorant or antiperspirant? The aluminum compounds in antiperspirants may be helpful in reducing the amount of sweat, limiting bacterial growth. In addition to, or instead of, deodorant, wash daily with antibacterial soaps. Shaving your armpits also tends to reduce odor. Prescription drugs that supposedly reduce sweating, such as those that contain aluminum chloride, whether applied to the skin or taken by mouth, may help some people. Your health care provider can also let you know if any new treatment techniques have been developed.

Alice

Flatulence

Dear Alice,
This is rather embarrassing, so I'm going to you for answers before I have to talk to anyone face to face about it. I have recently in the last two months developed a chronic gas problem. My stomach churns all day and night. To say the least, it is extremely embarrassing in class or in social situations. The other day I let one out in the middle of statistics and several people turned and looked at me. I have tried everything over the counter to put an end to the odorous problem. I haven't changed my diet in any significant way, so I'm really at a loss as to what would be causing this. What can I do?

SIGNED, FLATULENT

Dear Flatulent,
Okay, who among us hasn't "let one out" in a similar situation? Let them cast the first stone; of course, it's those people who turn and stare who have blamed their gaseous outbursts on the dog, their shoes, or their chair cushions.

Stomach upsets and gas usually can be attributed to excess food and alcohol, smoking, and certain kinds of food. You say you haven't changed your diet in any significant way, but maybe your body has changed in its ability to digest some of the foods in your diet. Think about your diet in terms of these foods that cause gas: beans, fruits (e.g., pears, apples, peaches), whole grains, veggies (e.g., broccoli, cabbage, onions, asparagus), milk and dairy products, carbonated drinks, some dietetic foods, sugar-free candies, and gum.

It sounds like you may be under more stress than usual right now. How you eat, versus what you eat, can affect intestinal gas, too. Are you taking enough time to eat at meals? Eating fast and not chewing your food thoroughly can cause you to take in too much air. So does chewing gum, eating hard candies, and smoking. More air going in equals more gas in the intestinal tract, and more air coming out.

To decrease gas, cut down on foods that cause gas and swallow less air when eating, chewing gum, etc. Eliminate foods that cause gas, one at a time, so that you'll be able to identify which ones make a difference. Start with the most likely foods first: milk and dairy, then beans, and then some of the others that Alice has listed. At the same time, concentrate on chewing your food well and on eating slowly. This may be a big drag if your daily schedule is hectic—but meals may become a welcome break in your day, instead of unwanted "breaks of wind."

Instead of the over-the-counter remedies you've used, try activated charcoal tablets or capsules available at health food stores. They may be effective for gas and upset stomach without knocking your bowel movements off balance.

Remember, too, that gas is normal. Many people think they have too much gas, mainly because of the social stigma attached to "letting one out" or belching in public. Use discretion, and, if worse comes to worse, say "excuse me" or go into another well-ventilated room before it happens, and, as a last resort, laugh, because the world is laughing with you.

Alice

Foot Odor

Dear Alice,

Thanks for the column and past advice. My wife recently began complaining of foot odor (her own). I suggested washing her feet several times a day and to use a deodorant. She's done this for about a week now but still complains about the odor. Please solve this dilemma. Thanks a bunch!

MARRIED TO BIGFOOT

Dear Married to Bigfoot,
Perspiration usually has a distinctive odor, but not an offensive one. Offensive odor could be caused by bacteria on skin and clothing. Your wife could wash her feet with antibacterial soap. If her feet are sensitive to one product, she can try another. Dusting cornstarch on her feet before getting into socks and shoes helps to keep them dry (moisture encourages bacteria to grow and flourish), or she can try soaking them daily in warm water with white vinegar or Epsom salts added.

Other tips include wearing cotton socks instead of nylons or other synthetic materials; changing the pads in the bottom of her shoes; wearing leather footwear; and a good, strong foot massage by a loving husband or partner to relax the feet. If the problem really bothers her, and she's tried various home remedies, a trip to the doctor could be in order.

Alice

Control Body Hair?

Dear Alice,
I'm only eighteen, but I have a lot of hair on my chest. I'm afraid of letting women see me with my shirt off because I don't want them to be turned off. How can I get rid of this rug and keep it under control without shaving daily? Also, is there a way to slow down my beard growth? Shaving more than once a day can be very irritating to my face, but I hate looking so dirty.

HARRY

Dear Harry,
If you still feel uncomfortable with the amount of hair you have, you could cut it, trim it, shave, wax, or use a chemical hair removal product. For beard growth, you may need to change your shaving cream or moisturizer and/or change your razor blade if you usually shave twice a day (which some men do). Talk with a health care provider about your hormone levels; or for other ideas about keeping your hair in check, make an appointment with your health care provider.

The truth is, the way you feel about your chest hair is up to you. Some women and men see a hairy man as masculine and sexy. They are turned on by thick body hair and an interesting hair pattern. It's truly a matter of individual taste.

Alice

Hairless Models: What's Their Secret?

Hey Alice,
How is it that all the guys I see in magazines and on TV have these per-

fectly hairless bodies? Most of us are not born with a smooth back, legs, and ass. What is it they use?

HAIRY AND CURIOUS

Dear Hairy and Curious,
Can you say waxing and computers? You're right: body hair removal isn't just for Olympic swimmers and cyclists anymore. A once quasi-weird practice reserved for increasing one's racing speed in a swimming pool or on a bike, it is now splashed on almost every ad featuring male skin from the neck down. Many male models (and nonmodels, for that matter) have their body hair professionally removed (waxed) because . . . well, someone on Madison Avenue must have decided that this look should be in. Or is it that bald boys appear more muscular and Adonislike, thus sparking a trend (i.e., Michael Jordan)? Who knows?

But don't be fooled, Alice's hairy and curious reader—computer technology also now makes hair removal, as well as skin blemish cover-up, wrinkle-smoothing, tanning, and even face and body proportion alterations, including fat reduction, possible with the simple click of a mouse (don't try this at home, kids). Some ads and movies even pass off two or three humans as one. What? Yes, part your nose hair and smell the coffee: computers enable body parts to be pieced together to make the "perfect" puzzle. If a supermodel's breasts or basket aren't so "super," they can easily be replaced by those of full-cupped gals and guys. The irony here is that advertisers try to convince us that we should look like these models who aren't all there themselves. Alice is sure you get the picture: No one's perfect, and that's okay.

Maybe the new millennium will bring a dramatic reaction to the current cutbacks: chest and pubic hair corn-rowing, perhaps. Until then, be a smart media consumer: Don't believe everything you see.

Alice

Nail Biting

Alice,
I have bitten my nails for as long as I can remember. It is a very nervous habit, and, obviously, made worse by stress. After graduation, I would like to make my first real effort to stop. Judging by the condition of my fingernails now, however, I do not think this will just be a matter of "letting them grow." They are hopelessly thin and soft, not to mention misshapen. I know it would help if I began my efforts with a professional manicure, but I am afraid a professional manicurist would run screaming out of the salon if asked to work on my hands. I am wondering if there are any resources available for nail-biters, or nail salons which specialize in treating them. I am trying to find something

more than the traditional drugstore products. Also, if you have any advice on breaking such a tough habit, I would be happy to hear it. Thank you.

Edward Scissorhands

Dear Edward Scissorhands,
Your idea of going for manicures is smart. Manicurists have undoubtedly seen all kinds of cuticles in crisis. Ask their advice. One suggestion they'll probably have is to use a clear polish, which can be buffed to look natural.

Taking care of your nails in this way can have positive results for you since it helps develop pride and a healthy change in behavior. Stress management techniques can also help, as can hypnosis for some people.

Alice

Nose Picking

Dear Alice,
I am an avid nose-picker. Is this bad for my nose?

Nose-picker

Dear Nose-picker,
Thanks for sharing. Sure, some will say, "Alice, must you post and respond to such an obscure and disgusting question?" Alice says yes, because like many other touchy topics and matters that are close to home, nose picking is a more common pastime than most folks, big and small, would like to admit. Alice bets some of you are picking and clicking right now! Besides, this act, however revolting it may seem, carries health risks that compel Alice to take a swipe at your inquiry.

Because the nose, mouth, throat, and sinuses are fertile territory for the development of infections, your picking finger can act like the Space Shuttle, delivering bacteria from a door knob or public telephone, let's say, directly into your body. (Of course, this route of transit works in the reverse direction, too.) Cuts in the nasal passage are another hazard that can result from your fingernails, whether they're well-clipped or not. Even microscopic lacerations that draw no visible blood can open the door even wider to bacteria and infections. Avid nose-pickers, such as yourself, may see more pimples in and around the nose due to increased oil deposits from the fingers. For a very small minority of the nostril-inclined, the consequences of their behavior have been nothing to sneeze at. Alice knows of one vigorous young nose-picker who broke a blood vessel that required cauterization (a burning process that deadens tissue) to halt the bleeding that resulted. And she never picked again.

So far, Alice has focused on possible self-inflicted nose-picking consequences, but what about secondhand effects? Alice would bet that most people, even closeted nose-pickers, would not relish watching others picking, or, God forbid, dipping, sticking, or flicking. Public pickers everywhere (as well as belchers and spitters too, for that matter), keep this in mind.

As always, safer nose picking is best done with a tissue. But if you must pick without protection: wash up, go easy, and keep it to yourself.

Alice

Could It Be ... Hemorrhoids?

Dear Alice,
I have this problem and I am too embarrassed to ask a doctor about it. I am a nineteen-year-old male and have this growth in my anus. It popped up about one week ago. It is about the size of a pea. Could it be hemorrhoids? If not, what can it be? Should I be worried, and what should I do about it?

THANK YOU, PEA-BOY

Dear Pea-Boy,
Although it can be embarrassing, it is important for you and your peace of mind to get your anal bump diagnosed by a health care provider. For example, if it is a wart, you do not have to treat it with a hemorrhoid medication.

Hemorrhoids, enlarged veins in the lower rectum and anus, are common and not serious. Straining to have a bowel movement, constipation, a low-fiber diet, pregnancy, overuse of laxatives, and prolonged sitting can cause hemorrhoids. Once hemorrhoids develop, they tend to persist, although they may not cause major problems. Discomfort and swelling may come and go, usually lasting between three to five days.

Common symptoms of hemorrhoids include:

- pain or itching near the growth in the anus
- bright red blood at the end of a bowel movement or on the toilet paper
- excessively moist anal area

If you have hemorrhoids, try the following to alleviate symptoms:

- Apply cold compresses of witch hazel for ten minutes, three to four times a day.
- Use an ice bag for ten minutes.
- Soak for ten to fifteen minutes in a warm bath a few times a day.

- Lay on your stomach or back instead of sitting on the old rear end.
- After a bowel movement, pat with toilet paper or gently wipe with witch hazel pads.
- Avoid scratching, which often increases discomfort.
- Stay away from anti-itch creams and lotions with "-caine" in their names—the local anesthetic in these products can make the irritation worse.
- Don't use products that advertise the ability to shrink swollen hemorrhoids because they're not very effective.
- Have larger hemorrhoids surgically removed or medically treated.

Either way, add fiber (such as fruits, vegetables, whole grains, beans, nuts, and peas) and lots of fluids (at least two quarts of water and juices) to your diet. Fiber adds bulk and moisture to the stool. If you want to increase fiber in your diet, do it slowly—too much fiber at once can cause gas and stomach cramping. Exercising regularly may help because it improves abdominal muscle tone and makes bowel movements more regular and frequent. If you are significantly overweight, weight loss can also help.

Remember, don't strain too hard or sit on the toilet for too long in order to have a bowel movement. On the other hand, if you gotta go—go! Holding the stool in the bowel tends to make it become hard and dry, and then it may be difficult to excrete.

Alice

Computer Hazards

Alice,
What is an unhealthy amount of time to spend in front of a computer terminal? It seems like everything I do, from workstudy work to classwork to play, entails sitting in front of a computer terminal for hours on end. Any feedback on this would be much appreciated.

GOING BLIND, STERILE, OR OTHERWISE?

Dear Going Blind, Sterile, or Otherwise?,
Since you're still going to work and class, and presumably eating and seeing your friends, these are good signs that you are not spending all of your time in front of a computer terminal. Eye care specialists have noticed problems related to extensive use of video display terminals (VDTs). If you are farsighted, you may experience blurred vision and discomfort while using a VDT. If you have astigmatism, working at a VDT can cause aching eyes, headache, and fatigue.

Another common problem associated with computer work is repetitive stress injury (RSI), such as carpal tunnel syndrome. RSIs occur when a certain muscle or tendon is repeatedly overused or kept in an awkward position. If you spend long hours at a computer, you might want to take some of the following steps to prevent RSIs:

- Use a firm, adjustable, and comfortable chair. Adjust chair height so that your thighs are horizontal, your feet flat on the floor, and the backs of your knees are slightly higher than the seat of your chair. The back of the chair should support your lower back. Stretch your lower back by standing up and pulling each knee to your chest, holding that position for a few seconds.
- Relax your shoulders. Your upper arms and forearm should form a right angle, with your wrist and hand in roughly a straight line.
- Use the computer as you would play the piano, with fingers up and down. Don't rest your wrists and move your fingers sideways to type.
- Position the mouse at the same height as your keyboard. When you slide the mouse around, move your entire arm and not just your wrist.
- Take breaks of at least five to ten minutes every hour or so.

"Playing" can happen off-line, too, so make sure your social life is balanced with real friends and activities—not just virtual ones.

Alice

SIGHT SAVERS

- Take frequent breaks.
- Reduce glare and reflections—clean your screen and block out excessive sunlight and reflections of lamps, etc., from the screen.
- Maintain high contrast between characters and screen background—use indirect room lighting.
- Prevent eyestrain—the top of your screen needs to be at, or slightly below, eye level; find a comfortable distance between your eyes and the screen (usually eighteen to twenty-eight inches).
- Gently massage your eyes, cheeks, forehead, etc., from time to time to keep blood flowing and muscles loose.

Loud Music and Ear-Ringing

Dear Alice,
I went to a club one night and the music was really loud. I've been going to clubs for a while now and the loud music usually makes my ears ring, but the ringing usually disappears in the morning. Well, this time, the ringing has lasted for several days. Is this a problem I should be worried about?

Dear Reader,
The ringing you hear could be tinnitus. Tinnitus, often associated with hearing loss, causes a ringing, buzzing, or other noise heard in the ear in the absence of any outside noises that can be annoying, irritating, bothersome, and/or infuriating to the person affected. Tinnitus can also be a symptom of other hearing and ear disorders.

Listening to loud music at concerts and clubs, or at home with headphones, can lead to temporary or permanent loss of hearing, sometimes referred to as "rock-and-roll deafness."

Perhaps the music on one night was particularly loud, you stayed longer than usual, you were near the amplifiers, or there's already some ear damage, and that's why the ringing in your ears lasted longer than it normally does. See your health care provider since you've noticed a change.

If you have tinnitus, your ears would benefit from not listening to loud music and noises. However, if music and the club scene are a significant part of your life, you may find it difficult to go to clubs less often. In that case, use disposable earplugs, which come in a variety of shapes, sizes, textures, and colors. To reduce the risk of an ear infection, replace your earplugs with a new pair after a few wears. Also, position yourself away from the amplifiers.

Finally, consider the usually smoky atmosphere at clubs and concerts. Some medical literature supports the association between smoking and hearing loss. RES

Alice

Do I Have a Learning Disability?

Dear Alice,
I am a college student who reads your page frequently. I wanted to know if there was some test that I could do to see if I have a learningdisability. I have a hard time reading and understanding things, and many times must read a sentence several times to understand it. I also very frequently read things wrong (like mixing up two sentences in a book—that is, taking words from two adjacent lines and mixing them

up). I also sometimes have difficulty hearing properly (I'm not sure if this is significant). And lastly, I have a hard time concentrating on one thing. I would like to find out whether I do have some sort of disability as this serves as a great deal of frustration for me.

THANK YOU, TRYING TO UNDERSTAND

DECIBEL (dB) DATA

- Normal conversation: 65 dB
- Live concert: 120 dB
- Pain threshold for average human ear: 130 dB

Dear Trying to Understand,

Learning disabilities include many of the characteristics that you experience. Learning disabilities are included in the Americans with Disabilities Act (ADA)—this means that, in most cases, academic, professional, and commercial institutions must provide "reasonable accommodations" to help disabled people perform to their potential.

Learning disabilities are usually identified through a series of standardized IQ (intelligence quotient) tests and psychoeducational and neuropsychological measures, as well as tests of basic academic achievement (e.g., tests of reading comprehension and reading rate). Your college may have an office of disability services that might either administer these tests or refer students to area testing services. Most public and private schools (K–12 and post-secondary) have services for people with disabilities, including testing and rehabilitation. Check the phone book under "disabilities," ask your health care provider for resources, or call the Association on Higher Education and Disability (AHEAD).

If you do have a learning disability, your school's disabilities services office (if your college has one) may work with you to make your reading, studying, and test-taking easier and more productive. Before taking the previously mentioned tests, make an appointment with a counselor at your school's counseling service. While a counselor cannot determine if you have a learning disability without formal testing, an initial screening may help you rule out, or rule in, other factors that contribute to learning difficulties, and assess the appropriateness of a formal evaluation. Talk to your health service about getting your hearing tested, as this may play a part in your inability to concentrate. This may sound like a lot to do, but once you get the appropriate diagnosis and help you deserve, your frustration will diminish and the quality of your life will improve.

Bravo to you for investigating your concerns and for considering the many resources available to you. **RES**

GOOD LUCK,
Alice

Always Tired

Dear Alice,

I'm always tired. I get plenty of rest (at least eight hours a night), eat healthy, and exercise regularly. I went to my doctor and he took blood only to conclude that I am perfectly healthy. But every day, I am exhausted constantly to the point that if affects my everyday activities. Any suggestions as to what I can do?

Dear Reader,

Glad to hear you went to your doctor to investigate your chronic tiredness. You covered many of the bases that Alice would have suggested: sleep, diet, exercise, and blood tests that check for anemia, hypoglycemia, Epstein-Barr virus, mononucleosis, Lyme disease, and other serious energy-drainers. You might consider seeking a second medical opinion.

You did not mention your psychological health. Are you pleased with your home life, job, friends, mates, finances, etc? Even occasional and mild sadness, not to mention stress, can cause prolonged fatigue. Dysthymia, the clinical diagnosis for mild depression, is common and claims tiredness as one of its primary symptoms. Mild and more serious forms of depression affect millions of people of all ages in every career, financial bracket, and lifestyle. Unfortunately, only a fraction of depressed people seek help in the form of counseling and/or medication. For too long, this common and highly treatable disorder has been stigmatized by our society, and unfairly dismissed as moodiness and laziness.

You may not be "down and out" or depressed, but Alice thinks it's worthwhile for everyone to think about these issues now and then. Talking with a counselor can be useful.

Alice

Energy Boosters

Dear Alice,

I lack energy. What tips can you give me to increase my energy levels?

Dear Reader,

First, rule out any medical conditions that could be making you feel de-energized. Here are some energy boosting tips to help you feel more like that battery-powered bunny:

Sleep: Get an adequate amount of sleep each and every night. Although this varies from person to person, try to sleep at least seven or eight hours a night. In addition, depending on the individual, "power" naps may either revive you or leave you feeling more tired. In the latter case, add that nap time to your nightly sleep so you will wake up feeling more rested.

Exercise: Exercise regularly three to four times a week for at least thirty minutes each time, but preferably every day for thirty minutes. Exercise may make you feel tired initially if you have not exercised or do not exercise regularly, but your body will adjust and feel more invigorated. Exercise outdoors, not only to get away from the sweaty smell of gyms, but also to breathe in fresh air and get some sun, which can help energize you (and make exercise seem less of a burden and more enjoyable).

Eat: Consume enough calories from a varied and healthy diet. Add more fresh fruits and vegetables to your diet, and also eat more complex carbohydrates, which will provide you with sustaining energy. Eat fewer simple carbohydrates (sugar from candy, for example), which give you a quick burst of energy, but soon leave you feeling tired from the sugar blues (hypoglycemia).

Enjoy Yourself!: Let your friends, partner(s), and family members know of your need to be energized so they can help motivate you to get involved and become more active. Their encouragement and support will help you follow through with your revitalization program. Also, being preoccupied can leave you stressed out and exhausted (physically and mentally). Instead, do something you enjoy. Have fun while improving your physical and emotional energy levels to help lift your spirits.

Lastly, another great energy booster you may want to try is meditation. (See 263.)

Carpe diem!

Alice

Meditation

Dear Alice,
How do you learn to meditate?

Dear Reader,
Meditation is a two-thousand-year-old technique that originated in the Far East as a means of communicating with one's spiritual and religious gods. Since then, it has taken many different forms—some still maintaining a religious connection, while others having only relaxation as a goal. Whatever the type, almost all forms of this ancient discipline are woven with the common thread of focused attention on a repetitive, or unchanging, sound or image.

No one really knows why this seemingly simple process produces increased energy, improved quality of sleep, greater resistance to common stressors, heightened concentration, greater dream recall, and other rewards for individuals who meditate every day. Meditation is challenging for most who try it; and it may not be the best relaxation technique if you can't sit still when you're not meditating. But it certainly doesn't hurt to give meditation a try. Sometimes practice makes perfect.

More and more universities, hospitals, health clubs, adult education programs, and corporations are offering meditation classes as acceptance of complementary medicine increases by leaps and bounds in the West. Call around to find the program that best suits your interests and schedule. For example, there are formal meditation programs that require a few weeks of time, and a few hundred dollars to register. Other one-time, low-cost classes provide, at a minimum, an introduction to meditation. If you are a student, your school or college may offer a stress management program that could include meditation. Or call your local YM/YWCA or community center. Meditation books and tapes are also available at major and alternative bookstores.

Here's a basic meditation guide:

(1) Choose a quiet place. Limit potential distractions by putting a "Do Not Disturb" sign on your door, unplugging your phone, and switching on a fan to block outside noise.

(2) Sit in a chair with firm lower back support and rest your feet on the floor. Or, sit on the floor with your back against a wall and legs uncrossed.

(3) Choose a simple word or sound, like *ing* (also called a *mantra*). You will repeat this sound to yourself during your meditation session.

(4) Close your eyes and sit quietly for one or two minutes. Then, begin to repeat your mantra in a rhythmic and relaxed way. You will soon realize that you are no longer reciting the mantra: this is fine, as it is impossible to keep your attention focused on any one thing for more than a very short time. At this point, once again, calmly bring your mantra back into focus.

(5) Try this *meditation cycle* for ten to twenty minutes, once a day— always before a meal, like breakfast or dinner. If you benefit from meditation (this can take a few weeks of regular practice), you can expand it to twenty to thirty minutes, twice daily.

(6) Use a silent clock, or watch, to time your meditation; and remain seated for at least a minute before you rise from your chair or the floor. (adapted from *The Stress Manager's Manual with Cassette Trainer* by Jordan Friedman)

If this process seems weird and/or complicated, know that it produces real benefits, and it gets easier over time.

Ing, ing, ing. . . .　　**RES**

Alice

Colds, Aches, and Pains

Cold Won't Go Away

Dear Alice,
I have been under quite a bit of stress lately and cannot seem to shake a cough and swollen gland. Every time I start to feel better, it starts all over again. Also, I hate to admit this, but I smoke. Do you think the stress has anything to do with the long period of time I seem to have had this "cold"? It's been going on about two months.

Dear Reader,
Even if you are a smoker and stressed out, two months is unusually long to have the "common" cold. Because your cold has lasted for so long, it could be sinusitis, bronchitis, walking pneumonia, a lung infection, allergies, or something else. People can have "consecutive colds"—never really feeling better—which seem like one *long* cold. See your health care provider to find out the cause of your symptoms and the best treatment(s).

Smokers can experience colds of longer duration, increased severity, and with more complications. This may be a good time for you to quit smoking.

Stress could also be a factor because it increases susceptibility to illness by suppressing your immune system. Stress-reduction therapies, such as aerobic exercise, meditation, yoga, and tai-chi, could help boost your energy levels and immune response. Regular exercise and rest can also be of some benefit.

Alice

What to Do for Headaches?

Alice,
What do I have to do to get rid of my headache?

THROBBING

Dear Throbbing,
Headaches can have many causes: tension, sinus, eyestrain, migraine, vascular (increased blood flow), or a brain tumor in *rare* cases. In addition, there are many kinds of pain: shooting, throbbing, dull, constant, sharp, etc.

Depending on the frequency and severity of your headaches, the following information may be useful:

Self-Care Tips for Headaches

- Apply ice packs or heat on your neck and head.
- Gently massage the muscles of your neck and scalp.
- Use relaxation exercises.
- Take aspirin, or an aspirin substitute, such as ibuprofen or acetaminophen.
- Use a decongestant medication, if you have nasal congestion.
- Reduce emotional and physical stressors, such as anger, eyestrain, or continuous loud noise.
- Avoid foods that may trigger headaches, such as aged cheeses, chocolate, nuts, red wine, alcohol, avocados, figs, raisins, or pickled foods.

Hope you find some relief. If none of these work, see a health care provider who can help you determine a cause and manage the pain. S/he might refer you to a headache clinic.

Alice

HEADACHE ALERT

SEE A PHYSICIAN IMMEDIATELY IF:

- You have an unusually severe headache.
- Your headache is accompanied by fever and a very stiff neck.
- You have had a recent head injury, and are experiencing slurred speech, visual disturbances, and/or numbness in your face, arms, or legs.
- Your headaches persist for more than three days, or increase in severity or frequency.

Tense Back

Dear Alice,
The muscles in my back become extremely tense/tight throughout the term as I am cramped down studying all the time. What should I do?

Posturing?

Dear Posturing?,
Stress and discomfort in your back are signals to you to change your posture or position for sleeping, lifting, sitting, etc. Emotional tension, strenuous activities, and poor posture when standing, sitting, or lying down can strain muscles and ligaments in the back and cause pain.

When you are sitting and studying, your lower back needs to be flat or slightly rounded outward. Your knees need to be slightly higher than your hips, with both feet planted firmly on the floor. A footrest can help keep your knees at a comfortable position. Be sure your computer setup is comfortable for your eyes, arms, and back as well.

When you're studying, take frequent breaks and stretch your body every fifteen or twenty minutes. Also, rest your eyes and change your position often. If you're in pain, see a health care provider.

Alice

CHECK YOUR POSTURE

1. Stand with your back to a wall. Press your heels, backside, shoulders, and head against the wall. If you feel any space between the small of your back and the wall, your back is arched too much.
2. Move your feet forward and bend your knees so that your back slides a few inches down the wall. Now tighten your abdominal and buttocks muscles so that you can flatten your lower back against the wall.
3. Hold this position and "walk" your feet back so that you slide up the wall.
4. Standing straight, walk away from the wall and around the room.
5. Return to the wall and back up to it to make sure you've kept proper posture.

Mono?

Alice,
My roommate infected me with some kind of virus that he had (actually still has it) and I got over it in one day. He, on the other hand, went out with his friends, drank insanely, stayed out all night, and consequently got sicker and sicker. Now, he's left for a few days to recover at home. I was wondering, since he got so sick (he was ill for over eight days, was coughing, vomiting, etc.), is it possible that he may have contracted mono, or even pneumonia? And if it is, should I be concerned for myself?

SIGNED, CURIOUS

Dear Curious,
Alice definitely can't diagnose your friend's illness through your letter, but his symptoms do not appear to match mono. It sounds as though he needs a trip to his health care provider.

Infectious mononucleosis (or mono) is caused by the Epstein-Barr virus. In developed countries, where individuals are not exposed as children, the peak years for mono infection are fourteen to eighteen (most adults are probably immune). The period during which mono is contagious is not completely clear. Most people with mono don't know where or from whom they got it. Although it used to be called the "kissing disease," mono is probably spread by close contact (not necessarily sexual) with an infected person, and symptoms appear approximately three weeks after contact. Symptoms include severe sore throat with a painful swelling of lymph nodes in the neck, lethargy, a fever, and, occasionally, a rash. An enlarged spleen (on the left side in your abdomen) may also develop and can be dangerous. Antibiotics have no effect on the disease, which is usually self-limited. This means that the person will get better without any intervention. Infected people may be troubled by fatigue for weeks, or even for several months. However, mono does not deserve its reputation as a prolonged illness. *Most* people get better quickly, often within two weeks, and some people have such a mild case that they are hardly sick at all.

Pneumonia, on the other hand, is a viral, bacterial, or even fungal infection that causes fever, shortness of breath, a persistent cough, and chest pains. Pneumonia is hard to catch from another person unless s/he coughs on you a lot.

You were perceptive in noticing the dramatic difference between the two courses of illness (yours and your friend's). You and your roommate could have had the same virus. You could have had different viruses. Immune response can definitely be influenced by lifestyle and behaviors. Research has shown that the number of T-cells (cells that carry out immune response) rises and falls inversely with stress. Stress ranges from emotional stressors, such as anger, anxiety, depression, and grief, to physical stressors, such as poor nutrition, sleep deprivation, overexertion, smoking, drinking, and other drug use. Your experience, combined with research, makes it clear that if one starts to feel a bit sick, s/he is better off taking it easy right from the beginning, instead of pushing oneself and risking a recurring, or prolonged, illness.

If you continue to feel okay, you probably don't have much to worry about—even when your roommate returns. Try to stay healthy by managing your stress, eating well, and keeping your hands clean, to name a few key strategies.

Alice

Lyme Disease vs. Chronic Fatigue

Alice,

I'm wondering about Lyme disease and chronic fatigue syndrome—the differences and similarities?

TIRED

Dear Tired,

Lyme disease and chronic fatigue syndrome (CFS) are two completely different conditions. Lyme disease is caused by a specific organism transmitted to humans by the bite of certain ticks. The tick is most commonly found living on deer and mice. The disease is most common in the northeastern and midwestern United States, but has also been reported in other parts of the United States and abroad.

Lyme disease usually is not difficult to recognize, particularly if there is a rash. The rash has a reddish bull's-eye or red spot appearing at the site of the tick bite that gradually expands into a larger reddened area, which can be several inches across. Other symptoms of Lyme disease at this stage can include flulike symptoms, fever, headache, and lethargy. Untreated, or unsuccessfully treated, people may experience complications of Lyme disease weeks to months after contact with the tick, including such things as partial facial paralysis, heart rhythm abnormalities, and arthritis, as the nervous, cardiovascular, and musculoskeletal systems are affected.

Exposure to Lyme disease can be indicated by a blood test; however, the blood test can still show up as positive after treatment. Lyme disease is treated with antibiotics. Once inflammation has set in, anti-inflammatory drugs, in addition to the antibiotics, are used to treat the condition. If the disease goes untreated, or is unsuccessfully treated, it can last for years. In pregnant women, Lyme disease may cause fetal damage or death to the fetus at any stage of the pregnancy, but this rarely happens.

Chronic fatigue syndrome, on the other hand, has an unknown cause and no known cure. Laboratory tests cannot confirm its presence in an individual. Diagnosis of CFS consists of identifying symptoms, ruling out diseases with similarities (such as lupus), a physical examination, and a patient history. CFS may be confused with depression as well. CFS is characterized by severe and debilitating fatigue and muscle pains that can persist for months or years, as well as mild fever, sore throat, painful lymph nodes, sleep disturbances, headaches, confusion, and forgetfulness. CFS affects previously healthy, active people with no history of the symptoms described.

The first episode of chronic fatigue syndrome is often the worst in terms of its debilitating nature; and CFS can significantly affect people's capacity to function, interfering with working and socializing. In the mid-1980s, CFS was referred to as "yuppie flu"; but over time, it gained legitimacy as a physical illness through continued in-depth research by both the National Institutes of Health (NIH) and the Centers for Disease Control and Prevention (CDC). Many people with CFS are viewed with skepticism by their family, friends, colleagues, and even health care providers, since many people question whether the syndrome actually exists, and many people who have some of the symptoms do not have CFS. This can add a psychological strain to an already confusing situation.

Fatigue could also be caused by an iron deficiency (especially in women), stress, insufficient sleep, a poor diet, alcohol or other drug abuse, or an inactive lifestyle.

For more information about Lyme disease, you can contact the Lyme Disease Foundation or the National Organization for Rare Disorders. For information on chronic fatigue syndrome, call the Chronic Fatigue and Immune Dysfunction Syndrome (CFIDS) Association of America. Also, various support groups exist to help validate and share symptoms, treatments, feelings, successes, and resources. **RES**

Alice

Skin Conditions

Antibiotics and Acne

Dear Alice,
I am a high school student, and have gotten acne. I got it for more than two years, and would like to find a way to cure it. I currently use Neutrogena's Acne face wash, Neutrogena's overnight acne treatment, and some face washers. They have decreased, but I really want them to be gone.

I also read that fatty foods don't contribute to acne, but in any case, I still eat low-fat foods for healthy reasons.

I hope you can help me. Thanks a lot for your help.

ANXIOUS ABOUT ACNE

Dear Anxious about Acne,
With the onset of adolescence, the body is bombarded with hormonal changes. The sebaceous glands (glands in our skin that produce and excrete sebum, a fluid that helps keep our skin lubricated) often overproduce sebum. The end result is the enlargement and clogging of the glands of the face, shoulders, chest, and back; and a pimple or blackhead is formed.

Over-the-counter products, such as those you mentioned, are sufficient for many people to control their acne. Generally, these products come in only one strength or dosage, which may work for a while (or not at all), but, in the future, may fail to control acne. If these don't work, stronger medications are available. Ask your health care provider or dermatologist. Be aware that one visit may not be enough to remedy your acne. Acne medications tend to affect people differently depending on skin type, classification, and severity of acne. You may, therefore, need to experiment with a few treatments before finding the "formula" that works for you.

Astringents, benzoyl peroxides, retinoic acids, and glycolic acids all work to prevent pores from clogging. Antibiotics, either taken orally or applied topically, can be used to control some types of acne. For really bad cases of acne, talk with your health care provider about stronger medications. If you are a woman, certain birth control pills may help, too. Dermatologic surgery, such as incision and drainage or freezing, can also help unclog and clear pores, as well as reduce inflammation.

You're right, it is a myth that certain foods, like chocolate or potato chips, will induce and/or aggravate acne. However, if you notice that your acne flares up more often when you eat a particular food, then don't eat it. It is also a myth that dirt causes acne, and that scrubbing your face with a buffer will help control it.

Alice

ACNE CONTROL AND PREVENTION SUGGESTIONS

HERE ARE SOME TIPS TO KEEP YOUR PORES CLEAN AND OPEN:
- Avoid oil-based cosmetics and/or facial lotions—look for products labeled "non-comedogenic."
- If you wear a headband, baseball hat, and/or helmet when you exercise or play sports, make sure you wash the sweat-soaked things each time you wear them.
- Stress also plays a role in pimple promotion, so try to reduce it in ways that work best for you.

"Cure" for Cellulite?

Dear Alice,

My sister has cellulite, especially in her legs. She went to one of these health clubs to look for a treatment and they put her on something like "lymphatic draining," and gave her some type of algae (Asiatic star or something like that), which is in a spray form that she has to apply to her legs once a week, and in pills once a day. The lymphatic draining worked as follows: they put a gel on her legs and then they covered them with a pair of "air trousers" which was inflating and deflating periodically, like massaging her legs.

Do you have any idea what this is about? Do these treatments really work? I mean, do they eliminate the fat accumulated on local spots, or do they merely "redistribute" it? Thank you.

Dear Reader,

Cellulite is fat—plain ol' ordinary fat. What is termed "cellulite" is actually a dimpling effect of fat caused by the way fat cells lie in or between connective tissue in the body, primarily in the hips-thighs-buttocks region. Connective tissue extends from the skin to the muscle below. Fat cells, especially when they get bigger, "push up" against the tissue to create the dimpling.

Regardless of whether or not it is deemed unsightly and abnormal, cellulite is normal for many adult women, and some men. The dimpling effect is less obvious in people who have thicker skin, like men and some women. The thickness of skin is determined by our genes. Skin tends to become thinner with age, and we cannot do anything to change it.

Your sister's treatment probably tightens the skin briefly to reduce the appearance of cellulite; that is what all the creams and lotions you can buy over the counter will do. Lymphatic draining sounds very medical and technical—the truth is that the body does its own lymphatic draining without the help of air trousers, and this has nothing to do with the dimpling effect of fat cells in a person's thighs. Cellulite is fat, and it seems to be harder to lose than other areas of fat on the body; this may stem from the way fat cells are embedded in connective tissues. To reduce the amount of fat that is absorbed, stored, or burned by the body eat less fat, consume fewer calories, and exercise.

Alice

CELLULITE: FACT OR FICTION?

The term "cellulite" came to the United States via *Vogue* magazine in the early 1970s. Before that time, cellulite was simply known as fat, and was considered a normal feature of adult female skin.

Almost twenty years ago, the *Journal of the American Medical Association (JAMA)* stated that "there is no medical condition known or described as cellulite in this country." Not being a medical condition or problem, can there be a cure or treatment? Apparently, yes, as is evidenced by the bazillion-dollar industry that supplies creams, gels, lotions, pills, various treatments, and even surgery (liposuction) to rid, or "cure," the body of cellulite. It may not be a bona fide medical problem—in fact, it's quite natural—but cellulite has certainly been made into a cosmetic problem of the worst degree.

Dry Skin and Eczema Help

Alice:

I have a long history of severely uncomfortable and troubling eczema. During the worst outbreaks, I have visited several different dermatologists, and all have prescribed topical hydrocortisones, such as Hytone or Topicort, as well as anti-itching pills, such as Atarax. One prescribed Diprolene ointment, which I used for a year, until my next dermatologist dismissively told me it was far too strong and could be damaging.

I would like to know once and for all how damaging the extensive and long-term use of any of these creams is. Please give me one of your straightforward answers; I have been frustrated by the differing views and lack of concern among the dermatologists I have visited. I am tired of being told it is "just eczema." I already use the gentlest cleansing products available, tons of moisturizing cream, rinse all my clothes twice, wear soft fabrics, etc. I am still absolutely tortured by itching, often resorting to scratching at my skin with a hairbrush. The eczema reappears without fail in the same places, even on my face, and is particularly bad after stress periods, when I absolutely cannot control my itching or scratching. Isn't there anyone anywhere doing research on this? Is there anything else I can try? I am not averse to vitamin, holistic, or homeopathic therapies, if there are any. Please help. This is really a very ugly and upsetting problem.

HELPLESSLY ITCHY

Dear Helplessly Itchy,

Eczema (a.k.a. "atopic dermatitis") is a skin disease with red, blistering, oozing, scaly, brownish, thickened, and itchy skin lesions. Eczema runs in families with allergies, such as hay fever or asthma. Eczema causes constant itching in a vicious itch-scratch-rash-itch cycle. Stress, dry skin, environmental temperature and/or humidity changes, bacterial skin infections, and wool and synthetic garments often make the condition worse.

No one knows what causes eczema. There is no cure, but several treatments for eczema are available. It is impossible to know exactly how any one treatment will affect each and every patient. Treatment involves a good deal of trial and error.

Corticosteroid creams or ointments applied topically are the most effective medications known. They vary widely in strength, however (the first two you name are quite mild hydrocortisones, whereas the last treatment you mention is strong and can be damaging). The major hazard of topical steroids is skin atrophy. This results from regular use of stronger creams, especially on the face, but this would be unusual with hydrocortisone. The other problem with long-term use is potential ineffectiveness after a time, which can be avoided by using simple emollients (moisturizers) for a week or more, after which the cream may again become effective.

Emollients, sedating antihistamines at night, antibiotics, bandaging, and avoidance of irritants, such as certain detergents, clothing, fabrics, perfumes, dyes, and metals, among other things, are other treatments. Phototherapy—exposure to ultraviolet radiation in gradually increasing increments—and a diet which eliminates potentially irritating foods can help some people. The most common foods eliminated are nuts, tomatoes, milk, eggs, and cereals. A dermatologist and/or nutritionist may be able to help with this approach. If your eczema continues to bother you, seeing a dermatologist regularly may help.

Acupuncture, Chinese herbs, and evening primrose oil (applied topically) are other possible treatments. Since stress can exacerbate eczema, you could sign up for a stress reduction/relaxation course. **RES**

Alice

RELIEF FROM DRY SKIN

Dry or sensitive skin can leave many of us itching and scratching, too, especially in the winter. There are some ways, however, to get relief. For one, water dries out skin. Taking shorter showers and baths in warm (not hot) water and patting yourself dry can help. Also, use soaps and moisturizers that won't dry your skin—look for ones that are hypo-allergenic and unscented, and avoid antibacterial products. In the winter, keep the air in your home moist by using a humidifier or vaporizer, or placing pans of water on the radiator.

Mole = Melanoma?

Dear Alice,
I have a mole that has appeared sometime in the last two years. It is underneath my pubic hair and it is about half an inch long with one raised area. I'm worried about it because it is larger than any others I have, and because I didn't have it as a child. It is NOT an STD, according to my ob/gyn. Could it be melanoma? Thanks.

Dear Reader,
Since you are concerned your mole could be melanoma, make an appointment with a dermatologist right away. A dermatologist can tell you if this mole is skin cancer. Melanoma can spread, some faster than others. It can be cured when caught early.

Compare your "mole" to the description of melanoma given by the American Cancer Society (ACS) and the American Academy of Dermatology.

The ABCDs of Melanoma Identification

- Asymmetry—Both sides of the growth do not match each other in terms of shape and/or size.
- Border Irregularity—The edges of the growth are ragged, notched, or blurred (versus smooth and well-defined edges).
- Color—The pigmentation is not uniform. Shades of tan, brown, and black are present. Dashes of red, white, and blue add to the mottled appearance.
- Diameter—The size of the growth is greater than 6 mm in diameter (roughly the size of a pencil eraser). Any enlargement of the growth should also be noted.

Less common warning signs include changes in the surface of a mole; scaliness, oozing, bleeding, or the appearance of a bump or nodule; spread of color from the border of the growth into surrounding skin; and itchiness, tenderness, or pain. Of course, regardless of whether or not your "mole" fits any of these descriptions, have it looked at.

`RES`

Alice

Sunscreen: What SPF Should I Use?

Dear Alice,
I'd like to get a healthy tan this summer. My question has to do with the level of sunscreen one should use. I've heard that if your natural skin color is brown (I'm South Asian), you can use a lower SPF (solar protection factor) sunscreen. Is this true, or should I be using SPF-15 regardless of my skin color?

Dear Reader,
People with dark brown or black skin tend to develop skin cancer much less often than fairer-skinned folks. However, the American Cancer Society recommends at least SPF-15 for anyone, regardless of skin color, who spends any time in the sun. Research also suggests using sunblock with both UVA and UVB protection. Everyone who spends significant amounts of time in the sun can develop skin cancer. Today's healthy-looking tans can lead to tomorrow's skin cancer.

Beware—the sun's powerful rays can make it through layers of clouds and three feet of water. And "fake baking" with tanning beds, sunlamps, and tanning pills can cause just as much harm as the sun.

For the "healthy" tan you crave, tan gradually by "laying out" only a little each day and follow the ACS guidelines to lower your risk for skin cancer.   **RES**

Alice

AMERICAN CANCER SOCIETY'S GUIDELINES FOR SKIN CANCER PREVENTION

- Avoid or limit exposure to the sun between 10 A.M. and 4 P.M., when its ultraviolet rays are strongest.
- Cover up with clothing, or at least a hat, to keep some of the sun from reaching your face.
- Use at least SPF-15 sunscreen; reapply after swimming and sweating.
- Apply sunscreen fifteen to thirty minutes before going out in the sun for maximum effectiveness.

Athlete's Foot

Dear Alice,

I have a common problem with a weird twist. I have athlete's foot, but only on one foot. I try to keep my shower clean, and if my shower was causing the problem, wouldn't my other foot have athlete's foot also? How do I get rid of it? I've tried Lotrimin AF and it seems to work, and then the AF returns. What is the best course of action to rid myself of the AF?

THANKS, ITCHY FOOT

Dear Itchy Foot,

Athlete's foot is a common skin condition caused by a fungus where the skin between the toes becomes itchy and sore, and may blister, crack, and peel. The skin cracks can also become infected by bacteria. Athlete's foot is associated with wearing shoes and sweating—so, you might try wearing 100 percent cotton socks; or socks made from wicking materials, usually found at sporting goods stores; or sandals, at least some of the time. Dry your feet thoroughly after a shower or bath, and use a medicated foot powder after bathing.

One of your feet may be more susceptible to fungus than the other. No one knows why. Over-the-counter antifungal lotions and creams usually work well when you follow the directions, using them for *four to six weeks*. Cleaning and ventilating the shower stall can help prevent the spread of fungus. Wash and dry your sneakers and socks thoroughly, too. If your discomfort continues, see a health care provider who will determine the cause and prescribe appropriate medication.

Alice

How Do Tattoos Work?

Alice,

How do tattoos work? I mean, if human skin cells are always shedding and reproducing themselves, how are the pigments of a tattoo able to stay in the skin for so long?

MOM

Dear MOM,

Tattoos are made by inserting ink into the deepest layers of the skin, which shed cells at a slower rate than layers closer to the surface. That is why tattoos can last a lifetime.

Alice

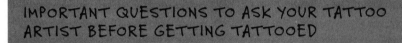

IMPORTANT QUESTIONS TO ASK YOUR TATTOO ARTIST BEFORE GETTING TATTOOED

DO YOU:

- thoroughly wash your hands with antibacterial solution immediately before and after each tattoo application?
- wear latex gloves during the tattooing procedure?
- use single-service materials and equipment (i.e., each needle and tube set is individually packaged, dated and sealed, and autoclave sterilized), and set up and open them in front of the client?
- use sterile disposable needles?
- have an FDA-regulated autoclave on site?
- sanitize your work space with an Enviornmental Protection Agency–approved viricidal disinfectant, preferably one that kills tuberculosis, before and after each client?
- thoroughly rinse tube/needle set from tattoo machine using an ultrasonic tank before discarding?
- properly dispose of contaminated materials?

Nose Piercing

Dear Alice,
I am a first-year student and I want to get my nose pierced. This isn't just a whim; I've wanted a nose ring for a long time. However, I know that there will come a time when the ring will look juvenile on me. My question: will such a hole close up fairly quickly, without leaving an ugly scar?

HOLY, HOLY, HOLIE

Dear Holy, Holy, Holie,
When you choose to get your nose pierced, have the piercing done with a needle, instead of a piercing gun; the piercing gun causes more trauma to the nose tissue and will result in a more difficult healing process. Use a nose ring versus a nose stud, as the rings are generally made with hypoallergenic material (i.e., surgical steel), which is not always the case with the stud. The stud also has the potential to sink into the tissue and cause infection. Once you get your nose pierced, do not remove the ring for six to eight weeks, giving your nose time to heal. Also, to prevent infection while it is healing, regularly clean the area, as directed, using a topical antibacterial cleanser, and apply an antibiotic cream or ointment. Make sure to dry the site, too. When you're ready to remove it for good, the amount of time it will take to close up completely depends on your body and your individual healing processes. If there is any scar, it should be minimal and barely noticeable to others.

Alice

Latex Allergies

Alice,
Can you tell us about latex allergies for condoms?

Dear Reader,
Certainly. A small percentage of the population is either sensitive, or allergic, to a natural rubber protein found in latex—the material of most condoms.

Sometimes, a latex allergy can resemble, and be mistaken for, a reaction to spermicide (e.g., nonoxynol-9) or lube, a vaginal or anal infection, or an STD. People who are allergic to latex experience a strong reaction immediately upon contact or exposure. Generally, reactions to latex in condoms tend to be less severe than reactions to latex in gloves. Symptoms usually include one or more of the following: skin rash, dryness, itching, eczema, and, in rare cases, welts. At the extreme, a person could experience difficulty breathing, and even go into anaphylactic shock. Severe latex allergies, however, are rare.

If you think you might be allergic, talk with your health care provider to determine the cause of the allergy: latex, spermicide (nonoxynol-9), lube, or an infection. If you're pretty sure that you are allergic to latex, try nonlatex condoms. If your sole concern is the prevention of pregnancy, lambskin condoms could be an option for you. Lambskin condoms do NOT prevent the transmission of sexually transmitted viruses. While it may seem challenging, some people wear two condoms—a latex condom over a lambskin one (or vice versa, depending on who is allergic to latex).

The U.S. Food and Drug Administration (FDA) has given approval to plastic polyurethane condoms (male and female) for people with latex sensitivities. These female and male condoms can be ordered by mail and may be available at your local drugstore.

If none of these clear up the problem, you may have an infection of some sort. In this case, it would be best to talk with your health care provider about it.   **RES**

Alice

Sleep

Insomnia

Alice,
I have recurring insomnia which lasts for about eight to twelve days. It seems to begin at about the same time each month. What are the common causes of sleep disturbance? Any suggestions?

SLEEPLESS IN SALT LAKE

Dear Sleepless in Salt Lake,
Insomnia is probably the most common sleep-related complaint along with daytime drowsiness. As with fever, it is not a disease, but a symptom. Insomnia affects nearly everyone at some point in their lives. Anxiety about a presentation or exam, psychological stress, environmental factors (such as noise, temperature changes, etc.), and pain can cause any person to have changes in her/his sleeping patterns. Is there anything that's happening at the same time every month that is causing you extra anxiety or stress? Women and men go through hormonal cycles that may possibly affect sleeping patterns. Look for clues in your own life that may suggest why the insomnia begins and ends at the same time each month. It is only you who knows your lifestyle best and is able to judge what's causing your sleeplessness.

A little-known fact about insomnia is that laboratory testing shows that insomniacs average only thirty minutes less sleep a night than normal sleepers, and they usually fall asleep within fifteen minutes after going to bed! But, obviously, people with insomnia think they're missing a lot more sleep than that.

Alice

Sleeping Too Much

Alice,

Since final exams, I have been sleeping way more than I did during the semester. Normally, I can get by on six to eight hours a night, with maybe one morning to sleep late, if I've been leaning to the six-hour end for too many nights. And I would sometimes even wake up in the A.M. before any alarm clock and just get up since I would be wide awake. (Which was a good thing . . .)

But lately, I've been sleeping for eight to twelve hours a night, and still feel groggy when I do get up. I'm not doing anything noticeably different now than during the spring semester and don't think I'm depressed about anything. I would like to get up at seven or eight A.M. like I'm used to doing, but I just can't drag myself out of bed.

ANY SUGGESTIONS?

Dear Any Suggestions?,

We each have a system of biological clocks that dictate our physiology and behavior. These internal clocks are usually well synchronized with each other and with the external clocks we have come to accept in society, so we are most often unaware of their existence. Circadian rhythms are cycles of biological functions regulated by your internal clock that run for a period of about twenty-four hours. These natural internal rhythms can become desynchronized when disturbed by stressors, such as flying across several time zones, or erratic sleeping and waking habits that many college students frequently experience.

Once your biological rhythms are out of phase with one another, you are more prone to feel stress in the form of irritability, exhaustion, and lowered resistance to illness. Many individuals cannot adapt their sleep schedules to the schedules they would like.

If your sleepiness continues, see a health care provider. Alice is glad you mentioned depression, because mild depression can be related to sleepiness. You could also explore this with a counselor.

Alice

Stop Snoring!

Dear Alice,

Do you have any hints to stop snoring?

HELP

Dear Help,

Snoring is noisy breathing through the open mouth during sleep. It is produced by vibrations of the soft palate. Snoring is usually caused by

SLEEP REGULATORS

ALICE'S SUGGESTIONS TO HELP REGULATE SLEEPING PATTERNS

- Get up at the same time every day. If you need to, change the time you go to bed to make sure you get enough sleep.
- Sleep in a cool, dark, and quiet room. Wear earplugs or create white noise with a fan to screen out external interruptions.
- Sleep only at night.
- Avoid alcohol before bedtime. It can interrupt REM (rapid eye movement) sleep, the most important part of the sleep cycle.
- Limit caffeine and sugar intake prior to sleep.
- Try not to drink a lot of any kind of liquid at night so you won't need to wake up and pee.
- Avoid heavy meals near bedtime.
- Don't exercise aerobically for several hours before bedtime.
- Ease into sleep by doing something pleasurable for thirty to sixty minutes before slumber: reading, watching TV, talking with a friend, holding a mate, etc.

conditions that interfere with breathing through the nose, such as a common cold, allergies, or enlarged adenoids. It is more common while sleeping on your back, when the lower jaw tends to drop open. As long as your doctor determines that your snoring is not stemming from apnea (a disorder where the snorer stops breathing for seconds, or even minutes) or any other serious condition, here are some tips for alleviating your predicament:

- Sew an object (i.e., a tennis ball) into the pajama top near the small of your back in order to make it uncomfortable to sleep on your back.
- For at least two to three hours before bedtime, don't drink alcohol or take sleeping pills, antihistamines, or tranquilizers. They depress the central nervous system and make your tongue floppy and throat muscles loose.
- Add some humidity to your bedroom. A dry throat tends to vibrate more than one that's moist. Try putting a container of water near your radiator.
- Use extra pillows to raise your head and align your airway.
- Try not to eat dairy products before bedtime because some people notice a buildup of mucus that can interfere with breathing.

- Try taking honey (chew honeycomb or swallow a couple of spoonfuls of liquid) daily for a few weeks.
- Have someone you sleep with, or your roommate, roll you over onto your side when you start to snore.

GOOD NIGHT,
Alice

Go to Alice at www.goaskalice.columbia.edu for more General Health Q & A's, including these:

- Altitude Sickness
- Are Doctors Turned on by Their Patients?
- Bad Stomachache
- Benefits of a Sauna
- Chocolate Cravings and PMS
- Clammy Hands and Feet?
- Do Whitening Toothpastes Work?
- Does Alice Smoke Pot?
- Hair Condition: Oily or Dry?
- Hair Loss
- Indoor Air Quality
- Knuckle Cracking
- Liposuction—Permanent Fat Removal?
- Melatonin—Jet Lag?
- Migraine Headaches
- More on Bad Breath (Halitosis)
- Naive Nose Blower
- Natural Ulcer Remedies?
- Problems Urinating in Public/"Pee-shy"
- Uncomfortable with College Stresses
- Unmanageable Hair

Alice's Resources RES

(The following list of resources is accurate and up-to-date at the time of this printing. This information is subject to change.)

RELATIONSHIPS

Center for the Prevention of Sexual and Domestic Violence (CPSDV)
936 North 34th, Suite 200
Seattle, WA 98103
Phone: (206) 634-1903
Fax: (206) 634-0115
Web site: http://www.cpsdv.org/
E-mail: cpsdv@cpsdv.org

A Different Light Bookstore
A gay, lesbian, bisexual, and transgender-oriented bookstore with three locations, plus a mail order service through which you can order titles published on these issues.
Mail Order Line: (800) 343-4002
Phone: (212) 989-4850
Fax: (212) 989-2158
Web site: http://www.adlbooks.com
E-mail: adl@adlbooks.com

Domestic Violence Hotlines
Provide crisis intervention, safe and confidential counseling, and referrals and information about services in your area (24 hours a day, 7 days a week).
3616 Far West Blvd., Suite 101-297
Austin, TX 78731
National Bilingual Hotline: (800) 799-SAFE (7233)
(plus translation services for over 130 languages)
TTY: (800) 787-3224
New York State Hotline: (800) 942-6906 (English)
(800) 942-6908 (Spanish)
Web site: http://www.inetport.com/~ndvh/
E-mail: ndvh@inetport.com

The Eulenspiegel Society (TES)
The oldest bondage, discipline, sadism, and masochism (BDSM) support group in the U.S.
P.O. Box 2783
New York, NY 10163
Phone: (212) 388-7022
Web site: http://www.tes.org/
E-mail: TES@tes.org

The Gay and Lesbian Switchboard of New York
Provides volunteer counseling and other information over the phone.
Phone: (212) 777-1800 [10am–midnight (EST), 7 days a week]
National Coalition Against Domestic Violence (NCADV)
P.O. Box 18749
Denver, CO 80218-0749
Phone: (303) 839-1852
Fax: (303) 831-9251
Web site: http://www.webmerchants.com/ncadv/
E-mail: ncadv1@ix.netcom.com
National Coalition Against Sexual Assault (NCASA)
Provides referrals to centers which aid survivors of sexual assault; membership info is available as well.
125 North Enola Dr.
Enola, PA 17025
Phone: (717) 728-9764
(800) 692-7445
Web site: http://www.cs.utk.edu/~bartley/ncasa/ncasa.html
E-mail: ncasa@redrose.net
The National Coming Out Project
An educational service of the Human Rights Campaign, the country's largest lesbian, gay, and bisexual political organization.
Phone: (800) 866-6263
The National Lesbian and Gay Health Association (NLGHA)
1407 S Street, N.W.
Washington, D.C. 20009
Phone: (202) 939-7880
Fax: (202) 234-1467
Web site: http://www.nlgha.org
E-mail: nlgha@aol.com
National Resource Center on Domestic Violence
Phone: (800) 537-2238
New York City Gay and Lesbian Anti-Violence Project
647 Hudson St.
New York, NY 10014
24-hour Bilingual Hotline: (212) 807-0197
Office phone: (212) 807-6761
Fax: (212) 807-1044
Web site: http://www.avp.org/
!OUTPROUD!
The National Coalition for Gay, Lesbian, Bisexual, and Transgender Youth.
Web site: http://www.outproud.org
E-mail: info@outproud.org
P-FLAG: Parents and Friends of Lesbians and Gays
Website: http://www.pflag.org
E-mail: info@pflag.org
Rape, Abuse, and Incest National Network (RAINN)
A nonprofit organization founded by singer/songwriter Tori Amos that operates a national toll-free hotline for survivors of sexual assault.
252 Tenth Street, N.E.
Washington, DC 20002

Hotline: (800) 656-HOPE (4673)
Web site: http://www.rainn.org/
E-mail: RAINNmail@aol.com
The Renaissance Education Association
Offers information and outreach support group for transgender people.
P.O. Box 1263
King of Prussia, PA 19406
Safety Net—Domestic Violence Resources
Web site: http://www.cybergrrl.com/planet/dv/
E-mail: cybergrrl@cgim.com
Violence Against Women Office (VAWO) of the U.S. Department of Justice (USDOJ)
VAWO
USDOJ
Room 5302
Tenth & Constitution Ave., N.W.
Washington, DC 20530
Web site: http://www.usdoj.gov/vawo/

Links
Barnard/Columbia Women's Handbook
Gopher Menu: gopher://gopher.cc.columbia.edu:71/11/publications/women
Queer Infoservers—Colleges and Universities
Web site: http://shemp.bucks.edu/~opendoor/college.htm
Sexual Assault Information Page
Web site: http://www.cs.utk.edu/~bartley/saInfoPage.html
Youth Assistance Organization (YAO)
Web site: http://youth.org/

Books
Alman, Isadora. *Let's Talk Sex: Q & A on Sex and Relationships.* Freedom, CA: The Crossing Press, 1993. (As well as other titles)

Berzon, Betty. *Setting Them Straight: You Can Do Something about Bigotry and Homophobia.* New York: Penguin Books, 1996.

Berzon, Betty. *Permanent Partners: Building Gay and Lesbian Relationships That Last.* New York: Penguin Books, 1988.

Borhek, Mary. *Coming Out to Parents: A Two-Way Survival Guide for Lesbians and Gay Men and Their Parents* (2nd ed.). Cleveland: The Pilgrim Press/The United Church Press, 1993.

Brame, Gloria G., William D. Brame, and Jon Jacobs. *Different Loving: The World of Sexual Dominance and Submission.* New York: Random House, 1996.

Brooks, Michael. *Instant Rapport.* New York: Warner Books, 1990.

Clark, Don. *Loving Someone Gay* (3rd ed.). Berkeley, CA: Celestial Arts Publishing Co., 1997.

Crohn, Joel. *Mixed Matches: How to Create Successful Interracial, Interethnic, and Interfaith Relationships.* New York: Fawcett Book Group, 1995.

de Biexedon, S. Yevette. *Lovers and Survivors: A Partner's Guide to Living with and Loving a Sexual Abuse Survivor.* San Francisco, CA: Robert D. Reed Publishers, 1995.

Fairchild, Betty, and Nancy Hayward. *Now That You Know: What Every Parent Should Know about Homosexuality.* New York: Harcourt Brace Jovanovich, 1989.

Kramer, Peter D. *Should You Leave? A Psychiatrist Explores Intimacy and Autonomy and the Nature of Advice.* New York: Simon & Schuster Trade, 1997.

Lerner, Harriet G. *The Dance of Intimacy: A Woman's Guide to Courageous Acts of Change in Key Relationships.* New York: HarperCollins Publishers, 1990.

Lerner, Harriet G. *Dance of Anger: A Woman's Guide to Changing the Patterns of Intimate Relationships.* New York: HarperCollins Publishers, 1989. (As well as other titles)

Levy, Barrie (editor). *Dating Violence: Young Women in Danger.* Seattle, WA: Seal Press, 1998.

Lobel, Kerry (editor). *Naming the Violence: Speaking Out about Lesbian Battering.* Seattle, WA: Seal Press, 1986.

Marcus, Eric. *Is It a Choice? Answers to Three Hundred of the Most Frequently Asked Questions about Gays and Lesbians.* San Francisco: Harper San Francisco, 1993. (As well as other titles)

Martin, Del and Phyllis Lyon. *Lesbian-Woman, 1991.* Volcano, CA: Volcano Press, Inc., 1991.

Monette, Paul. *Becoming a Man: Half a Life Story.* San Francisco, CA: Harper San Francisco, 1993.

Nicarthy, Ginny. *Getting Free: You Can End Abuse & Take Back Your Life.* Seattle, WA: Seal Press, 1997.

Nicarthy, Ginny, and Sue Davidson. *You Can Be Free: An Easy-to-Read Handbook for Abused Women.* Seattle, WA: Seal Press, 1997.

Parrot, Andrea, and Laurie Bechhofer (editors). *Acquaintance Rape: The Hidden Crime.* New York: John Wiley & Sons, Inc., 1991.

Penn, Robert E. *The Gay Men's Wellness Guide: The National Lesbian and Gay Health Association's Complete Book of Physical, Emotional, and Mental Health and Well-Being.* New York: Henry Holt & Co., 1998.

Rabin, Susan, and Barbara J. Lagowski. *101 Ways to Flirt: How to Get More Dates and Meet Your Mate.* New York: NAL/Dutton, 1997.

Roiphe, Katie. *The Morning After: Sex, Fear, and Feminism on Campus.* Boston: Little, Brown and Company, 1993.

Rollins, C. E. *52 Ways to Get Along with Your College Roommate.* Nashville, TN: Thomas Nelson, 1994.

Russo, Vito. *The Celluloid Closet.* New York: Harper & Row Publishers, 1981.

Scherer, Migael. *Still Loved by the Sun: A Rape Survivor's Journal.* New York: NAL/Dutton, 1993.

Shyer, Marlene, and Christopher Shyer. *Not Like Other Boys, Growing Up Gay: A Mother and Son Look Back.* Boston: Houghton Mifflin Co., 1996.

Signorile, Michaelangelo. *Outing Yourself.* New York: Simon & Schuster Trade, 1996.

Tannen, Deborah. *You Just Don't Understand: Women & Men in Conversation.* New York: Ballantine Books, 1991.

Van Daves, Prentiss. *Roommates, College Sublets, and Living in the Dorm.* St. Louis, MO: Jordan Enterprises Publishing Company, 1989.

Warshaw, Robin. *I Never Called It Rape: The Ms. Report on Recognizing, Fighting, and Surviving Date Rape.* New York: HarperCollins Publishers, 1991.

White, Jocelyn C., and Marissa C. Martinez (editors). *The Lesbian Health Book: Caring for Ourselves.* Seattle, WA: Seal Press, 1997.

Films

The Accused (1988): Jodie Foster and Kelly McGillis star in this movie about a women who is gang raped and finds herself battling the legal system.

All Over Me (1997): Film about two teenage girls and how their friendship and love for each other are threatened when one of them falls for a drug dealing punk. Also deals with drug use and questioning sexuality.

Beautiful Thing (1996): An independent British film about the coming out struggles and joys of two teenage boys and their families.

Boys Life (1994): Three short independent films which relate different male coming out experiences.

Boys Life 2 (1996): Another series of short independent films about gay men's experiences, including "Trevor," an Academy award–winning short film that follows the coming out story of a male high school student in the 1980s.

The Brothers McMullen (1995): Edward Burns, Mike McGlone, and Maxine Bahns star in this romantic comedy about love and relationship struggles among three Irish-American brothers in New York.

The Burning Bed (1984): Farrah Fawcett stars in this made-for-television movie about an abused woman who decides to end the violence against her.

Chasing Amy (1997): Film about the relationships and sexual explorations of young people in NYC and NJ that is presented with wit, wide-ranging emotion, and candor.

The Color Purple (1985): Whoopi Goldberg, Danny Glover, and Oprah Winfrey star in this film adaptation of the Alice Walker novel about the life and empowerment of a black woman growing up in the South.

Crossing Delancey (1988): Amy Irving and Peter Riegert star in this film about a woman finding love where she least expects it.

Double Happiness (1995): An independent American film about a young woman who struggles with her identity as a Chinese-Canadian, being torn between her family's traditional values and expectations and her more Westernized lifestyle, including her budding relationship with a non-Asian man.

Fried Green Tomatoes (1991): Jessica Tandy, Kathy Bates, Mary Stuart Masterson, and Mary Louise Parker star in this movie exploring the relationships of two pairs of women, in the past and present, and the empowerment of Bates's character.

Go Fish (1994): Independent film about lesbian relationships takes a quirky, "real life" approach.

The Incredibly True Adventures of 2 Girls in Love (1995): An independent American film about two teenage girls and their struggles and fun as their relationship develops.

Love Jones (1997): Larenz Tate, Nia Long, and Bill Bellamy star in this romantic comedy about the search for love among a group of young African American professionals in Chicago.

A Reason to Believe (1995): This independent American film is about the events surrounding the rape of a college woman at a fraternity party.

Sling Blade (1996): Billy Bob Thornton stars as Karl Childers, a mentally challenged man, who comes to terms with the domestic violence situation of a young friend.

Spanking the Monkey (1994): Jeremy Davies stars in this disturbing black comedy about the relationship between a mother and her teenage son that deals with masturbation and mother-son incest.

Swingers (1996): Independent American comedy that deals with gender stereotypes and relationships.

This Boy's Life (1993): Leonardo Di Caprio, Robert DeNiro, and Ellen Barkin star in this disturbing drama, based on the semiautobiographical novel by Tobias Wolff, about a mother and son living in an abusive household.

The Truth about Cats and Dogs (1996): Janeane Garofalo and Uma Thurman star in this romantic comedy that revolves around a young professional woman's relationships, her struggles with her body image, and her search for love.

The Wedding Banquet (1993): Taiwanese film about the family dynamics and struggles which arise around an interracial, gay male relationship.

When Harry Met Sally (1989): Billy Crystal and Meg Ryan star in this comedy about what can happen when friends become lovers.

SEXUALITY

American Association of Sex Educators, Counselors, and Therapists (AASECT)
For a referral list of sex counselors and therapists in your state, send a self-addressed, stamped envelope to:
P.O. Box 238
Mount Vernon, IA 52314
Phone: (319) 895-8407
Fax: (319) 895-6203
Web site: http://www.aasect.org/
E-mail: Info@aasect.org
Good Vibrations
A twenty-year-old worker-owned distributor of products, materials, and information based in California, but will ship anywhere.
"The Sexuality Library" Mail Order:
938 Howard St.
San Francisco, CA 94103
Mail Order Line: (415) 974-8900
(800) BUY-VIBE (289-8423)
Mail Order Fax: (415) 974-8989
Mail Order Web site: http://www.goodvibes.com
Mail Order E-mail: goodvibe@well.com
Phone: (415) 974-8980
National Rehabilitation Information Center (NARIC)
A resource for people with spinal cord injury and their families that provides info on research and rehabilitation, including sexuality issues.
8455 Colesville Rd., Suite 935
Silver Spring, MD 20910
Phone: (301) 588-9284
(800) 346-2742
TTY: (301) 495-5626
Fax: (301) 587-1967
Web site: http://www.naric.com/naric
Sexuality Information and Education Council of the United States (SIECUS)
130 West 42nd Street, Suite 350
New York, NY 10036
Phone: (212) 819-9770
Fax: (212) 819-9776
Web site: http://www.siecus.org
E-mail: SIECUS@siecus.org

Books

Alman, Isadora. *Let's Talk Sex: Q & A on Sex and Relationships*. Freedom, CA: The Crossing Press, 1993. (As well as other titles)

AMWA Staff. *The American Medical Women's Association Guide to Sexuality*. New York: Dell Publishing Co., Inc., 1996.

Barbach, Lonnie G. *For Each Other: Sharing Sexual Intimacy*. New York: NAL/Dutton, 1984. (As well as other titles)

Barbach, Lonnie G. *For Yourself: The Fulfillment of Female Sexuality*. New York: Doubleday & Company, Inc., 1976. (As well as other titles)

The Boston Women's Health Book Collective Staff. *The New Our Bodies, Ourselves*. Magnolia, MA: Peter Smith Publisher, Inc., 1996.

Dobkin, Rachel, and Shana Sippy. *The College Woman's Handbook*. New York: Workman Publishing Company, Inc., 1995.

Dodson, Betty. *Sex for One: The Joy of Self-Loving*. New York: Crown Publishing Group, 1996.

Ducharme, Stanley H. and Kathleen M. Gill. *Sexuality after Spinal Cord Injury: Answers to Your Questions*. Baltimore: Paul H. Brookes Publishing Co., 1996.

Friday, Nancy. *My Secret Garden*. New York: Pocket Books, 1991.

Friday, Nancy. *Men in Love, Male Sexual Fantasies: The Triumph of Love over Rage*. New York: Dell Publishing Co., Inc., 1983. (As well as other titles)

Haseltine, Florence P., Sandra S. Cole, and David B. Gray (editors). *Reproductive Issues for Persons with Physical Disabilities*. Baltimore, MD: Paul H. Brookes Publishing Company, 1993.

Heiman, Julia, and Joseph LoPiccolo. *Becoming Orgasmic: A Sexual and Personal Growth Program for Women*. New York: Simon & Schuster, 1987.

Hite, Shere. *The Hite Report*. New York: Dell Publishing Company, Inc., 1987. (As well as other titles)

Katzman, John, and Cynthia Brantley. *Sex on Campus: The Naked Truth about the Real Sex Lives of College Students*. New York: Random House, 1997.

Klein, Erica L., and Ken Kroll. *Enabling Romance: A Guide to Love, Sex, and Relationships for the Disabled (And the People Who Care about Them)*. Bethesda, MD: Woodbine House, Inc., 1995.

Ladas, Alice K., Beverly Whipple, and John D. Perry. *The G Spot*. New York: Dell Publishing Company, Inc., 1983.

Loulan, Jo Ann. *Lesbian Passion: Loving Ourselves and Each Other*. Duluth, MN: Spinsters Ink, 1987.

Mauro, Robert. *Finding Love and Intimacy*. Bloomington, IL: Accent Special Publications, Cheever Publishing, 1994.

Morin, Jack. *Anal Pleasure and Health: A Guide for Men and Women*. San Francisco: Down There Press, 1998.

Morin, Jack. *The Erotic Mind: Unlocking the Inner Sources of Sexual Passion and Fulfillment*. New York: HarperCollins Publishers, 1996.

Penn, Robert E. *The Gay Men's Wellness Guide: The National Lesbian and Gay Health Association's Complete Book of Physical, Emotional, and Mental Health and Well-Being*. New York: Henry Holt & Co., 1998.

Stoltenberg, John. *Refusing to Be a Man: Essays on Sex and Justice*. New York: Meridian Books, The Penguin Group, 1989.

Valins, Linda. *When a Woman's Body Says No to Sex: Understanding and Overcoming Vaginismus*. New York: Viking Penguin, 1992.

Westheimer, Ruth K. *Sex for Dummies*. Indianapolis, IN: IDG Books Worldwide, Inc., 1995. (As well as other titles)

Winks, Cathy and Anne Semans. *The New Good Vibrations Guide to Sex: How to Have Fun Safe Sex*. San Francisco, CA: Cleis Press, 1997.

Wolf, Naomi. *Promiscuities: The Secret Struggle for Womanhood*. New York: Random House, 1997.

Zilbergeld, Bernie. *The New Male Sexuality*. New York: Bantam Books, 1992.

Films

Coming Home (1978): John Voight plays a Vietnam veteran with a spinal cord injury who develops an intimate relationship with a married woman played by Jane Fonda.

Stealing Beauty (1996): Film about a young American woman's coming-of-age in the Italian countryside.

The Waterdance (1992): Eric Stoltz and Helen Hunt star in this film about the dynamics and struggles of an intimate relationship when one partner becomes disabled from a spinal cord injury.

SEXUAL HEALTH

The Alan Guttmacher Institute
An independent, not-for-profit organization for reproductive health research, policy analysis, and public education.
NY Address:
120 Wall Street
New York, NY 10005
Phone: (212) 248-1111
Fax: (212) 248-1951
Web site: http://www.agi-usa.org/home.html
General Info E-mail: info@agi-usa.org

American Liver Foundation
Provides information on hepatitis and other liver diseases.
1425 Pompton Ave.
Cedar Grove, NJ 07009
Phone: (800) GO-LIVER (465-4837)
(800) 223-0179
Web site: http://www.liverfoundation.org
E-mail: webmail@liverfoundation.org

American Medical Women's Association (AMWA)
801 N. Fairfax St., Suite 400
Alexandria, VA 22314
Phone: (703) 838-0500
Fax: (703) 549-3864
Web site: http://www.amwa-doc.org/
E-mail: info@amwa-doc.org

American Social Health Association (ASHA)
P.O. Box 13827
Research Triangle Park, NC 27709
Fax: (919) 361-4855
Web site: http://sunsite.unc.edu/ASHA
E-mail: hivnet@ashastd.org

All Services:
TTY: (800) 243-7889

[10am–10pm (EST), M–F]
Spanish Hotline: (800) 344-7432
[8am–2am (EST), 7 days a week]
CDC's National HIV/AIDS Hotline: (800) 342-AIDS (2437)
CDC's National STD Hotline: (800) 227-8922
National Herpes Hotline: (919) 361-8488
For written material requests: (800) 230-6039
For recorded info about STDs: (800) 653-4325
Herpes Resource Center:
(info on Herpes and HPV, including subscriptions to *HPV News*, a quarterly
  newsletter about genital warts)
Phone: (800) 230-6039

Breast Cancer Information Clearinghouse (BCIC)
NYSERNet, Inc.
200 Elwood Davis Rd., Suite 103
Liverpool, NY 13088
Phone: (315) 453-2912 (x225)
Fax: (315) 453-3052
Web site: http://nysernet.org/bcic/
E-mail: kennett@appliedtheory.com

The Canadian Women's Health Network
The Canadian Women's Health Network
c/o Women's Health Clinic, Second Floor
419 Graham Ave.
Winnipeg, Manitoba R3C 0M3
CANADA
Phone: (204) 947-2422 (x134)
Fax: (204) 943-3844
Web site: http://www.cwhn.ca/index.html
E-mail: cwhn@cwhn.ca

Condomania
A full service retail and mail order company.
Mail Order Phone: (800)-9-CONDOM (926-6366) [9am–5pm (PT), M–F]
Web site: http://www.condomania.com

Emergency Contraception Hotline
Provides information regarding various forms of emergency contraception and referrals to providers in your area.
Hotline: (888)-NOT-2-LATE (668-2-5283)
Web site: http://opr.princeton.edu/ec/

Endometriosis Association International
Endometriosis Association International Headquarters
8585 North 76th Place
Milwaukee, WI 53223
Voice mail: (800) 992-3636
Phone: (414) 355-2200
Fax: (414) 355-6065
Web site: http://www.endometriosisassn.org/

The Female Health Company
Manufactures, markets, and distributes the female condom, Reality.
875 North Michigan Avenue, Suite 3660
Chicago, IL 60611
For free samples and information: (800) 274-6601
Mail Order Phone: (800) 635-0844

Office Phone: (312) 280-1119
Fax: (312) 280-9360
Web site: http://www.femalehealth.com
Gay Men's Health Crisis (GMHC)
The oldest and largest not-for-profit AIDS organization in the United States is also affiliated with The David Geffen Center for HIV Prevention and Health Education, which provides confidential HIV testing by appointment, as well as pre-, during, and post-counseling for HIV testing.
   119 West 24th Street
   New York, NY 10011
   AIDS Hotline: (212) 807-6655 [10am–9pm (EST), M–F]
   TTY: (212) 645-7470
   GMHC Phone: (212) 367-1000
   Geffen Center Phone: (212) 367-1100
   Fax: (212) 367-1220
   Web site: http://www.gmhc.org/
   Geffen Center E-mail: geffnctr@gmhc.org
HIV/AIDS Treatment Information Service (ATIS)
Provides information about federally approved treatment guidelines for HIV and AIDS.
   P.O. Box 6303
   Rockville, MD 20849-6303
   Phone: (800)-HIV-0440 (448-0440)
   TTY: (800) 243-7012
   International Phone: (301) 519-0459
   Fax: (301) 519-6616
   Web site: http://www.hivatis.org/
   E-mail: atis@cdcnac.org
HIV Center for Clinical and Behavioral Studies at the NY State Psychiatric Institute
   722 West 168th St.
   New York, NY 10032
   Phone: (212) 543-5969
   Web site: http://www.hivcenternyc.org
London International
Distributes the male polyurethane condom.
   Mail Order Phone: (888) 266-3660
March of Dimes Birth Defects Foundation
Has information regarding birth defects and how to have healthier babies, including information about pre-pregnancy and pregnancy, genetics, and drug use and environmental hazards during pregnancy.
   1275 Mamaroneck Avenue
   White Plains, NY 10605
   Phone: (888)-MODIMES (663-4637)
   TTY: (914) 997-4764
   Fax: (914) 997-4763
   Web site: http://www.modimes.org
   E-mail: resourcecenter@modimes.org
National Abortion and Reproductive Rights Action League (NARAL)
   1156 Fifteenth Street, N.W.
   Washington, DC 20005
   Legal, Library, and Information Line: (202) 973-3018
   Phone: (202) 973-3000
   Web site: http://www.naral.org/
   E-mail: naral@newmedium.com

National Alliance of Breast Cancer Organizations (NABCO)
NABCO
9 East 37th Street, 10th Floor
New York, NY 10016
Phone: (212) 889-0606
Web site: http://www.nabco.org/
E-mail: NABCOinfo@aol.com
National Lesbian and Gay Health Association (NLGHA)
1407 S Street, N.W.
Washington, DC 20009
Phone: (202) 939-7880
Fax: (202) 234-1467
Web site: http://www.nlgha.org
E-mail: nlgha@aol.com
National Women's Health Network
*A nonprofit organization which provides advocacy and information, aiming to aid women
in having a greater voice in the health care system.*
514 Tenth St., N.W.
Suite 400
Washington, DC 20004

For info regarding legislation, etc.:
Phone: (202) 347-1140
Fax: (202) 347-1168

For comprehensive information about any women's health issue, or referrals to
other appropriate organizations:
Information Clearinghouse Line: (202) 628-7814
The Norplant Foundation
P.O. Box 25223
Alexandria, VA 22313-5223
Phone: (800) 760-9030 [9am–5pm (EST), M–F]
Planned Parenthood
Planned Parenthood Federation of America, Inc.
810 Seventh Avenue
New York, NY 10019
To connect you with the Planned Parenthood in your area: (800) 230-PLAN (7526)
Office Phone: (212) 541-7800
Web site: http://www.igc.apc.org/ppfa/
The Susan G. Komen Breast Cancer Foundation
5005 LBJ Freeway, Suite 370
Dallas, TX 75244
National Breast Care Help Line: (800) I'M-AWARE (462-9273)
Phone: (972) 855-1600
Fax: (972) 855-1605
Web site: http://www.breastcancerinfo.com
U.S. Public Health Service—Office on Women's Health (U.S. PHS OWH)
National Women's Health Information Center
Information Line: (800) 994-WOMAN (96626)
Web site: http://www.4woman.org
Y-ME National Breast Cancer Organization
Provides peer counseling with breast cancer survivors, written info, and referrals.
212 W. Van Buren
Chicago, IL 60607

Information Hotline: (800) 221-2141 (24 hours a day, 7 days a week)
[This number can also connect you with the "Men's Hotline," where male family
members and significant others of women with breast cancer can speak with other
men in a similar position.]
*Hearing Impaired can "relay" through an operator
Spanish Hotline: (800) 986-9505 [9am–5pm (CT), M–F]
Fax: (312) 294-8598
Web site: http://www.y-me.org/index.html
E-mail: help@y-me.org

Links

Barnard/Columbia Women's Handbook
Gopher Menu: gopher://gopher.cc.columbia.edu:71/11/publications/women
Café Herpé
A Web site with lots of herpes info
Web site: http://www.cafeherpe.com
CDC National AIDS Clearinghouse
Web site: http://www.cdcnac.org/
**The Columbia University College of Physicians and Surgeons Complete Home
Medical Guide**
Web site: http://cpmcnet.columbia.edu/texts/guide/
Community Breast Health Project
Web site: http://www-med.Stanford.EDU:80/CBHP/
Feminist Majority Foundation—Women's Health Links
Web site: http://www.feminist.org/gateway/h_exec2.html
GYN 101
Web site with detailed information to help women with the process of seeing a gynecologist.
Web site: http://www.gyn101.com
Healthtouch On-line
*Covers many areas of health, including men's and women's health, as well as prescription
and over-the-counter drug info.*
Web site: http://www.healthtouch.com
Johns Hopkins University STD Research Information for Patients
Web site: http://www.jhustd.org/pub/jhustd/patinfo.htm
**Journal of the American Medical Association HIV/AIDS Information
Center**
Web site: http://www.ama-assn.org/special/hiv/hivhome.htm
The Male Health Center
Web site: http://www.malehealthcenter.com/

Books

American Medical Association Staff. *The American Medical Association Encyclopedia
of Medicine.* New York: Random House, 1989.
American Medical Women's Association Staff. *The Women's Complete Healthbook.*
New York: Dell Publishing Company, Inc., 1997.
American Medical Women's Association Staff. *The American Medical Women's Asso-
ciation Guide to Fertility and Reproductive Health.* New York: Dell Publishing
Company, Inc., 1996.
Baron-Faust, Rita. *Breast Cancer: What Every Woman Should Know.* New York:
Hearst Books, 1995.
Berger, Gilda. *PMS: Premenstrual Syndrome: A Guide for Young Women.* Alameda,
CA: Hunter House, 1991.

The Boston Women's Health Book Collective Staff. *The New Our Bodies, Ourselves.* Magnolia, MA: Peter Smith Publisher, Inc., 1997.

Chaitow, Leon. *Candida Albicans: Could Yeast Be Your Problem?* Rochester, VT: Inner Traditions International, Ltd, 1989.

Crook, William G. *The Yeast Connection.* Jackson, TN: Professional Books/Future Health, Inc., 1989. (As well as many other titles)

Dobkin, Rachel, and Shana Sippy. *The College Woman's Handbook.* New York: Workman Publishing Company, Inc., 1995.

Ebel, Charles. *Managing Herpes: How to Live and Love with a Chronic STD.* Research Triangle Park, NC: American Social Health Association, 1994.

Guren, Denise and Nealy Gillette. *The Ovulation Method—Cycles of Fertility.* Anchorage: The Ovulation Method Teachers Association, 1984.

Harrison, Michelle. *Self-Help for Premenstrual Syndrome.* New York: Random House, 1998.

Haseltine, Florence P., Sandra S. Cole, and David B. Gray (editors). *Reproductive Issues for Persons with Physical Disabilities.* Baltimore, MD: Paul H. Brookes Publishing Company, 1993.

Hatcher, Robert A., James Trussell, Felicia Stewart, Gary K. Stewart, Deborah Kowal, Felicia Guest, Willard Cates, Jr., and Michael S. Policar. *Contraceptive Technology* (17th ed., rev.). New York: Irvington Publishers, Inc., 1998.

Lark, Susan M. *PMS Self-Help Book.* Berkeley, CA: Celestial Arts Publishing Company, 1995. (As well as other titles)

Love, Susan M. *Dr. Susan Love's Breast Book.* Reading, MA: Addison Wesley Longman, Inc., 1995.

McCoy, Kathy, and Charles Wibbelsman. *The New Teenage Body Book.* New York: Berkley Publishing Group, 1992.

Merck and Co., Inc. Staff. *The Merck Manual of Medical Information: Home Edition.* Rahway, NJ: Merck & Company, Inc., 1997.

Morgentaler, Abraham. *The Male Body: A Physician's Guide to What Every Man Should Know about His Sexual Health.* New York: Simon & Schuster Trade, 1993.

Oppenheim, Michael. *The Man's Health Book.* Paramus, NJ: Prentice Hall, 1994.

Pasquale, Samuel A., and Jennifer Cadoff. *The Birth Control Book: A Complete Guide to Your Contraceptive Options.* New York: Ballantine Books, 1996.

Physicians' Desk Reference and David W. Sifton (editor-in-chief). *The PDR Family Guide to Women's Health and Prescription Drugs.* Montvale, NJ: Medical Economics, 1994.

Pinsky, Laura and Paul Harding Douglas. *The Essential AIDS Fact Book, Newly Revised and Updated.* New York: Simon & Schuster, 1996.

Planned Parenthood Federation of America, Inc., Staff. *The Planned Parenthood Women's Health Encyclopedia.* New York: Crown Publishing Group, 1996.

Tapley, Donald F., Thomas Q. Morris, Lewis P. Rowland, and Jonathan Lapook (Editors). *The Columbia University College of Physicians and Surgeons Complete Home Medical Guide.* New York: Crown Publishers, Inc., 1995.

White, Jocelyn C., and Marissa C. Martinez (editors). *The Lesbian Health Book: Caring for Ourselves.* Seattle, WA: Seal Press, 1997.

Films

If These Walls Could Talk (1996): Demi Moore, Sissy Spacek, and Cher star in this cable television movie about a woman's right to choose abortion during three different decades in America.

A Private Matter (1992): Sissy Spacek and Aidan Quinn star in this cable television movie about a couple's decision to have an abortion during the pre–Roe vs. Wade era.

Silverlake Life: The View From Here (1993): A documentary made by a gay filmmaker chronicling his devastating death from AIDS.

EMOTIONAL HEALTH

American Association of Suicidology (AAs)
4201 Connecticut Avenue, N
Suite 310
Washington, DC 20008
Phone: (202) 287-2280
Fax: (202) 287-2282
Web site: http://www.cyberpage.org/aas.htn
E-mail: amyjomc@ix.netcom.com
American Psychiatric Association
1400 K. Street, N.W.
Washington, DC 20005
Phone: (202) 682-6220
Fax: (202) 682-6255
Web site: http://www.psych.org (click on "public information" for various fact sheets)
American Psychological Association (APA)
Offers a practice directory for referrals to psychological services.
750 First St., N.E.
Washington, DC 20002-4242
Phone: (800) 374-2721
(202) 336-5500
TTY: (800) 374-2721 (x6123)
Fax: (202) 336-5708
Web site: http://www.apa.org/
Anxiety Disorders Association of America (ADAA)
11900 Parklawn Dr., Suite 100
Rockville, MD 20852
Phone: (301) 231-9350
Web site: http://www.adaa.org/
E-mail: anxdis@aol.com
The ANXIETY-PANIC Internet Resource (tAPir)
Web site: http://www.algy.com/anxiety/
E-mail: tapir@algy.com
Center for Environmental Therapeutics, Inc. (CET)
CET Executive Office
Georgetown, CO 80444-0532
Phone & Fax: (303) 569-0910
Web site: http://www.cet.org/cet1996/
E-mail: ccneely@csn.net
Center for Mental Health Services (CMHS)
5600 Fishers Lane
Rockville, MD 20857
Phone: (800) 789-2647
(301) 443-2792
Fax: (301) 443-5163
Web site: http://www.samhsa.gov/cmhs/cmhs.htm

CMHS National Mental Health Services Knowledge Exchange Network (KEN)

Provides mental health info via phone, electronic bulletin board, and publications.

P.O. Box 42490

Washington, DC 20015

Phone: (800) 789-CMHS (2647) [8:30 am–5pm (EST), M–F]

TTY: (301) 443-9006

Fax: (301) 984-8796

Electronic Bulletin Board System: (800) 790-CMHS (2647)

Web site: http://www.mentalhealth.org/

E-mail: ken@mentalhealth.org

The Centre for Living with Dying

A non-profit organization providing emotional support, crisis intervention, and education to individuals, families, professionals, and the community facing the issues of loss, trauma, life-threatening illness, stress, or grief.

554 Mansion Park Drive

Santa Clara, CA 95054

Phone: (408) 980-9801

Fax: (408) 980-9838

Web site: http://www.thecentre.org

E-mail: support@thecentre.org

Dr. Bob's Mental Health Links

Web site: http://uhs.bsd.uchicago.edu/dr-bob/mental.html

E-mail: dr-bob@uchicago.edu

Dr. Ivan's Depression Central

Web site: http://www.psycom.net/depression.central.html

E-mail: Psydoc@PsyCom.Net

GriefNet

Offers links to a variety of resources related to death, dying, bereavement, and major emotional and physical losses, including discussion and support groups.

Web site: http://www.rivendell.org/

E-mail: griefnet@griefnet.org

Growth House, Inc.

An international site of resources for life-threatening illness and end-of-life issues.

Phone: (415) 255-9045

Web site: http://www.growthhouse.org/

E-mail: info@growthhouse.org

National Adolescent Suicide Hotline

Hotline: (800) 621-4000

National Alliance for the Mentally Ill (NAMI)

200 North Glebe Rd., Suite 1015

Arlington, VA 22203-3754

Help Line: (800) 950-NAMI (6264)

Front Desk Phone: (703) 524-7600

TTY: (703) 516-7991

Fax: (703) 524-9094

Web site: http://www.nami.org/

National Association of Social Workers, Inc. (NASW)

Provides referrals to social workers and services.

National Address:

750 First Street, N.E.

Suite 700
Washington, DC 20002-4241
Phone: (202) 408-8600
Fax: (202) 336-8310
Web site: http://www.naswdc.org
National Depressive and Manic Depressive Association (NDMDA)
Has several educational programs in support of individuals, couples, and families coping with depressive and manic-depressive illness.
730 N. Franklin Street, Suite 501
Chicago, IL 60610-3526
Phone: (800) 826-3632
Fax: (312) 642-7243
Web site: http://www.ndmda.org
National Empowerment Center
Promotes recovery and self-help strategies. Offers information on hundreds of topics, such as holistic alternatives, symptom treatment, and support groups.
20 Ballard Road
Lawrence, MA 01843
Phone: (800) 769-3728
Fax: (508) 681-6426
National Institutes of Mental Health (NIMH),
Information Resources and Inquiries Branch
Provides info about mental health disorders through written publications.
5600 Fishers Lane, Rm. 7C-02
Mail Code MSC 8030
Bethesda, MD 20892-8030
Phone: (301) 443-4513
Fax-on-Demand: (301) 443-5158
Fax: (301) 443-4279
Web site: http://www.nimh.nih.gov
E-mail: nimhpubs@nih.gov
nimhinfo@nih.gov

Additional Services:
National Institute of Mental Health Depression/Awareness, Recognition, and Treatment Program (D/ART):   *(800) 421-4211*
Anxiety Information Line: (888)-8-ANXIETY (826-9438)
Panic Information Line: (800)-64-PANIC (647-2642)
National Mental Health Association (NMHA)
1021 Prince St.
Alexandria, VA 22314-2971
24-hour NMHA Information Center Line: (800) 969-NMHA (6642)
(888) 836-6070 (to have info read or faxed to you)
Phone: (703) 684-7722
TTY: (800) 433-5959
Fax: (703) 684-5968
Web site: http://www.nmha.org/
E-mail: nmhainfo@aol.com

National Mental Health Consumers' Self-Help Clearinghouse
   1211 Chestnut St.
   Philadelphia, PA 19107
   Phone: (800) 553-4539
   Fax: (215) 636-6310
   E-mail: THEKEY@delphi.com
National Youth Crisis Hotline
Hotline: (800)-HIT-HOME (448-4663)
The Samaritans
Offers a twenty-four-hour suicide prevention hotline providing confidential, nonreligious support services and also provides public education and a support group for survivors called "Safe Place."
   P.O. Box 1259
   Madison Square Station
   New York, NY 10159
   NY Hotline (and Safe Place "Suicide Survivor" Support Groups Info):
      (212) 673-3000
   Volunteer Recruitment Information Line: (212) 673-3041
   Business Office Phone: (212) 677-3009
   Mental Health Net U.S. Mirror Site:
   http://www.mhnet.org/samaritans/
   International Web site for the depressed and suicidal seeking help:
   http://www.samaritans.org.uk/
   Anonymous E-mail: samaritans@anon.twwells.com
   Regular E-mail: jo@samaritans.org
Self-Abuse Finally Ends (S.A.F.E.) Alternatives Program, L.L.C.
Offers a variety of services for people who self-injure, including group and individual therapy, in- and out-patient treatment, and a partial/day hospital.
   S.A.F.E. Alternatives
   7115 W. North Avenue, Suite 319
   Oak Park, IL 60302
   Information Line: (800) DON'T-CUT (366-8288)
   Web site: http://www.selfinjury.com
Society for Light Treatment and Biological Rhythms (SLTBR)
Send a self-addressed stamped envelope for info about melatonin and other light-related issues to:
   10200 West 44th Avenue, Suite 304
   Wheat Ridge, CO 80033-2840
   Phone: (303) 424-3697
   Fax: (303) 422-8894
   Web site: http://www.websciences.org/sltbr/
   E-mail: sltbr@resourcenter.com
Suicide Awareness\Voices of Education (SA\VE)
   SA\VE
   P.O. Box 24507
   Minneapolis, MN 55424-0507
   Phone: (612) 946-7998
   Web site: http://www.save.org/
   E-mail: save@winternet.com

Survivors of Incest Anonymous (SIA)
World Service Office
P.O. Box 21817
Baltimore, MD 21222-6817
Phone: (410) 282-3400

Toastmasters International
Holds meetings to help people develop and strengthen their public speaking skills.
P.O. Box 9052
Mission Viejo, CA 92690
Information Line: (800) 993-7732
Phone: (714) 858-8255
Fax: (714) 858-1207
Web site: http://www.toastmasters.org/
E-mail: tminfo@toastmasters.org

Trichotillomania Learning Center
Provides information, support group referral, and other services regarding compulsive hair pulling.
1215 Mission St.
Santa Cruz, CA 95060
Phone: (408) 457-1004 [9am–3pm (PT), M–W]

VOICES (Victims Of Incest Can Emerge Survivors) In Action, Inc.
An international organization that provides assistance to survivors of incest and child sexual abuse.
VOICES In Action, Inc.
P.O. Box 148309
Chicago, IL 60614
Phone: (800) 7-VOICE-8 (786-4238)
(773) 327-1500
Web site: http://www.voices-action.org/
E-mail: voices@voices-action.org

Liïnks

Internet Mental Health
Web site: http://www.mentalhealth.com

Mental Health Net
Web site: http://www.mhnet.org/

PsychCentral: Dr. John Grohol's Mental Health Page
Web site: http://www.grohol.com/

The Substance Abuse and Mental Health Services Administration (SAMHSA) of the Department of Health and Human Services (DHHS)
Web site: http://www.samhsa.gov

Books

American Psychiatric Association. *Quick Reference to the Diagnostic Criteria from DSM-IV.* Washington, D.C.: American Psychiatric Press, Inc., 1994.

Appleton, William S. *Prozac and the New Antidepressants: What You Need to Know about Prozac, Zoloft, Paxil, Luvox, Wellbutrin, Effexor, Serzone, and More.* New York: NAL/Dutton, 1997.

Babior, Shirley, and Carol Goldman. *Overcoming Panic, Anxiety, & Phobias: New Strategies to Free Yourself from Worry and Fear.* Duluth, MN: Whole Person Associates, Inc., 1995.

Baron-Faust, Rita. *Mental Wellness for Women.* New York: William Morrow & Company, Inc., 1997.

Bass, Ellen, and Laura Davis. *The Courage to Heal: A Guide for Women Survivors of Child Sexual Abuse* (3rd ed.). New York: HarperCollins Publishers, 1994. (As well as other titles)

Benson, Herbert. *The Relaxation Response.* Avenal, NJ: Random House Value Publishing, Inc., 1992.

Burka, Jane B. *Procrastination: Why You Do It, What to Do about It.* Reading, MA: Addison-Wesley Publishing Co., Inc., 1990.

Caine, Lynn. *Being a Widow.* New York: Viking Penguin., 1990.

Carducci, Bernardo. *The Shy Life: Understanding, Hope & Healing.* New York: HarperCollins Publishers, 1998.

Carnegie, Dale. *The Leader in You: How to Stop Worrying and Start Living/ How to Win Friends and Influence People:* New York: Pocket Books, 1996.

Conterio, Karen, and Wendy Lader, with Jennifer Kingston-Bloom. *Bodily Harm.* New York: Hyperion, 1998.

Cronkite, Kathy. *On the Edge of Darkness: Conversations about Conquering Depression.* New York: Dell Publishing Company, Inc., 1995.

Daly, John A., James C. McCroskey, Joe Ayres, Tim Hopt, and Debbie M. Ayres (editors). *Avoiding Communication: Shyness, Reticence, and Communication Apprehension.* Cresskill, NJ: Hampton Press, Inc., 1997.

Davis, Laura. *Allies in Healing: When the Person You Love Was Sexually Abused as a Child, A Support Book for Partners.* New York: HarperCollins Publishers, 1991.

de Biexedon, S. Yevette. *Lovers and Survivors: A Partner's Guide to Living with and Loving a Sexual Abuse Survivor.* San Francisco, CA: Robert D. Reed Publishers, 1995.

Edelman, Hope. *Motherless Daughters: The Legacy of Loss.* New York: Dell Publishing Company, 1997.

Freedman, Rita. *That Special You: Feeling Good about Yourself.* White Plains, NY: Peter Pauper Press, Inc., 1994.

Friedman, Jordan. *The Stress Manager's Manual with Cassette Trainer.* New York: StressHelp Press, 1996.

Gabor, Don. *Talking with Confidence for the Painfully Shy.* New York: Crown Publishing Group, 1997.

Hales, Dianne and Robert E. Hales. *Caring for the Mind: The Comprehensive Guide to Mental Health.* New York: Bantam Books, 1996.

Hoff, Ron. *I Can See You Naked (A Fearless Guide to Making Great Presentations).* Kansas City, MO: Andrews & McMeel, 1992.

Jamison, Kay Redfield. *An Unquiet Mind.* New York: Random House, 1997.

Kramer, Peter D. *Listening to Prozac.* New York: Viking Penguin, 1997.

Krementz, Jill. *How It Feels When a Parent Dies.* Magnolia, MA: Peter Smith Publisher, Inc., 1993.

Kushner, Harold S. *When Bad Things Happen to Good People.* New York: Schocken Books, Inc., 1989.

Lee, Sharice A. *The Survivor's Guide: A Guide for Teenage Girls Who are Survivors of Sexual Abuse.* Thousand Oaks, CA: Sage Publications, Inc., 1995.

Levenkron, Steven. *Cutting: Understanding and Overcoming Self-Mutilation.* New York: W.W. Norton & Company, Inc., 1998.

Levenkron, Steven. *Obsessive-Compulsive Disorders: Treating and Understanding Crippling Habits.* New York: Warner Books, Inc., 1992.

Lew, Mike. *Victims No Longer.* New York: Harper & Row, 1990.

Loiselle, Mindy B. and Leslie B. Wright. *Shining Through: Pulling It Together after Sexual Abuse.* Brandon, VT: Safer Society Press, 1996.

Marshall, John R. *Social Phobia: From Shyness to Stage Fright.* New York: Basic Books, 1995.

McCoy, Kathy, and Charles Wibbelsman. *Life Happens: A Teenager's Guide to Friends, Failure, Sexuality, Love, Rejection, Addiction, Peer Pressure, Families, Loss, Depression, Change, and Other Challenges of Living.* New York: Berkley Publishing Group, 1996.

Mendel, Matthew P. *The Male Survivor: The Impact of Sexual Abuse.* Thousand Oaks, CA: Sage Publications, Inc., 1994.

Miller, Dusty. *Women Who Hurt Themselves: A Book of Hope and Understanding.* New York: Basic Books, 1995.

Parker, Jim. *Prozac: Pros and Cons.* Tempe, AZ: Do It Now Foundation, 1996.

Penn, Robert E. *The Gay Men's Wellness Guide: The National Lesbian and Gay Health Association's Complete Book of Physical, Emotional, and Mental Health and Well-Being.* New York: Henry Holt & Co., 1998.

Pipher, Mary. *Reviving Ophelia: Saving the Selves of Adolescent Girls.* New York: Ballantine Books, 1995.

Porat, Frieda, *Creative Procrastination: Organizing Your Own Life.* New York: Harper & Row, Publishers, 1980.

Rothstein, Larry, and Julia Thorne. *You Are Not Alone: Words of Experience and Hope for the Journey Through Depression.* New York: HarperCollins Publishers, 1993.

Sanford, Linda, and Mary Donovan. *Women & Self-Esteem.* New York: Viking Penguin, 1985.

Schneier, Franklin R., and Lawrence A. Welkowitz. *The Hidden Face of Shyness: Understanding & Overcoming Social Anxiety.* New York: Avon Books, 1996.

Seaward, Brian L. *Stand Like Mountain, Flow Like Water: Reflections on Stress and Human Spirituality.* Deerfield Beach, FL: Health Communications, Inc., 1997.

Selye, Hans. *The Stress of Life.* New York: The McGraw-Hill Companies, 1978.

Selye, Hans. *Stress without Distress.* New York: NAL/Dutton, 1975.

Spiegel, Jill. *Flirting for Success: The Art of Building Rapport.* New York: Warner Books, 1995.

Stevens, Jean A. *Say Good-Bye to Shy: Change Your Thinking, Change Your Life.* Newport Beach, CA: Sandpiper Press, 1995.

Styron, William. *Darkness Visible: A Memoir of Madness.* New York: Vintage Books, 1992.

Thompson, Tracy. *The Beast: A Journey through Depression.* New York: NAL/Dutton, 1996.

Wassmer, Arthur C. *Making Contact: A Guide to Overcoming Shyness.* New York: Henry Holt & Co., Inc. 1991.

Wegscheider-Cruse, Sharon. *Learning to Love Yourself: Finding Your Self-Worth.* Deerfield Beach, FL.: Health Communications Inc., 1987.

Westerlund, Elaine. *Women's Sexuality after Childhood Incest.* New York: W.W. Norton and Company, Inc., 1992.

Whybrow, Peter C. *A Mood Apart: Depression, Mania, and Other Afflictions of the Self.* New York: Basic Books, 1998.

Woolis, Rebecca. *When Someone You Love Has a Mental Illness: A Handbook for Family, Friends and Caregivers.* New York: Putnam Books, 1992.

Wurtzel, Elizabeth. *Prozac Nation: Young and Depressed in America.* New York: Berkley Publishing Group, 1997.

Zimbardo, Philip G. *Shyness.* Reading, MA: Addison-Wesley Longman, Inc., 1990.

Films

Dead Poets Society (1989): Robin Williams, Ethan Hawke, and Robert Sean Leonard star in this film about the relationship between a popular English teacher and his students, the tragic suicide of one of the students who is abused by a strict father, and how his roommate and friends deal with his sudden death.

Ordinary People (1980): Timothy Hutton, Mary Tyler Moore, and Donald Sutherland star in this drama about a young man's grief over his brother's tragic death and his troubled relationship with one of his parents.

Ponette (1996): This French film centers around how a girl copes with the loss of a parent.

Shadowlands (1993): Anthony Hopkins and Debra Winger star in this film about author C. S. Lewis's relationship with American poet Joy Davidman, who dies from breast cancer.

Shine (1996): Geoffrey Rush stars in this film about the life of pianist David Helfgott, who has a mental breakdown as a result of an abusive relationship with his stern father.

Surviving (1984): This made-for-television movie starring Molly Ringwald, Zach Galligan, Ellen Burstyn, Paul Sorvino, Marsha Mason, and Len Cariou deals with the suicide of a young couple and how their families and friends cope with the loss.

What's Eating Gilbert Grape? (1993): Johnny Depp, Leonardo Di Caprio, Juliette Lewis, and Mary Steenburgen star in this heartbreaking story centered around Depp's character, his family, and his younger, mentally challenged brother, played brilliantly by Di Caprio.

FITNESS AND NUTRITION

American Academy of Allergy, Asthma, and Immunology (AAAAI)
Has information on food allergies.
611 East Wells St.
Milwaukee, WI 53202
Physician Referral and Information Line: (800) 822-2762
Business Office Phone: (412) 272-6071
Web site: http://www.aaaai.org/

American Cancer Society (ACS) Call Center
Will direct your call to other affiliated services, refer you to physicians and cancer care centers, or provide written materials.
Main Headquarters:
1599 Clifton Road, N.E.
Atlanta, GA 30329-4251
Phone: (800) ACS-2345 (227-2345)
        (404) 320-3333
Web site: http://www.cancer.org

American Council on Exercise (ACE)
5820 Oberlin Drive, Suite 102
San Diego, CA 92121-3787
ACE Academy Hotline and Public Membership Information Line: (800) 825-3636
ACE Fit Facts or Frequently Requested ACE Documents Fax-on-Demand: (888)
    FIT-FAXX (348-3299)
Phone: (619) 535-8227
        (800) 529-8227

Fax: (619) 535-1778
Web site: http://www.acefitness.org/
American Diabetes Association (ADA)
1660 Duke St.
Alexandria, VA 22314
Phone: (800) DIABETES (342-2383) (English and Spanish)
(800) 232-3472
(703) 549-1500
Fax: (703) 549-6995
Web site: http://www.diabetes.org
The American Dietetic Association (ADA)
216 West Jackson Blvd., Suite 800
Chicago, IL 60606-6995
For a referral to a Registered Dietitian in your area, and for info regarding nutrition and healthy eating:
Nutrition Hotline: (800) 366-1655
Phone: (800) 877-1600
(312) 899-0040
Fax: (312) 899-1979
Web site: http://www.eatright.org/
American Heart Association (AHA) National Center
Provides referrals, distributes literature, and has information regarding diseases of the heart.
7272 Greenville Ave.
Dallas, TX 75231
Phone: (800) AHA-USA1 (242-8721)
(214) 373-6300
Web site: http://www.americanheart.org
Exercise/Physical Activity Web site: http://amhrt.org/heartg/exercise.html
American Institute for Cancer Research (AICR)
A nonprofit organization that publishes **The AICR Newsletter on Diet, Nutrition, and Cancer** and other informational publications—free for members and supporters.
1759 R Street, N.W.
Washington, D.C. 20009
Nutrition Hotline: (800) 843-8114 [9am–5pm (EST), M–F]
Phone: (202) 328-7744
Fax: (202) 328-7226
Web site: http://www.aicr.org/
E-mail: aicrweb@aicr.org
Center for Science in the Public Interest (CSPI)
A nonprofit education and advocacy organization that focuses on food safety, nutrition, and alcohol issues, and publishes the **Nutrition Action Healthletter** ten times a year.
1875 Connecticut Ave., N.W.
Suite 300
Washington, D.C. 20009-5728
Phone: (202) 332-9110
Fax: (202) 265-4954
Web site: http://www.cspinet.org/
E-mail: cspi@cspinet.org
Nutrition Action Healthletter E-mail: nah@cspinet.org
Subscription E-mail: circ@cspinet.org

Consumer Information Center of the U.S. General Services Administration
Offers online access to free federal consumer publications about food and nutrition, health, etc.
   Web site: http://www.pueblo.gsa.gov
   E-mail: catalog.pueblo@gsa.gov
Department of Health Fitness (DHF) and National Center for Health Fitness (NCHF)
   DHF (or NCHF)
   American University
   4400 Massachusetts Avenue, N.W.
   Nebraska Hall-Lower Level
   Washington, DC 20016-8037
   Phone: (202) 885-6275
   Fax: (202) 885-6288
   Web site: http://www.healthy.american.edu
   E-mail: dhfaa@american.edu
      nchfaa@american.edu
Institute of Food Science and Technology (IFST)
Has information on food quality and safety.
   5 Cambridge Court
   210 Shepherd's Bush Road
   London W6 7NL
   UK
   Web site: http://www.easynet.co.uk/ifst/
   E-mail: ifst@easynet.co.uk
International Food Information Council (IFIC) Foundation
   1100 Connecticut Ave., N.W.
   Suite 430
   Washington, DC 20036
   Web site: http://ificinfo.health.org/
   E-mail: foodinfo@ific.health.org
Melpomene Institute
A nonprofit research organization that has information on women's health and physical activity.
   1010 University Ave.
   St. Paul, MN 55104
   Phone: (612) 642-1951
   Fax: (612) 642-1871
   Web site: http://www.melpomene.org
   E-mail: melpomen@skypoint.com
National Cancer Institute (NCI)
Behind the Five-A-Day (five servings of fruits and vegetables) Campaign.
   NCI
   Office of Cancer Communications
   31 Center Dr., MSC 2580
   Bethesda, MD 20892-2580
   Cancer Information Service: (800) 4-CANCER (422-6237) [9am–4:30pm (EST), M–F]
   Cancer Fax-R (Cancer Facts Fax-on-Demand): (301) 402-5874
   Phone: (301) 496-5583
   TTY: (800) 332-8615

NCI Web site: http://WWW.NCI.NIH.GOV/
Cancernet-R Web site: http://cancernet.nci.nih.gov/
  gopher://gopher.nih.gov.
E-mail: cancermail@icicc.nci.nih.gov
  cancernet@icicc.nci.nih.gov

National Heart, Lung, and Blood Institute (NHLBI) Information Center

Provides written information regarding high blood pressure, cholesterol, obesity, exercise, heart attack, asthma, sleep disorders, and other related topics.

NHLBI Information Center
P.O. Box 30105
Bethesda, MD 20824-0105
Web site: http://www.nhlbi.nih.gov/nhlbi/nhlbi.htm

National Institute of Diabetes, Digestive, and Kidney Diseases (NIDDK) of The National Institutes of Health (NIH)

Fax: (301) 907-8906
Web site: http://www.niddk.nih.gov

National Diabetes Information (Clearinghouse):
1 Information Way
Bethesda, MD 20892-3560
Phone: (301) 654-3327

National Institute of Digestive Diseases (Clearinghouse):
2 Information Way
Bethesda, MD 20892-3570
Phone: (301) 654-3810

National Institute of Kidney Diseases (Clearinghouse):
3 Information Way
Bethesda, MD 20892-3580
Phone: (301) 654-4415

National Osteoporosis Foundation (NOF)

Provides professional education, patient education, advocacy, public awareness, and support for research.

1150 17th Street, N.W.
Suite 500
Washington, DC 20036-4603
Phone: (202) 223-2226
Web site: http://www.nof.org

Penn State Sports Medicine Newsletter

A monthly newsletter about athletic performance published by the Department of Kinesiology, College of Health and Human Development at Pennsylvania State University.

Penn State Sports Medicine Newsletter
P.O. Box 3000
Denville, NJ 07834
Customer Service Line: (800) 783-4903

Shape Up America!

Web site: http://www.shapeup.org/sua/index.html
E-mail: suainfo@shapeup.org

Surgeon General's Report on Physical Activity and Health
For a free copy of the Executive Summary, At-A-Glance, and/or Fact Sheets:
(888)-CDC-4NRG (232-4674)
Web site: http://www.cdc.gov/nccdphp/sgr/sgr.htm
Tufts University Health & Nutrition Letter
A monthly newsletter published by Tufts University.
Reader's Questions:
6 Beacon Street, Suite 1110
Boston, MA 02108

New Subscription Information:
P.O. Box 57857
Boulder, CO 80322-7857
Customer Service Line: (800) 274-7581 (National)
(303) 447-9330 (Colorado only)
Nutrition Navigator Web site: http://navigator.tufts.edu
E-mail: tufts@tiac.net
U.S. Centers for Disease Control and Prevention (CDC), Division of Nutrition and Physical Activity
Division of Nutrition and Physical Activity
National Center for Chronic Disease Prevention and Health Promotion
CDC
Mail Stop K-46
4770 Buford Highway, N.E.
Atlanta, Ga 30341-3724
Phone: (770) 488-6042
Fax: (770) 488-5473
Web site: http://www.cdc.gov/nccdphp/dnpa/readyset/
E-mail: ccdinfo@cdc.gov
U.S. Department of Agriculture (USDA) Food and Nutrition Information Center (FNIC)
Has info on the food pyramid, vegetarian nutrition, and other topics.
FNIC
Agricultural Research Service
USDA
National Agricultural Library, Room 304
10301 Baltimore Ave.
Beltsville, MD 20705-2351
Phone: (301) 504-5719
TTY: (301) 504-6856
Fax: (301) 504-6409
Web site: http://www.nal.usda.gov/fnic
E-mail: fnic@nal.usda.gov
U.S. Food and Drug Administration (FDA) Center for Food Safety and Applied Nutrition (CFSAN)
200 C Street, S.W.
Washington, DC 20204
Web site: http://vm.cfsan.fda.gov/list.html
University of California at Berkeley Wellness Letter
A monthly newsletter of nutrition, fitness, and stress management published by the UC Berkeley School of Public Health.

Health Letter Associates
P.O. Box 412
Prince Street Station
New York, NY 10012-0007

Subscription Inquiries Address:
P.O. Box 420148
Palm Coast, FL 32142
Phone: (904) 445-6414
Web site: http://www.enews.com/magazines/ucbwl/
The Vegetarian Resource Group (VRG)
P.O. Box 1463
Baltimore, MD 21203
Phone: (410) 366-8343
Web site: http://www.vrg.org
E-mail: vrg@vrg.org

Links

Dr. Stephen M. Pribut's Sports Pages
Has information on the prevention and treatment of running injuries.
Web site: http://www.clark.net/pub/pribut/spinjur.html
Dole 5-A-Day
Has lots of information about the health benefits of fruits and vegetables.
Web site: http://www.dole5aday.com/
Fitness Partner Connection Jumpsite!
Web site: http://primusweb.com/fitnesspartner/
The Medical Tent Section of the Sports Med Web (for endurance athletes)
Web site: http://www.rice.edu/~jenky/medtent.1.html

Books

American College of Sports Medicine Staff. *ACSM Fitness Book*. Champaign, IL: Human Kinetics Publishers, 1997.

American Medical Association Staff. *The American Medical Association Encyclopedia of Medicine*. New York: Random House, 1989.

American Medical Women's Association Staff. *The AMWA Guide to Nutrition and Wellness*. New York: Dell Publishing Company, Inc., 1996.

Anderson, Bob. *Stretch Yourself for Health and Fitness*. Columbia, MO: South Asia Books, 1993.

Anderson, Bob. *Stretching*. Bolinas. CA: Shelter Publications, Inc., 1980.

Bricklin, Mark, and Linda Konner. *Prevention's Your Perfect Weight*. Emmaus, PA: Rodale Press, 1995.

Brody, Jane. *Jane Brody's Good Food Book*. New York: Bantam Books, 1996.

Crocker, Betty. *Betty Crocker's Good & Easy Cookbook*. Old Tappan, NJ: Macmillan Publishing Company, 1996.

Duyff, Roberta Larson. *The American Dietetics Association's Complete Food and Nutrition Guide*. Minneapolis, MN: Chronimed Publishing, 1996.

Griffith, H. Winter. *Complete Guide to Vitamins, Minerals, and Supplements*. Tucson, AZ: Fisher Books, 1988.

Jacobson, Michael. F. *Safe Food*. New York: Berkeley Publishing Group, 1993.

Herbert, Victor, and Genell J. Subak-Sharpe. *Total Nutrition—The Only Guide You'll Ever Need*. New York: St. Martin's Press, 1995.

Krauss, Pam (editor). *Moosewood Restaurant Low-Fat Favorites*. New York: Crown Publishing Group, 1996.

Lappé, Frances Moore. *Diet for a Small Planet*. (20th anniversary ed.). New York: Ballantine Books, 1992.

McQuillan, Susan, and Edward Saltzman. *The Complete Idiot's Guide to Losing Weight*. New York: Alpha Books, 1998.

Pennington, Jean A.T. *Bowes and Church's Food Values of Portions Commonly Used* (17th ed.). Philadelphia: Lippincott-Raven Publishers, 1997.

Robertson, Laurel. *The New Laurel's Kitchen*. Berkeley, CA: Ten Speed Press, 1986.

Sindell, Cheryl. *Cooking Without Recipes*. New York: Kensington Books, 1997.

Travis, John W., and Regina S. Ryan. *Wellness Workbook*. Berkeley, CA: Ten Speed Press, 1993.

University of California at Berkeley Wellness Letter Editors. *The Wellness Encyclopedia of Food and Nutrition*. New York: Rebus, Inc., 1992.

Vegetarian Times Editors. *Vegetarian Times Complete Cookbook*. Old Tappan, NJ: Macmillan Publishing. Company, 1995.

Westmoreland, Susan (editor). *The Good Housekeeping Step-by-Step Cookbook*. New York: Hearst Books, 1997.

White, Timothy. *The Wellness Guide to Lifelong Fitness*. New York: Rebus, Inc., 1993.

Body Image and Eating Concerns (Including Eating Disorders)

About-Face!

A grassroots organization that educates about body image and body acceptance.

P.O. Box 77665

San Francisco, CA 94107

Phone: (415) 436-0212

Web site: http://www.about-face.org/

E-mail: info@about-face.org

American Anorexia/Bulimia Association, Inc. (AABA)

A national nonprofit organization dedicated to the prevention, treatment, and cure of eating disorders that helps people with eating disorders, as well as their families and friends. AABA offers various services, including public information, self-help/support groups, speakers bureau/outreach presentations, and nationwide referrals to therapists, centers, and support services.

165 West 46th Street, Suite 1108

New York, NY 10036

Phone: (212) 575-6200

Fax: (212) 278-0698

Web site: http://members.aol.com/amanbu/index.html

E-mail: amanbu@aol.com

Anorexia Nervosa and Bulimia Association (ANAB) [of Ontario, Canada]

Provides information, referral to doctors in Canada, support groups, and a quarterly Q&A newsletter.

767 Boxridge Dr.

P.O. Box 20058

Kingston, ON K7PICO

CANADA

Information and Support Line: (613) 547-3684

Web site: http://qlink.queensu.ca/~4map/anabhome.htm

Anorexia Nervosa and Related Eating Disorders, Inc. (ANRED)

ANRED

P.O. Box 5102
Eugene, OR 97405
Information Line: (541) 344-1144
Web site: http://www.anred.com
E-mail: jarinor@rio.com
National Eating Disorders Organization (NEDO)
NEDO
6655 South Yale Avenue
Tulsa, OK 74136
Phone: (918) 481-4044
Fax: (918) 481-4076
Web site: http://www.laureate.com/nedointro.html
Overeaters Anonymous (OA)
World Service Office Address:
6075 Zenith Ct., N.E.
Rio Rancho, NM 87124
Phone: (505) 891-2664
Fax: (505) 891-4320
World Service Web site: http://www.overeatersanonymous.org
NY Office Phone: (212) 206-8621
Northeast Web site: http://www.oaregion6.org

Links
Barnard/Columbia Women's Handbook
Gopher Menu: gopher://gopher.cc.columbia.edu:71/11/publications/women

Books
Alexander-Mott, Lee Ann, and D. Barry Lumsden (editors). *Understanding Eating Disorders: Anorexia Nervosa, Bulimia Nervosa, and Obesity.* Washington, D.C.: Taylor & Francis, 1994.

Andersen, Arnold E. *Males with Eating Disorders.* New York: Brunner/Mazel, 1990.

Brumberg, Joan J. *The Body Project: An Intimate History of American Girls.* New York: Random House, 1997.

Claude-Pierre, Peggy. *The Secret Language of Eating Disorders: The Revolutionary New Approach to Curing Anorexia and Bulimia.* New York: Random House, 1997.

Freedman, Rita. *Bodylove: Learning to Like Our Looks—and Ourselves.* New York: HarperCollins Publishers, 1990.

Hornbacher, Marya. *Wasted: A Memoir of Anorexia and Bulimia.* New York: HarperCollins Publishers, 1997.

Hutchinson, Marcia. *Transforming Body Image: Learning to Love the Body You Have.* Freedom, CA: The Crossing Press, Inc., 1985.

Johnston, Joni E. *Appearance Obsession: Learning to Love the Way You Look.* Deerfield Beach, FL: Health Communications, Inc., 1994.

Kano, Susan. *Making Peace with Food: Freeing Yourself from the Diet/Weight Obsession.* New York: Harper & Row, Publishers, 1989.

Levenkron, Steven. *Treating and Overcoming Anorexia Nervosa.* New York: Warner Books, Inc., 1997.

Orbach, Susie. *Fat Is a Feminist Issue.* New York: Berkeley Publishing Group, 1994.

Pipher, Mary. *Hunger Pains.* New York: Ballantine Books, 1997.

Rodin, Judith. *Body Traps: Breaking the Binds that Keep You from Feeling Good about Your Body.* New York: Quill/William Morrow, 1992.

Roth, Geneen. *Appetites.* New York: NAL/Dutton, 1997.

Roth, Geneen. *Breaking Free from Compulsive Eating*. New York: NAL/Dutton, 1993.

Roth, Geneen. *When Food Is Love: Exploring the Relationship Between Eating and Intimacy*. New York: NAL/Dutton, 1992. (As well as other titles)

Schroeder, Charles R. *Fat Is Not a Four-Letter Word*. Minnetonka, MN: Chronimed Publishing, 1992.

Siegel, Michelle, Judith Brisman, and Margot Weinshel. *Surviving an Eating Disorder: Strategies for Family and Friends*. New York: HarperCollins Publishers, 1997.

Stunkard, Albert J., and Eliot Stellar (editors). *Eating and Its Disorders*. Ann Arbor, MI: Books on Demand, 1984.

Wolf, Naomi. *The Beauty Myth: How Images of Beauty Are Used Against Women*. New York: Doubleday & Company, Inc., 1992.

Zerbe, Kathryn J. *The Body Betrayed: A Deeper Understanding of Women, Eating Disorders, and Treatment*. Carlsbad, CA: Gürze Books, 1995.

Films

The Best Little Girl in the World (1981): Jennifer Jason Leigh and Charles Durning star in this film about a family whose daughter is struggling with anorexia nervosa.

Eating (1990): Henry Jaglom's film is "a very serious comedy about women and food."

The Full Monty (1997): Robert Carlyle stars in this comedy about out-of-work steelworkers in England who are willing to strip to try to make ends meet. Among the issues the film focuses on are male bonding/relationships, male sexual stereotypes, body image, and impotence.

ALCOHOL, NICOTINE, AND OTHER DRUGS

AL-ANON and ALATEEN
Provides information, support, and resources to families and friends of alcoholics.
AL-ANON Family Group Headquarters, Inc.
World Service Office
1600 Corporate Landing Parkway
Virginia Beach, VA 23454-5617
24-hour Meeting Information Line: (800) 344-2666 (U.S.)
(800) 443-4525 (Canada)
For Free Introductory Literature Packet: (800) 356-9996 (U.S.)
(800) 714-7498 (Canada)
General Information and Literature Order Line: (757) 563-1600
World Service Office Web site: http://www.al-anon.org/
AL-ANON Member Volunteers-Sponsored Web site: http://www.al-anon-alateen.org/
E-mail: info@Al-Anon-Alateen.org
Alcohol National Hotline
A service of AdCare Hospital of Worcester, Inc., that is a free, confidential 24-hour-a-day help line that offers information on drug and alcohol abuse treatment services and support groups.
Hotline: (800) ALCOHOL (252-6465)
Alcoholics Anonymous (AA)
Offers a variety of services, including support group meetings and an AA book for beginners.
P.O. Box 459
Grand Central Station
New York, NY 10163
Phone: (212) 870-3400

Web site: http://www.alcoholics-anonymous.org
(lists AA meetings, local and national, in English, Spanish, & French)

American Cancer Society (ACS) Call Center
Will direct your call to other affiliated services, refer you to physicians and cancer care centers, or provide written materials.
Main Headquarters:
1599 Clifton Road, N.E.
Atlanta, GA 30329-4251
Phone: (800) ACS-2345 (227-2345)
(404) 320-3333
Web site: http://www.cancer.org

American Council for Drug Education (ACDE)
Develops and disseminates drug education materials to individuals, professionals, and organizations regarding drug use and abuse—especially geared toward helping children, adolescents, and their families.
Phone: (212) 595-5810 (x7860)
Web site: http://www.acde.org

American Lung Association (ALA)
1740 Broadway, 14th Floor
New York, NY 10019
Phone: (212) 315-8700
(800) 586-4872
Web site: http://www.lungusa.org
E-mail: info@lungusa.org

BACCHUS (Boost Alcohol Consciousness Concerning the Health of University Students) and GAMMA (Greeks Advocating for Mature Management of Alcohol) of the United States
Provide information over the phone and in written form to any interested party concerning all issues pertinent to the college-age population (i.e., alcohol and drug use, sexual assault, etc.).
P.O. Box 100430
Denver, CO 80250-0430
Phone: (303) 871-0901
Web site: http://www.bacchusgamma.org
E-mail: bachgam@aol.com

Center for Substance Abuse Research (CESAR)
CESAR
University of Maryland, College Park
4321 Hartwick Rd., Suite 501
College Park, MD 20740
Phone: (301) 403-8329
Fax: (301) 403-8342
Web site: http://www.bsos.umd.edu/cesar/cesar.html
E-mail: cesar@cesar.umd.edu

Center for Substance Abuse Treatment (CSAT)
National Drug and Alcohol Treatment Hotline: (800) 662-HELP (4357)
(choose from a touch-tone menu of information and services)
Web site: http://www.samhsa.gov/csat/csat.htm

Children of Alcoholics Foundation, Inc. (CoAF)
Helps individuals from alcoholic and/or substance-abusing families and provides educational materials, resources, and referrals to any individual or professional seeking information, but does not provide crisis counseling. However, will refer to appropriate services.
33 W. 60th St., 5th Floor

New York, NY 10023
Phone: (212) 757-2100 (x6370)
        (800) 359-2623
Fax: (212) 757-2208
E-mail: coaf@phoenixhouse.org
Cocaine Anonymous (CA)
Cocaine Anonymous World Service Office (CAWSO, Inc.)
P.O. Box 2000
Los Angeles, CA 90049-8000
National Help Line: (800) 347-8998
Phone: (310) 559-5833
Fax: (310) 559-2554
Web site: http://www.ca.org/
Public Information E-mail: pubinfo@ca.org
Other E-mail: cawso@ca.org
The Do It Now Foundation
Provides brochures on Ecstasy and other "club drugs."
P.O. Box 27568
Tempe, AZ 85285-7568
Phone: (602) 736-0599
Web site: http://www.doitnow.org/
E-mail: doitnow123@earthlink.net
Marijuana Anonymous (MA)
Web site: http://www.marijuana-anonymous.org
E-mail: info@marijuana-anonymous.org
Narcotics Anonymous (NA)
Provides referrals to drug treatment and people to talk with in your own community.
NA World Service Office
P.O. Box 9999
Van Nuys, CA 91409
Phone: (818) 773-9999
Fax: (818) 700-0700
Web site: http://wsoinc.com/
E-mail: info@wsoinc.com
National Association for Children of Alcoholics (NACoA)
Advocates "for all children and families affected by alcoholism and other drug dependencies."
11426 Rockville Pike, Suite 100
Rockville, MD 20852
To receive info about the association, locations of nearest meetings, or referrals
    and information about further help:
Phone: (301) 468-0985
        (888) 554-COAS (2627)
Fax: (301) 468-0987
Web site: http://www.health.org/nacoa
E-mail: nacoa@charitiesusa.com
National Cancer Institute (NCI)
NCI
Officer of Cancer Communications
31 Center Dr., MSC 2580
Bethesda, MD 20892-2580
Cancer Information Service: (800) 4-CANCER (422-6237)
    [9am–4:30pm (EST), M–F]
CancerFax-R (Cancer Facts Fax-on-Demand): (301) 402-5874

Phone: (301) 496-5583
TTY: (800) 332-8615
NCI Web site: http://WWW.NCI.NIH.GOV/
Cancernet-R Web site: http://cancernet.nci.nih.gov/
gopher://gopher.nih.gov
E-mail: cancermail@icicc.nci.nih.gov
cancernet@icicc.nci.nih.gov

The National Center on Addiction and Substance Abuse (CASA) at Columbia University
A national organization, comprised of all professional disciplines, that aims to study and combat all types of substance abuse as they affect all aspects of society.
152 West 57th Street
New York, NY 10019-3310
Phone: (212) 841-5200
Fax: (212) 956-8020
Web site: http://www.casacolumbia.org

The National Clearinghouse for Alcohol and Drug Information
Provides free information and resources about alcohol-related health topics, including disease and abuse prevention.
Box 2345
Rockville, MD 20847-2345
Phone: (301) 468-2600
(800) 729-6686
TTY: (800) 487-4889
Web site: http://www.health.org

National Council on Alcoholism and Drug Dependency, Inc. (NCADD)
Provides statistical information and resources related to drug abuse recovery, as well as information and referral services regarding alcohol and drug abuse.
12 West 21st Street
New York, NY 10010
24-Hour Hope Line: (800) NCA-CALL (622-2255)
Phone: (212) 206-6770
(800) 622-2255
(800) 467-4753
Fax: (212) 645-1690
Web site: http://www.ncadd.org
E-mail: national@ncadd.org

National Institute on Alcohol Abuse and Alcoholism (NIAAA), Distribution Center
P.O. Box 10686
Rockville, MD 20849-0686
Web site: http://www.niaaa.nih.gov

National Institute on Drug Abuse (NIDA)
Web site: http://www.nida.nih.gov/
E-mail: Information@lists.nida.nih.gov

National Organization for the Reform of Marijuana Laws (NORML)
Taking a liberal perspective, provides info on urine testing, laws, prohibition, and the movement to reform the current laws.
1001 Connecticut Ave., N.W.
Suite 1010
Washington, DC 20036

Phone: (202) 483-5500
Web site: http://www.norml.org
E-mail: natlnorml@aol.com
Nicotine Anonymous
Nicotine Anonymous World Services
P.O. Box 591777
San Francisco, CA 94159-1777
Phone: (415) 750-0328
Web site: http://www.nicotine-anonymous.org
E-mail: nica@onramp.net
Office for Substance Abuse Prevention
5600 Fishers Lane
Rockwall II
Rockville, MD 20857
Phone: (301) 443-0365
Web site: http://www.samhsa.gov/csap/index.html
E-mail: nnadal@samhsa.gov
Phoenix House
Education, prevention, and treatment association with 23 programs in New York, New Jersey, Texas, and California. Programs provide direct treatment and referrals for adolescents and adults, including residential long-term treatment, in-prison programs, outpatient programs, drug education and prevention programs, and "phoenix academies" (high school and residential treatment at the same time).
164 W. 74th St.
New York, NY 10023
Nationwide Hotline: (800) COCAINE (262-2463)
   (provides free, confidential treatment referrals and immediate crisis intervention, 24
      hours a day, 7 days a week, for any alcohol or other drug-related issue)
Web site: http://www.phoenixhouse.org

Links
Online Recovery Resources
   Web site: http://www.recovery.org/
Recovery Online
List links to various 12-step, religious, and secular self-help and other recovery groups.
   Web site: http://recovery.netwiz.net/index.html
The Substance Abuse and Mental Health Services Administration (SAMHSA) of the Department of Health and Human Services (DHHS)
   Web site: http://www.samhsa.gov

Books
Braun, Stephen. *Buzz: The Science and Lore of Alcohol and Caffeine.* New York: Penguin USA, 1997.

Carroll, Jim. *The Basketball Diaries.* New York: Penguin Books, 1995.

Friedman, Lawrence, Nicholas F. Fleming, David H. Roberts, and Steven E. Hyman (editors). *Source Book of Substance Abuse and Addiction.* Baltimore: Williams & Wilkins, 1996.

Jonnes, Jill. *Hep Cats, Narcs, and Pipe Dreams: A History of America's Romance with Illegal Drugs.* New York: Simon & Schuster Trade, 1996.

Knapp, Caroline. *Drinking: A Love Story.* New York: Dell Publishing Company, Inc., 1997.

Maximin, Anita, and Lori Stevic-Rust. *The Stop Smoking Workbook*. New York: Fine Communications, 1997.

McGovern, George. *Terry: My Daughter's Life and Death Struggle with Alcoholism*. New York: NAL/Dutton, 1997.

Sandmaier, Marian. *The Invisible Alcoholics: Women and Alcohol*. New York: TAB Books, 1997.

Stahl, Jerry. *Permanent Midnight*. New York: Warner Books, Inc., 1997.

Weil, Andrew, and Winifred Rosen. *From Chocolate to Morphine: Everything You Need to Know About Mind-Altering Drugs*. Boston: Houghton Mifflin Co., 1993.

Zimmer, Lynn and John P. Morgan. *Marijuana Myths, Marijuana Facts: A Review of the Scientific Evidence*. New York: Open Society Institute, 1997.

Films

The Basketball Diaries (1995): Leonardo Di Caprio stars in this film, adapted from the diary of the same title by Jim Carroll, about a young man's coming of age and experimentation with sex, drugs, and rock and roll on the tough NYC streets in the mid-1960s.

Basquiat (1996): This film is about Jean-Michel Basquiat's rise as an artist, but downfall and death due to drug addiction.

Clean and Sober (1988): Michael Keaton and Kathy Baker star in this drama as alcohol and drug abusers trying to get and stay clean and sober. Morgan Freeman also stars.

Drugstore Cowboy (1989): Matt Dillon and Kelly Lynch star in this film about a group of drug addict friends who resort to thieving to stay high.

Drunks (1997): This independent American drama details the lives of alcoholics in and out of recovery.

Nil by Mouth (1998): Written and directed by actor Gary Oldman, this film presents an unflinching portrayal of a London family rocked by alcohol and drug abuse.

The People vs. Larry Flynt (1996): Woody Harrelson stars as Larry Flynt, publisher of *Hustler* magazine, who challenges the First Amendment and deals with his wife's drug addiction.

Pulp Fiction (1994): Quentin Tarantino's award-winning film is a black comedy about the intertwined lives of various groups of people. Displays a particularly graphic and shocking scene revolving around heroin use and overdose.

Rush (1991): Jennifer Jason Leigh and Jason Patric star in this film about a narcotics officer who goes undercover to catch a drug dealer and gets hooked on drugs.

Sid and Nancy (1986): This film is about Sid Vicious of the rock group the Sex Pistols, who killed his girlfriend, Nancy Spungen, and later died of a heroin overdose.

Sweet Nothing (1995): Mira Sorvino stars in this film as the wife of a young man, played by Michael Imperioli, who descends from casual drug use to crack addiction.

Trainspotting (1995): This film starring Ewan McGregor is about Scottish youths and the dark side of heroin culture.

A Woman Under the Influence (1974): This John Cassavettes film starring Gena Rowlands is about a family dealing with a mother's mental and emotional deterioration due to her drinking problem.

GENERAL HEALTH QUESTIONS

Abledata
A resource for information on assistive devices, rehabilitative equipment, and the "assisted devices database."
8455 Colesville Rd., Suite 935
Silver Spring, MD 20910
Phone: (301) 608-8998
(800) 227-0216
TTY: (301) 608-8912
Fax: (301) 608-8958
Web site: http://www.abledata.com
E-mail: KABELKNAP@aol.com
Alliance of Professional Tattooists, Inc. (APT)
A non-profit educational and professional standards organization whose primary concerns are the continuing education of artists and their apprentices in the practice of infection control, the establishment of professional standards, and the implementation of professional practices with regard to health and safety in the tattoo industry.
428 Fourth Street
Unit 3
Annapolis, MD 21403
Phone: (410) 216-9630
Fax: (410) 760-1880
Web site: http://home.safetattoos.com/safetattoos/
E-mail: APThomeoffice@worldnet.att.net
America's Blood Centers
A network of 70 not-for-profit, independent community blood centers in 40 states.
725 Fifteenth St., N.W.
Suite 700
Washington, DC 20005
Phone: (202) 393-5725
Fax: (202) 393-1282
Web site: http://www.Americasblood.Org/
E-mail: ABC@americasblood.org
American Academy of Allergy, Asthma, and Immunology (AAAAI)
611 East Wells St.
Milwaukee, WI 53202
Physician referral and information line: (800) 822-2762
Business Office Phone: (414) 272-6071
Web site: http://www.aaaai.org/
American Academy of Dermatology (AAD)
930 North Meacham Rd.
Schaumburg, IL 60173-4965
Phone: (847) 330-0230
Fax: (847) 330-0050
Web site: http://www.aad.org/
American Cancer Society (ACS) Call Center
Will direct your call to other affiliated services, refer you to physicians and cancer care centers, or provide written materials.
Main Headquarters:
1599 Clifton Road, N.E.

Atlanta, GA 30329-4251
Phone: (800) ACS-2345 (227-2345)
(404) 320-3333
Web site: http://www.cancer.org
American Dental Association (ADA)
211 East Chicago Ave.
Chicago, IL 60611
Phone: (312) 440-2500
Fax: (312) 440-2800
Web site: http://www.ada.org/
E-mail: publicinfo@ada.org
American Diabetes Association (ADA)
1660 Duke Street
Alexandria, VA 22314
Phone: (800) DIABETES (342-2383) (English and Spanish)
(800) 232-3472
(703) 549-1500
Fax: (703) 549-6995
Web site: http://www.diabetes.org
American Heart Association (AHA) National Center
Provides referrals, distributes literature, and has information regarding diseases of the heart.
7272 Greenville Ave.
Dallas, TX 75231
Phone: (800) AHA-USA1 (242-8721)
(214) 373-6300
Web site: http://www.americanheart.org
American Institute for Cancer Research (AICR)
· *A nonprofit organization that publishes* **The AICR Newsletter on Diet, Nutrition, and Cancer** *and other informational publications—free for members and supporters.*
1759 R Street, N.W.
Washington, DC 20009
Nutrition Hotline: (800) 843-8114 [9 am–5pm (EST), M–F]
· *Phone: (202) 328-7744*
Fax: (202) 328-7226
Web site: http://www.aicr.org/
E-mail: aicrweb@aicr.org
American Lung Association (ALA)
1740 Broadway, 14th Floor
New York, NY 10019
Phone: (212) 315-8700
(800) 586-4872
Web site: http://www.lungusa.org
E-mail: info@lungusa.org
American Lyme Disease Foundation, Inc. (ALDF)
ALDF, Inc.
Mill Pond Offices
293 Route 1000
Somers, NY 10589
Phone: (914) 277-6970
Fax: (914) 277-6974
Web site: http://www.aldf.com
E-mail: Inquire@aldf.com

American Medical Association (AMA)
515 North State St.
Chicago, IL 60610
Main AMA Phone: (312) 464-5000
Library–Document Delivery Service Line: (312) 464-4855
AMA Answer Center answers general medical questions: (312) 464-4818
AMA Data Services Department provides written profiles of doctors for a fee:
  (312) 464-5199
  (800) 665-2882
Web site: http://www.ama-assn.org/
(When on home page, go to "physician select" area for limited info by doctor's name)

American Medical Women's Association (AMWA)
801 N. Fairfax St., Suite 400
Alexandria, VA 22314
Phone: (703) 838-0500
Fax: (703) 549-3864
Web site: http://www.amwa-doc.org/
E-mail: info@amwa-doc.org

American Paralysis Association (APA)
500 Morris Avenue
Springfield, NJ 07081
Phone: (800) 225-0292
  (973) 379-2690
Fax: (973) 912-9433
Web site: http://www.apacure.com
E-mail: Paralysis@aol.com

American Tinnitus Association (ATA)
Has information on tinnitus, or ringing in the ears.
ATA
P.O. Box 5
Portland, OR 97207-0005
Phone: (503) 248-9985
Fax: (503) 248-0024
Web site: http://www.teleport.com/~ata
E-mail: tinnitus@ata.org

Association on Higher Education and Disability (AHEAD)
AHEAD
P.O. Box 21192
Columbus, OH 43221-0192
Phone and TTY: (614) 488-4972
Fax: (614) 488-1174

Bone Marrow Foundation (BMF)
981 First Avenue, Suite 129
New York, NY 10022
Phone: (212) 838-3029
Lifeline Online Web site: http://www.bonemarrow.org/
E-mail: theBMF@aol.com

The Canadian Women's Health Network
The Canadian Women's Health Network
c/o Women's Health Clinic
Second Floor
419 Graham Ave.
Winnipeg, Manitoba R3C 0M3

CANADA
Phone: (204) 947-2422 (x134)
Fax: (204) 943-3844
Web site: http://www.cwhn.ca/index.html
E-mail: cwhn@cwhn.ca
Chronic Fatigue and Immune Dysfunction Syndrome (CFIDS) Association of America
Offers advocacy, information, research, support group referrals, and encouragement.
P.O. Box 220398
Charlotte, NC 28222-0398
Automated Voice Messaging System: (800) 442-3437
Fax: (704) 365-9755
E-mail: cfids@vnet.net
Cold Self-Care Center of the University of Rochester Health Services
Phone: (716) 273-5775
Web site: http://www.cc.rochester.edu/student-srvcs/uhs/CSCINTRO.HTM
Consumer Information Center of the U.S. General Services Administration
Offers online access to free federal consumer publications about food and nutrition, health, etc.
Web site: http://www.pueblo.gsa.gov
E-mail: catalog.pueblo@gsa.gov
Gilda's Club
A free, nonresidential cancer support community for people with cancer and their families and friends who join together to build social and emotional support as a supplement to medical care. Offers support and networking groups, lectures, workshops, and social events in a homelike setting, as well as a special children's program called Noogie Land.
195 West Houston Street
New York, NY 10014
Phone: (212) 647-9700
Fax: (212) 647-1154
Harvard Health Letter
A monthly newsletter published by the Harvard Medical School.
Harvard Health Letter
P.O. Box 420300
Palm Coast, FL 32142-0300
(include your mailing label)
Customer Service/Subscription Phone: (800) 829-9045 (U.S.)
(904) 445-4662 (Canada)
Web site: http://www.countway.harvard.edu/publications/Health_Publications
Job Accommodation Network (JAN)
Helps individuals with any disability find ways of accommodating their current jobs, and also aids employers and employees to review their rights.
Job Accommodation Network
West Virginia University
P.O. Box 6080
Morgantown, WV 26506-6080
Americans with Disabilities Act Info Phone & TTY: (800) ADA-WORK (232-9675)
Accommodation Info Phone: (800) 526-7234
(304) 293-7186
Fax: (304) 293-5407
Web site: http://janweb.icdi.wvu.edu (English and French)
E-mail: jan@jan.icdi.wvu.edu
Computer Bulletin Board System: (800) DIAL-JAN (342-5526)

The Lighthouse, Inc.

A not-for-profit vision rehabilitation organization that provides regional direct services for people who are partially sighted or blind, and, nationally, provides educational services—to health care professionals as well as those with impaired vision—research, advocacy, and national referral services.

111 E. 59th St.
New York, NY 10022
Bilingual Nationwide Information and Resource Line: (800) 334-5497
TTY: (212) 821-9713
Main Office Phone: (212) 821-9200
Fax: (212) 821-9707
Web site: http://www.lighthouse.org
E-mail: info@lighthouse.org

Lung Line Information Line at National Jewish Medical and Research Center

Choose from a touch-tone menu of options regarding lung, allergic, and immune diseases and their treatment.

Information Line: (800) 222-5864

Lupus Foundation of America

Provides a literature packet including in-depth information about lupus, book lists, membership info, and a list of additional services, including support groups.

Main Headquarters:
4 Research Place, Suite 180
Rockville, MD 20850-3226
Information Line: (800) 558-0121
Main Headquarters Phone: (301) 670-9292 [9am–5pm (EST), M–F]
Web site: http://www.lupus.org/lupus

The Lyme Disease Foundation

Provides written information, referral and support info, and research and prevention info for all tick-related diseases.

One Financial Plaza
Hartford, CT 06103-2610
24-hour Information Line: (800) 886-5963
Phone: (203) 525-2000

Mayo Clinic Health Letter

A monthly newsletter published by Mayo Foundation for Medical Education and Research.

Subscription Services
P.O. Box 53889
Boulder, CO 80322-3889
Phone: (800) 333-9037
        (303) 604-1465
Mayo Clinic Health O@sis Web site: http://www.mayo.ivi.com

The National Arthritis and Musculoskeletal and Skin Diseases Information Clearinghouse

Provides written materials and referrals to other related organizations.

NAMSIC
NIH
1 AMS Circle
Bethesda, MD 20892-3675
"NIAMS Fast Facts" fax service provides excerpts from information packets:
        (301) 881-2731
Phone: (301) 495-4484
TTY: (301) 565-2966

Fax: (301) 587-4352
Web site: http://www.nih.gov/niams/
National Cancer Institute (NCI)
NCI
Office of Cancer Communications
31 Center Dr., MSC 2580
Bethesda, MD 20892-2580
Cancer Information Service: (800) 4-CANCER (422-6237) [9am–4:30pm (EST), M–F]
CancerFax-R (Cancer Facts Fax-on-Demand): (301) 402-5874
Phone: (301) 496-5583
TTY: (800) 332-8615
NCI Web site: http://WWW.NCI.NIH.GOV/
Cancernet-R Web site: http://cancernet.nci.nih.gov/
gopher://gopher.nih.gov
E-mail: cancermail@icicc.nci.nih.gov
cancernet@icicc.nci.nih.gov
National Headache Foundation
An information resource providing written information, physician names for treatment through the mail, educational materials, and membership ($20 fee).
428 W. St. James Place, 2nd Floor
Chicago, IL 60614-2750
Headache Hotline: (800) 843-2256 [9am–5pm (CT), M–F]
Phone: (773) 388-6399
Fax: (773) 525-7357
Web site: http://www.headaches.org
National Health Information Center (NHIC) of the Office of Disease Prevention and Health Promotion (ODPHP)
A referral service to public and private resources for health information, including public library links across the U.S.
NHIC
Referral Specialist
P.O. Box 1133
Washington. D.C. 20013-1133
Phone: (301) 565-4167
(800) 336-4797 [9am–5pm (EST), M–F]
Fax: (301) 984-4256
Web site: http://nhic-nt.health.org/
E-mail: nhicinfo@health.org
National Heart, Lung, and Blood Institute (NHLBI) Information Center
Provides written information regarding high blood pressure, cholesterol, obesity, exercise, heart attack, asthma, sleep disorders, and other related topics.
NHLBI Information Center
P.O. Box 30105
Bethesda, MD 20824-0105
Web site: http://www.nhlbi.nih.gov/nhlbi/nhlbi.htm
National Institute of Allergy and Infectious Diseases (NIAID)
Provides info regarding Lyme disease, chronic fatigue syndrome, airborne and food allergies, parasitic diseases, and viral infections, such as the common cold, flu, and chicken pox, etc., over the phone or through written publications.
NIAID
Building 31, Rm. 7A50

Bethesda, MD 20892
Phone: (301) 496-5717
Web site: http://www.niaid.nih.gov/
National Institute of Diabetes, Digestive, and Kidney Diseases (NIDDK) of the National Institutes of Health (NIH)
Fax: (301) 907-8906
Web site: http://www.niddk.nih.gov

National Diabetes Information (Clearinghouse):
1 Information Way
Bethesda, MD 20892-3560
Phone: (301) 654-3327

National Institute of Digestive Diseases (Clearinghouse):
2 Information Way
Bethesda, MD 20892-3570
Phone: (301) 654-3810

National Institute of Kidney Diseases (Clearinghouse):
3 Information Way
Bethesda, MD 20892-3580
Phone: (301) 654-4415
National Institutes of Health (NIH)
Web site: http://www.nih.gov/
E-mail: nihinfo@od31tm1.od.nih.gov
NIH Office of Alternative Medicine (OAM)
9000 Rockville Pike
Building 31, Rm. 5B-38
Bethesda, MD 20892
Information Specialist Line & TTY: (888) 644-6226
Web site: http://altmed.od.nih.gov/

Information Clearinghouse can provide info by mail or by fax:
P.O. Box 8218
Silver Spring, MD 20907-8218
Fax Service: (301) 402-2466
National Institute for Occupational Safety and Health (NIOSH)
Robert A. Taft Laboratories
4676 Columbia Parkway
Cincinnati, OH 45226-1998
Info Service Line: (800) 35-NIOSH (64674) [9am–4pm (EST)]
Web site: http://www.cdc.gov/niosh/
The National Network of Libraries of Medicine
Connects you with the medical library in your area.
Phone: (800) 338-7657
National Organization for Rare Disorders, Inc. (NORD)
Has written materials on specific diagnosed rare disorders (first report is free; each additional will cost $5), referrals to other related organizations, and a member networking program.
100 Route 37
P.O. Box 8923
New Fairfield, CT 06812-8923
Phone: (800) 999-6673

(203) 746-6518
TTY: (203) 746-6927
Fax: (203) 746-6481
Web site: http://www.nord-rdb.com/~orphan
E-mail: orphan@nord-rdb.com

National Rehabilitation Information Center (NARIC)
A resource for people with spinal cord injury and their families that provides info on research and rehabilitation.

8455 Colesville Rd., Suite 935
Silver Spring, MD 20910-3319
Phone: (301) 588-9284
(800) 346-2742
TTY: (301) 495-5626
Fax: (301) 587-1967
Web site: http://www.naric.com/naric
E-mail: wendling@mindspring.com

National Sleep Foundation
Has info on sleep apnea and other sleep disturbances and resources for help.

729 Fifteenth St., N.W.
Fourth Floor
Washington, DC 20005
Web site: http://www.sleepfoundation.org/
E-mail: natsleep@erols.com

The National Spinal Cord Injury Association's Spinal Cord Org.
An international resource for people living with spinal cord injury.

Web site: http://www.erols.com/nscia/
Resource Center E-mail: NSCIRC2@aol.com
General E-mail: NSCIA3@aol.com

National Women's Health Network
A nonprofit organization that provides advocacy and information, aiming to aid women in having a greater voice in the health care system.

514 Tenth St., N.W.
Suite 400
Washington, DC 20004

For info regarding legislation, etc:
Main Office Phone: (202) 347-1140
Fax: (202) 347-1168

For comprehensive information about any women's health issue, or referrals to other appropriate organizations:
Information Clearinghouse Line: (202) 628-7814

Occupational Safety and Health Administration (OSHA)
Provides info on occupational safety and health hazards.

Room N 3647
U.S. Dept. of Labor
200 Constitution Ave., N.W.
Washington, DC 20210
Phone: (202) 219-8151
Web site: http://www.osha.gov/

Office of Minority Health Resource Center
Phone: (800) 444-6472
Web site: http://www.omhrc.gov/
E-mail: info@omhrc.gov
The Richard and Hinda Rosenthal Center for Complementary and Alternative Medicine
The Richard and Hinda Rosenthal Center for Complementary and Alternative
Medicine
Columbia University
College of Physicians and Surgeons
630 W. 168th St.
New York, NY 10032
Phone: (212) 543-9542
Web site: http://cpmcnet.columbia.edu/dept/rosenthal/
Society for the Advancement of Women's Health Research
1828 L. Street, N.W.
Suite 625
Washington, DC 20036
Phone: (202) 223-8224
Fax: (202) 833-3472
Web site: http://www.womens-health.org/
E-mail: info@womens-health.org
Stanford Center for Research in Disease Prevention, Health Promotion Resource Center (HPRC)
Has a library and information center offering reference requests, information referrals, current awareness, and computer searching (via various databases and an electronic bulletin board system, HPRCNET).
Stanford Center for Research in Disease Prevention
HPRC
Stanford University School of Medicine
1000 Welch Road
Palo Alto, CA 94304-1825
General Phone: (415) 723-1000
Library Phone: (415) 725-8993
General Fax: (415) 725-6906
U.S. Centers for Disease Control and Prevention (CDC)
Has recorded information by phone or by fax regarding many health issues, including international travel concerns, AIDS, the flu, Lyme disease and other tick-related diseases, childhood viruses such as measles and mumps, injury, smoking and tobacco, chronic disease, and many other health concerns.
1600 Clifton Rd., N.E.
Atlanta, GA 30333
24-hour CDC Voice and Fax Information System: (888) 232-3228 [for all disease and health risk information]
Fax-on-Demand: (888) CDC-FAXX (232-3299)
Phone: (404) 639-3311
CDC Web site: http://www.cdc.gov/
CDC Travel Health Information Web site: http://www.cdc.gov/travel/travel.html
E-mail: netinfo@cdc.gov

U.S. Food and Drug Administration (FDA)
Center for Drug Evaluation and Research:
Web site: http://www.fda.gov/cder/index.html

Office of Consumer Affairs:
Has general information on FDA-regulated products.

5600 Fishers Lane, HFE88
Rockville, MD 20857
Consumer Inquiries Information Line: (301) 827-4420 [10am–4pm (EST), M–F]
Office of Cosmetics and Colors Automated Information Line: (800) 270-8869
    [24 hours a day, 7 days a week]
Web site: http://www.fda.gov

U.S. Public Health Service—Office on Women's Health (U.S. PHS OWH)
National Women's Health Information Center
Information Line: (800) 994-WOMAN (96626)
Web site: http://www.4woman.org

University of Pennsylvania Cancer Center
Oncolink Web site: http://cancer.med.upenn.edu
E-mail: editors@oncolink.upenn.edu

World Health Organization (WHO)
The WHO Headquarters
CH-1211 Geneva 27
SWITZERLAND
WHO Web site: http://www.who.ch/Welcome.html
WHO International Travel and Health Web site:
    http://jupiter.who.ch/programmes/emc/yellowbook/yb_home.htm

YMCA of the U.S.A.
For information about YMCA programs and locations near you:
101 North Wacker Drive
Chicago, IL 60606
National Phone: (800) 872-9622
            (312) 977-0031
National Fax: (312) 977-9063
Web site: http://www.ymca.net

YWCA of the U.S.A.
The mission of the largest and oldest women's organization in the U.S. is to empower women and girls and to work to eliminate racism. Provides shelter; child care; employment training and job placement services for women; health care referrals, screening, and educa- tion services for breast cancer; racial justice; sports and physical fitness programs; youth development; women's leadership training; and world relations. For information about YWCA programs and locations near you:
YWCA of the U.S.A.
Empire State Building
Suite 301
New York, NY 10118
Phone: (800) YWCA-US1 (992-2871)
          (212) 273-7800
Fax: (212) 465-2281
Web site: http://www.ywca.org

Links

American Academy of Family Physicians (AAFP)
Has a web site with a variety of health information derived from their patient brochures.
Web site: http://www.aafp.org/patientinfo/

Barnard/Columbia Women's Handbook
Gopher Menu: gopher://gopher.cc.columbia.edu:71/11/publications/women

The Carol Ann Schwartz Cancer Education Initiative
Web site: http://cpmcnet.columbia.edu/dept/rosenthal/cancer/info/infosheets.html

The Columbia University College of Physicians and Surgeons Complete Home Medical Guide
Web site: http://cpmcnet.columbia.edu/texts/guide/

DermInfo-Net
Provides information regarding medical issues of the skin, hair, and nails.
Web site: http://www.derminfo-net.com/

Feminist Majority Foundation—Women's Health
Web site: http://www.feminist.org/gateway/h_exec2.html

Healthfinder
Consumer health and human services info from the U.S. government.
Web site: http://www.healthfinder.gov
(includes 550 links to web pages and 500 medical documents)

Healthtouch Online
Covers many areas of health, including men's and women's health, as well as prescription and over-the-counter drug info.
Web site: http://www.healthtouch.com

The Male Health Center
Web site: http://www.malehealthcenter.com/

Medical College of Wisconsin (MCW) International Travelers Clinic
Web site: http://www.intmed.mcw.edu/travel.html

Medicine Net
A free medical reference on the Web
Web site: http://www.medicinenet.com/

Office of Disease Prevention and Health Promotion (ODPHP)
Web site: http://odphp.osophs.dhhs.gov/

Pharmaceutical Information Network
Web site: http://www.pharminfo.com/

U.S. Department of Health and Human Services (DHHS)
Web site: http://www.os.dhhs.gov/

Books

American Medical Association Staff. *The American Medical Association Encyclopedia of Medicine.* New York: Random House, 1989.

American Medical Women's Association Staff. *The Women's Complete Healthbook.* New York: Dell Publishing Company, Inc., 1997.

Ancoli-Israel, Sonia. *All I Want Is a Good Night's Sleep.* St. Louis, MO: Mosby-Year Book, 1996.

Bell, David S. *Curing Fatigue.* New York: Berkley Publishing Group, 1996.

Bell, David S. *The Doctor's Guide to Chronic Fatigue Syndrome: Understanding, Treating & Living with CFIDS.* Reading, MA: Addison Wesley Longman, Inc., 1995.

The Boston Women's Health Book Collective Staff. *The New Our Bodies, Ourselves.* Magnolia, MA: Peter Smith Publisher, Inc., 1996.

Carlinsky, Dan. *Stop Snoring Now.* New York: St. Martin's Press, 1987.

Carskadon, Mary A. (editor). *Encyclopedia of Sleep and Dreaming*. Old Tappan, NJ: Macmillan Library Reference, 1996.

Dobkin, Rachel, and Shana Sippy. *The College Woman's Handbook*. New York: Workman Publishing Company, Inc., 1995.

Insel, Paul M. and Walton T. Roth. *Core Concepts in Health*. Mountain View, CA: Mayfield Publishing Company, 1997.

Kryger, Meir H., Thomas Roth, and William C. Dement. *Principles and Practice of Sleep Medicine*. Philadelphia, PA: W.B. Saunders Company, 1993.

Lang, Denise. *Coping with Lyme Disease*. New York: Henry Holt & Co., 1996.

MacKie, Rona M. *Healthy Skin: The Facts*. New York: Oxford University Press, 1992.

McCoy, Kathy, and Charles Wibbelsman. *The New Teenage Body Book*. New York: Berkley Publishing Group, 1992.

Merck and Co., Inc. Staff. *The Merck Manual of Medical Information: Home Edition*. Rahway, NJ: Merck & Company, Inc., 1997.

Micozzi, Marc S. (editor). *Fundamentals of Complementary and Alternative Medicine*. New York: Churchill Livingstone, Inc., 1996.

Moyers, Bill. *Healing and the Mind*. New York: Doubleday, 1993.

Nadakavukaren, Anne. *Our Global Environment: A Health Perspective*. Prospect Heights, IL: Waveland Press, Inc., 1995.

New York University Medical Center Women's Health Service, Division of Cardiology Physicians Staff, and Rita Baron-Faust. *Preventing Heart Disease: What Every Woman Should Know*. New York: Hearst Books, 1995.

Oppenheim, Michael. *The Man's Health Book*. Paramus, NJ: Prentice Hall, 1994.

Penn, Robert E. *The Gay Men's Wellness Guide: The National Lesbian and Gay Health Association's Complete Book of Physical, Emotional, and Mental Health and Well-Being*. New York: Henry Holt & Co., 1998.

Physicians' Desk Reference and David W. Sifton (editor-in-chief). *The PDR Family Guide to Women's Health and Prescription Drugs*. Montvale, NJ: Medical Economics, 1994.

Piver, M. Steven, and Gene Wilder. *Gilda's Disease: Personal Experiences and Authoritative Medical Advice on Ovarian Cancer*. New York: Bantam Doubleday Dell Publishing Group, Inc., 1998.

Planned Parenthood Federation of America, Inc. *The Planned Parenthood Women's Health Encyclopedia*. New York: Crown Publishing Group, 1996.

Silverstein, Alvin, and Robert Silverstein. *Overcoming Acne: The How and Why of Healthy Skin Care*. New York: William Morrow & Co., Inc., 1990.

Tapley, Donald F., Thomas Q. Morris, Lewis P. Rowland, and Jonathan Lapook (editors). *The Columbia University College of Physicians and Surgeons Complete Home Medical Guide*. New York: Crown Publishers, Inc., 1995.

United States Pharmacopoeia Staff. *Complete Drug Reference, 1998 Edition*. Yonkers, NY: Consumer Reports Books, 1997.

Weil, Andrew. *Health and Healing*. Boston: Houghton Mifflin Co., 1995. (As well as other titles)

White, Jocelyn C., and Marissa C. Martinez (editors). *The Lesbian Health Book: Caring for Ourselves*. Seattle, WA: Seal Press, 1997.

Films

Awakenings (1990): Robin Williams and Robert DeNiro star in this moving film based on psychiatrist Oliver Sachs's work with patients suffering from Parkinson's disease.

Beaches (1988): Bette Midler and Barbara Hershey star as childhood friends in this film about how one woman copes with the other's losing battle with a terminal illness.

Lorenzo's Oil (1993): Nick Nolte and Susan Sarandon star in this poignant and powerful drama about a couple who proactively search for a cure for their son's debilitating disease.

Steel Magnolias (1989): Julia Roberts and Sally Field star in this film about a young woman with diabetes and her desire to have a baby knowing the risk to her health.

Terms of Endearment (1983): Shirley MacLaine, Jack Nicholson, Debra Winger, John Lithgow, and Jeff Daniels star in this moving drama centering on the relationship between a mother and daughter, who later discovers she has cancer.

Unstrung Heroes (1995): Andie MacDowell, John Turturro, and Michael Richards star in this heartbreaking drama about how a father and son deal with MacDowell's terminal lung cancer.

Index